THE JOY*ful* TABLE

Gluten & Grain Free, Paleo Inspired Recipes
for Good Health and Well-Being

SECOND EDITION

SUSAN JOY

Copyright ©2019 Second Edition Susan Joy

ISBN: Softcover   978-0-6487140-2-6

All rights reserved. No part of this book may be reproduced or transmitted in any form or by any means, electronic or mechanical, including photocopying, recording, or by any information storage and retrieval system, without permission in writing from the copyright owner.

Disclaimer: This is my personal story and what has worked for me. All information and material in this book is for informational purposes only and is not intended to replace or substitute advice of a qualified Health Care Practitioner. If you have health concerns always seek medical attention immediately. If you have allergies or food intolerances to any foods mentioned in this book please do not consume. Neither the author or publisher shall be liable for any negative consequences to anyone reading or following the information in this book.

CONTENTS

Dedication vi
Foreword vii
A Little About Myself ix
Introduction 1
My Personal Journey 3
What is a Paleo lifestyle? 6
Breakfast 16
Soups 44
Breads, Crackers & Crusts 62
Salads & Vegetables 88
Snacks & Dips 118
Lunch & Light Meals 136
Main Meals 166
Gravy, Sauces and Dressings 202
Muffins, Cakes and Slices 214
Desserts 256
Toppings & Spreads 278
Basics 292
Acknowledgements 308
Index 309

DEDICATION

To my beautiful grandchildren, whom I love with all my heart, Emily, Harrison, Ruby and to my grandchildren still to come. You have been blessed with mothers that have given you real food with minimal processing, my prayer is that you will be able to continue this on in your own lives and in the lives of your own children. As a result we will see healthier people with less food intolerances and illnesses.

To my best friend, who happens to be my darling husband, you have been a wonderful taste tester and the best dishwasher anyone could have wished for throughout my adventure of producing this book. Thank you.

FOREWORD

"There are many recipe books available which are essentially variations of the same theme in their approach to food. However, this recipe book is different, it was conceived when the author was trying to address multiple health concerns. As a result of the author's difficult and ultimately empowering journey, has led to a plethora of useful knowledge contained in this book. Sue has in the process diligently sought the best ingredients for her recipes. I have personally known Sue for over twenty years, and her inspiring journey of discovery has created a fantastic recipe book that will improve your diet and more importantly your long term health. This book is an invaluable aid to help with the prevention of illness or disease. It has been a delight to review this book and I can personally attest to the time, energy and commitment required to bring this work to fruition. This book is much more than a recipe book, it is a recipe for good health."

Dr. William A Taylor

BAppSc (Clinical Science) RMIT University School of Health Sciences

BCSc, RMIT University School of Health Sciences

PostGradDip (Therapeutics) Cardiff University School of Medicine

MSc (Clinical Management of Pain & Headache Disorders) University of Edinburgh Medical School

A LITTLE ABOUT MYSELF

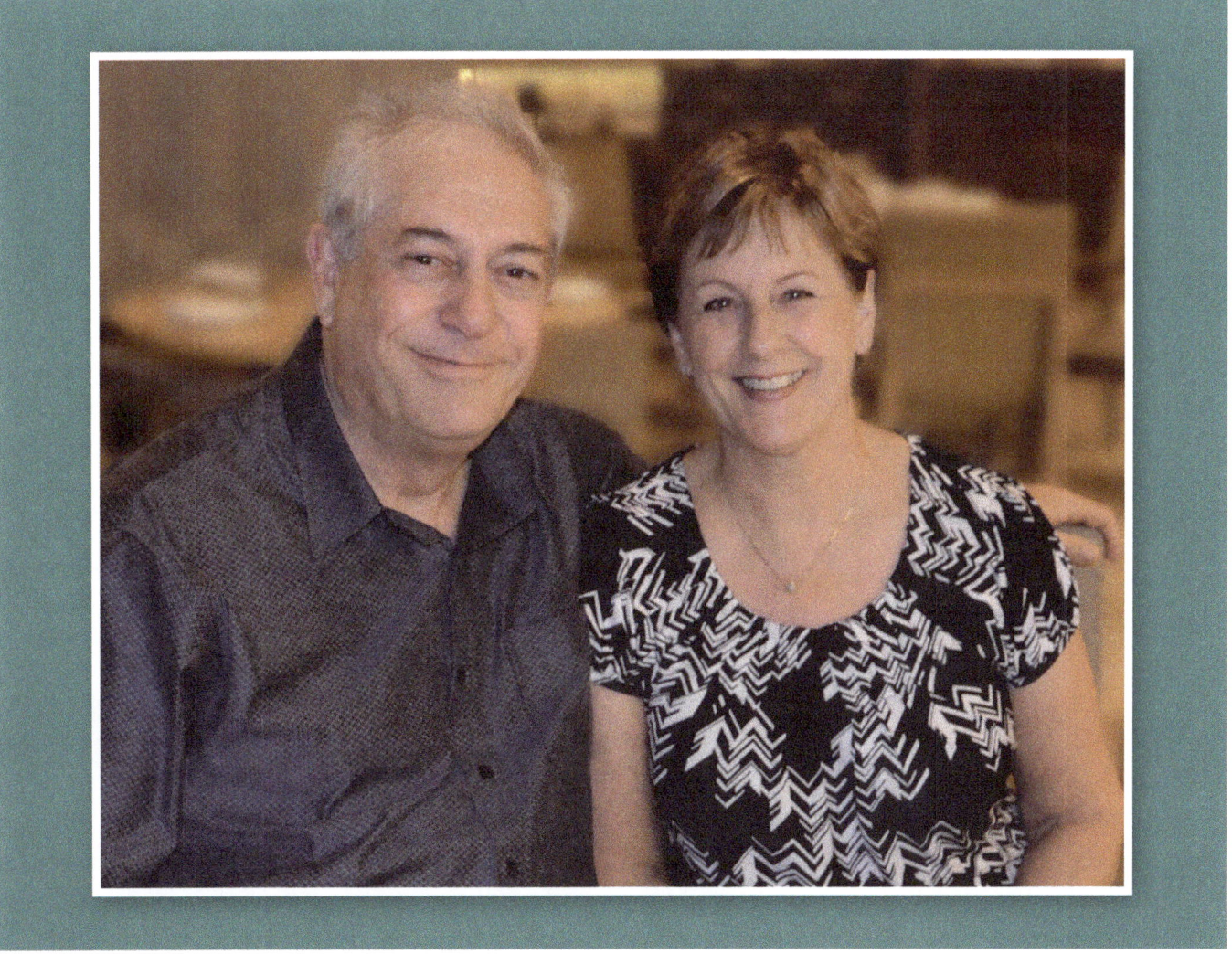

Family is one of my greatest pleasures in life. I have been married to my soul mate, Bryan for over 40 wonderful years. Together we have 3 adult sons, 3 gorgeous daughters in law and the icing on the cake, is our precious grandchildren. I have lived my whole life in Perth, Western Australia. We are involved with our local Baptist Church where I have the pleasure of teaching Sunday School to children aged from 5 to 8 years.

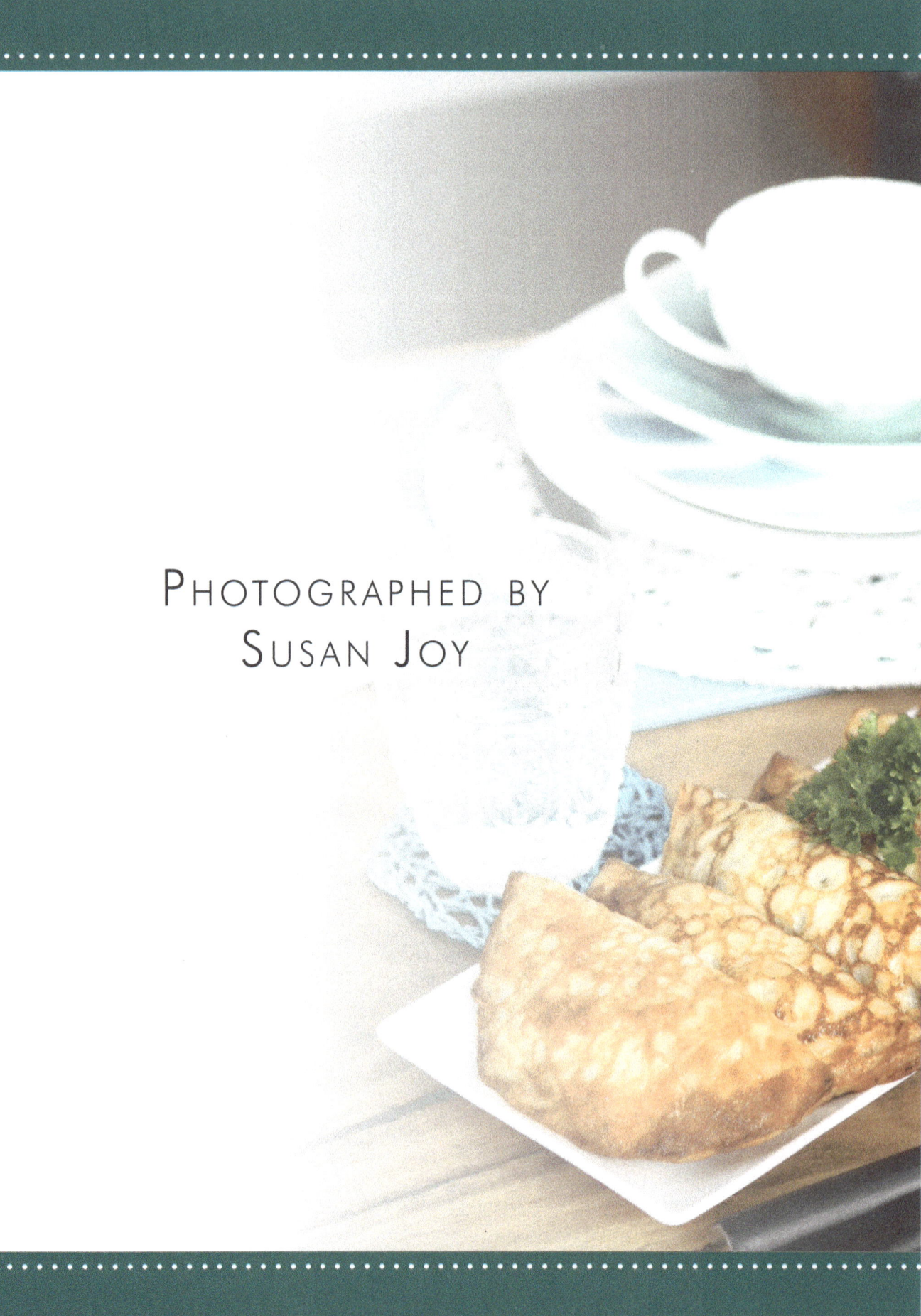

PHOTOGRAPHED BY
SUSAN JOY

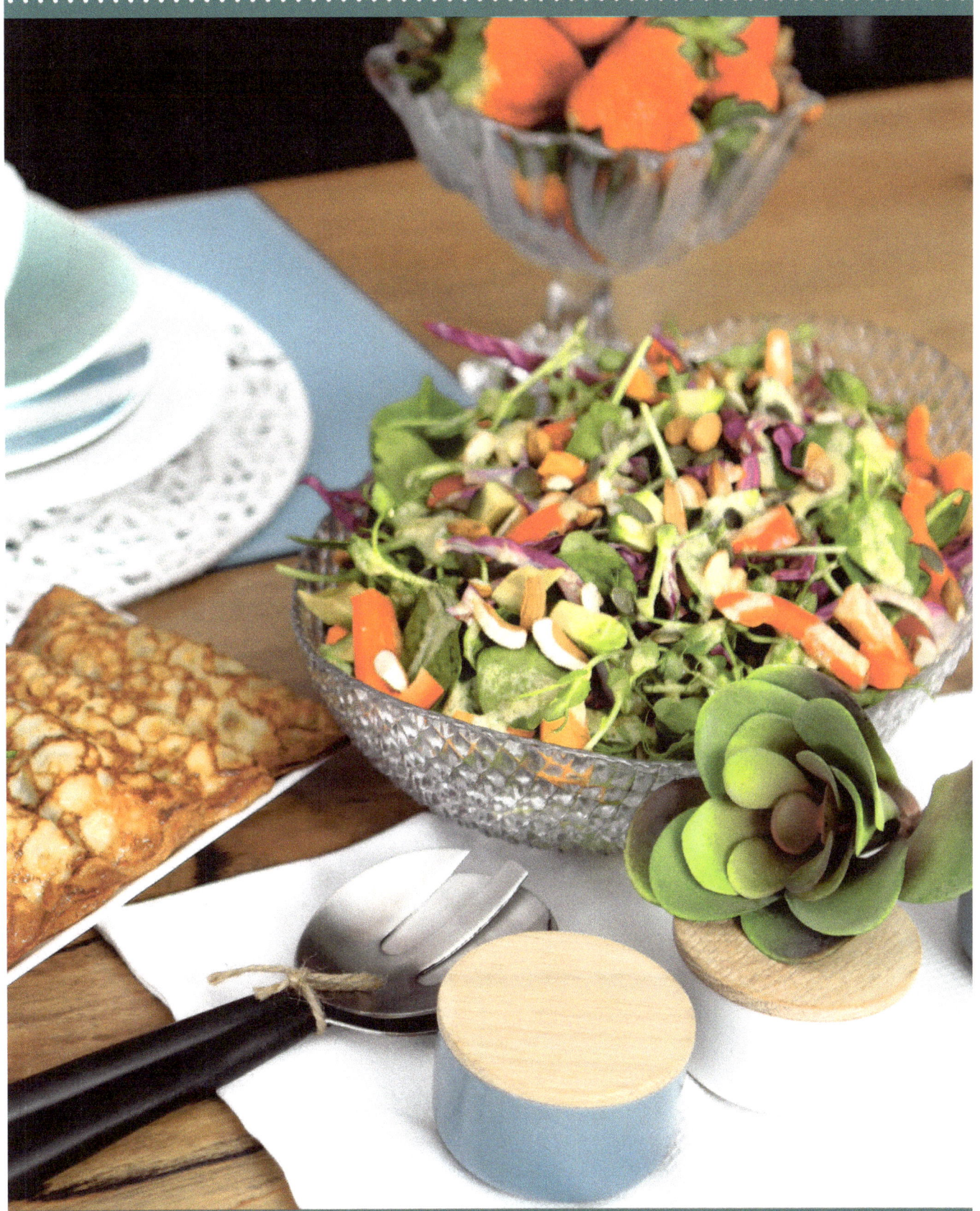

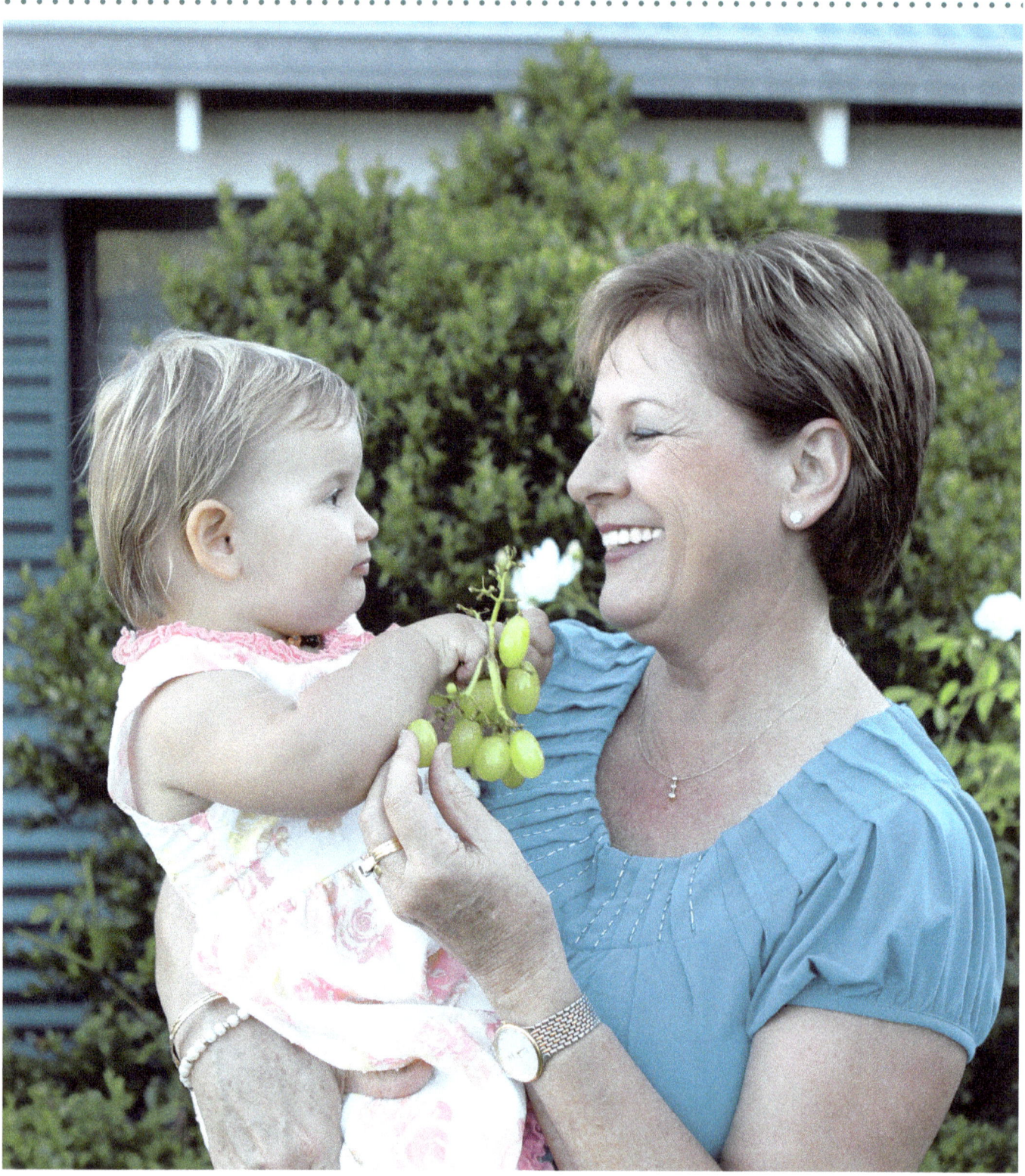

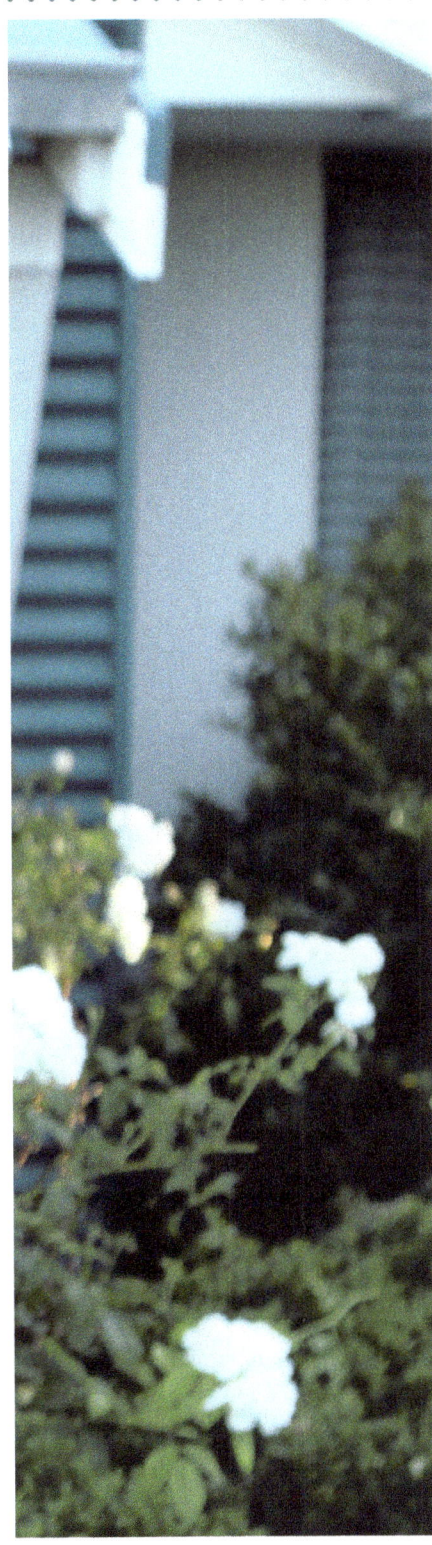

INTRODUCTION

Hello!

I am delighted you have chosen my book. That means you are looking to change your diet or you have health issues. I've been there and at that time there was a lack of tasty unprocessed, wheat free recipe books, so I started playing around with different ingredients in an effort to create recipes that I could eat and enjoy with my family.

Most of us lead busy lives, time is short. Food companies have provided us with quick and easy meals but at a cost to our health. What we eat does matter! A diet full of processed foods based on grains, refined sugars, preservatives and additives like colours and flavours, does not equal good health. I believe we need to nourish our bodies and let food be our medicine.

I have been pleased to have helped friends, acquaintances and family, encouraging them to change their eating habits and regain their health. As I created recipes, shared them and gave samples, I found them encouraging me to put my recipes into a book. My desire is for you to be able to eat tasty, healthy food that you can be proud to serve up to guests.

Eating healthy does require effort, it means reading food labels so you only consume real food. Look at the ingredients not the nutrition information. An excellent book to read on this subject is 'Changing Habits Changing Lives' by Cyndi O'Meara. Her website has a lot of very good information to help you decipher food labeling.

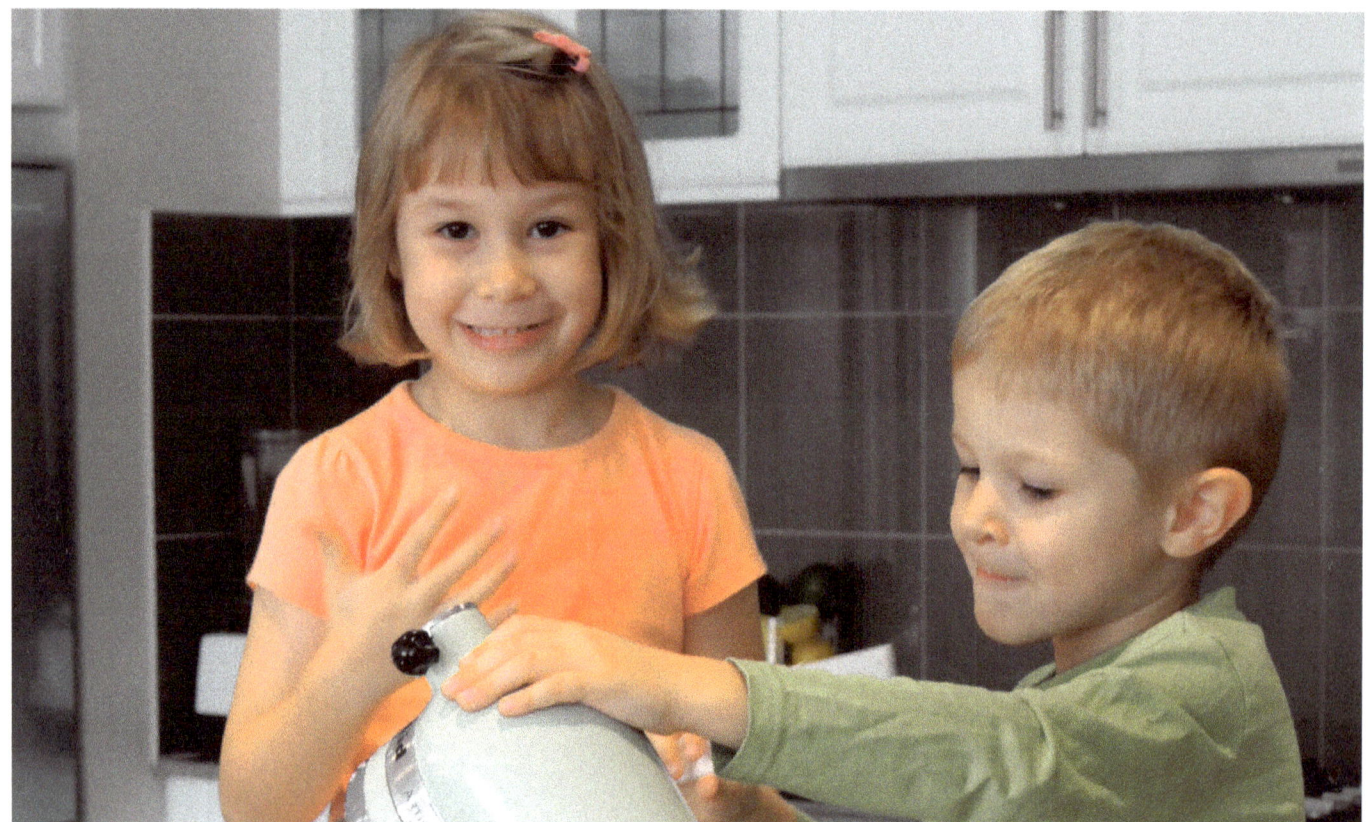

One of the biggest concerns most people have about changing to a grain-free diet is that they won't be able to eat their favourite foods. One of my desires was to reproduce our family favourites without thinking we were deprived or missing out. I encourage you to experiment and if things don't work out, keep trying, make it fun, laugh about your failures, but don't give up. Get your children involved in dinner preparations. Talk about real foods and why you choose them. Kids take in a lot. Educate from a young age and prevent food related illness manifesting later in their lives.

For a very long time, I battled with Chronic Fatty Liver Disease, an Autoimmune Thyroid Disease (Hashimotos), Arthritis and digestive issues. After many visits to various Doctors and Specialists, I decided to conduct my own research on what food choices could help my condition.

These choices culminate under what is termed a Paleo Lifestyle and it is that; a lifestyle rather than a diet. The dictionary definition of Paleo means 'old' or 'ancient' and in terms of this lifestyle, it takes into account a simpler time where food came from natural sources and where they weren't genetically modified or saturated with chemicals. Different people have their own definition of what Paleo is but for me, it's about choosing unprocessed foods. By choosing to follow this lifestyle, I have not only reversed my Chronic Fatty Liver Disease but have also reduced the symptoms of my Arthritis, Thyroid Disease and other health issues.

We are so fortunate to have such an abundance of food to choose from in our modern world, we just need the correct guidelines to help us make wise and healthy food choices with the highest nutritional value.

MY PERSONAL JOURNEY

For many years Doctors had no answer to my unhealthy liver function tests. To cut a long story short, I eventually had to have a liver biopsy, which proved Fatty Liver disease. My Specialist sent me to a dietician who placed me on a low GI diet full of whole grains and low fat dairy etc., there was no improvement. Since then I have discovered that they were the worst foods for my Fatty Liver disease. I also know now that the low fat diet that I followed for 18 years was probably the starting point of my liver deterioration.

Then I was diagnosed with Hashimotos, an autoimmune thyroid disease. I was also having hormone issues, so I sought advice from another medical doctor, who is a member of the Australasian College of Nutritional and Environmental Medicine. He requested a full set of blood and saliva tests. When my liver function test came back, he explained that if something wasn't done straight away, scar tissue would form and result in cirrhosis of the liver. That day he gave me a book by Dr Sandra Cabot "Fatty Liver Disease, You Can Reverse It". He told me to follow it word for word, as there wouldn't be much of a chance that I would receive a liver transplant at my age. I had to cut out grains containing gluten, in addition to high carbohydrate foods like rice, corn, white potatoes, sugar, high fructose corn syrup, ice cream and processed foods. After 6 months there was some improvement in my liver function test results but I still had a way to go.

It was very hard to find recipes as I was working long hours managing a busy Chiropractic Clinic. I then made the decision to retire and concentrate on my health, food and spend time with my precious grandchildren. My passion was to create tasty, appealing food for myself and my family.

As I researched food to help with Liver and Thyroid diseases, I started eliminating all grains (not just gluten ones). As information regarding the Paleo lifestyle started to immerge, I realized that I was already adhering to this type of diet. A further five months passed and my liver function test results were all reading within the normal ranges. This was a very exciting time for me (as it had been at least 6 years since I had a normal reading). I currently take medication for my Thyroid disease but cope well without many symptoms from my other conditions; which I put down to my Paleo lifestyle.

Over the course of researching the internet and reading every book I could put my hands on, it was very evident that the food I had been eating for so many years had made me sick. However, the revelation that the right foods can heal my body and become my medicine is incredible.

Food is a very important part in the Joy family's life. We are very close and most gatherings revolve around food. Every Sunday lunchtime and usually one night through the week, our house is filled with our children and grandchildren around the dinner table. Cooking for them, and watching their interactions, laughter and jokes as they all eat, is the greatest pleasure for me. I found myself cooking two meals. One for me and one for the rest of the family, the job was getting harder plus I wanted to keep my loved ones healthy too. So

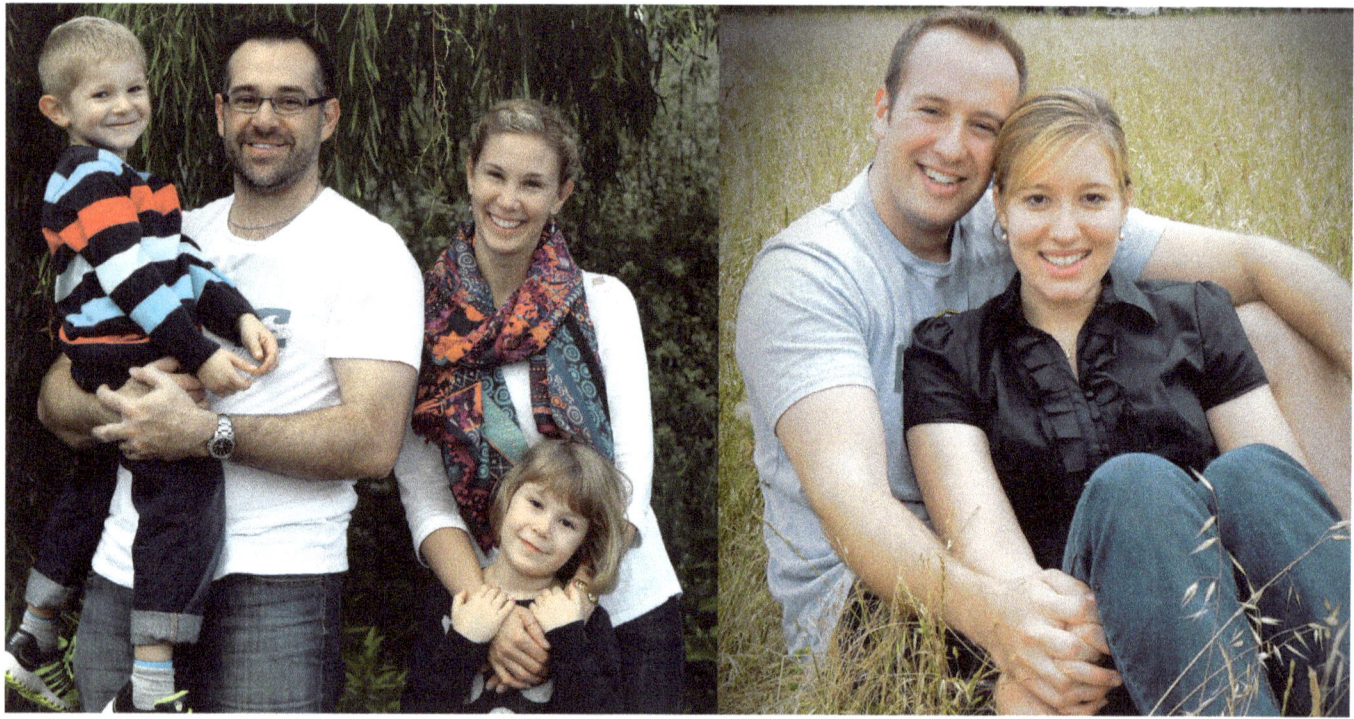

this was the start of getting more creative with food. After a new recipe everyone would give their verdict. My biggest critic was my granddaughter Emily. If I got her approval that was a bonus.

As the New Year started, my husband Bryan asked me what was I wanting to achieve this year? While I ponded, he surprised me by saying; maybe this is the year you write your recipe book. That is all the encouragement I needed. He may regret it now though. He is an amazing man, walks in the door from work and straight to the dirty dishes from that days cooking adventures. His philosophy is, a happy wife, means a happy husband, plus his health has improved dramatically since he has now come off gluten and grains. A huge migraine sufferer from a small child is now migraine free.

I suggest through experience that you follow the Paleo diet strictly to start healing and repairing your body. After several months I found I could occasionally consume small amounts of good quality dairy. You will be the best person to judge how your body reacts. If you add a food back into your diet and an old symptom returns like joint pain, headaches, bloating, reflux, constipation, cough, congestion, weight gain, skin rash etc. you know straight away you must avoid it.

So here is my book, filled with family friendly food, that is gluten free, grain free, refined sugar free, additive free, and mostly dairy free. It was made with love for my family and friends and I am now sharing it with you, I really hope you enjoy it and are blessed by it.

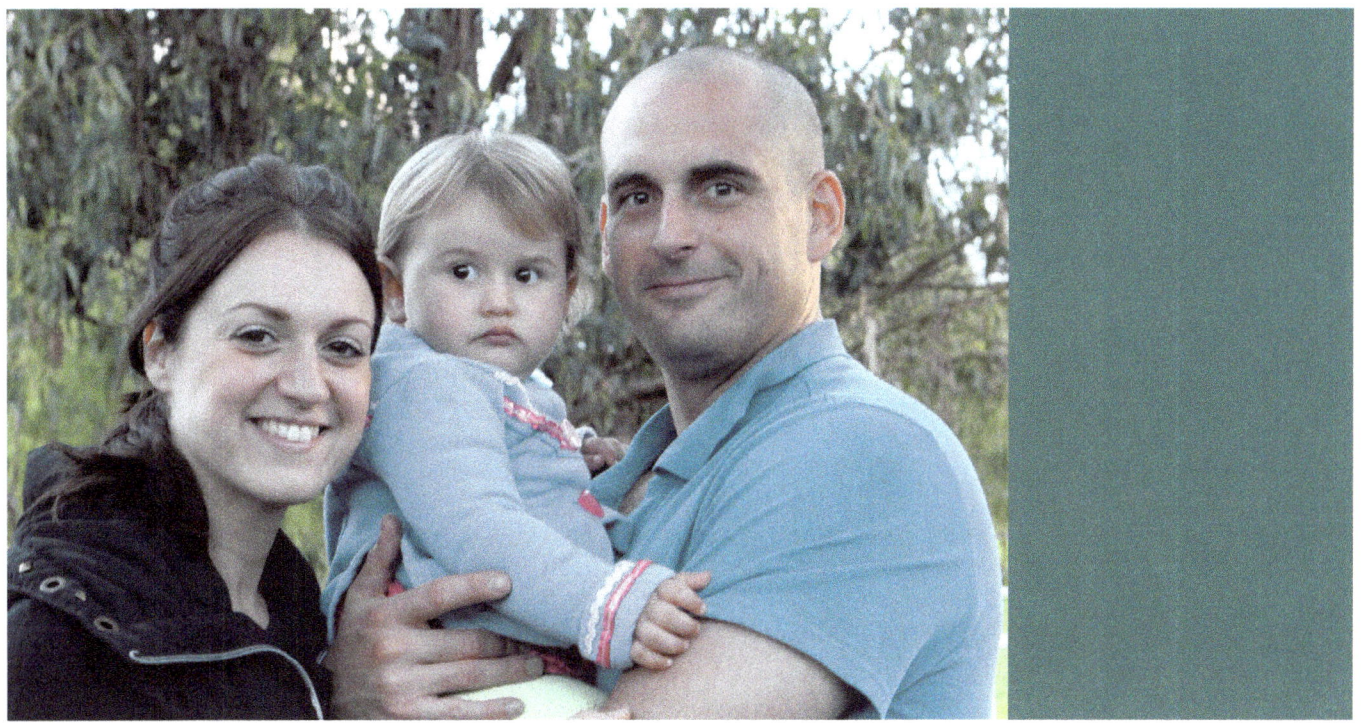

Happy and Joyful cooking to you all,

Love Sue

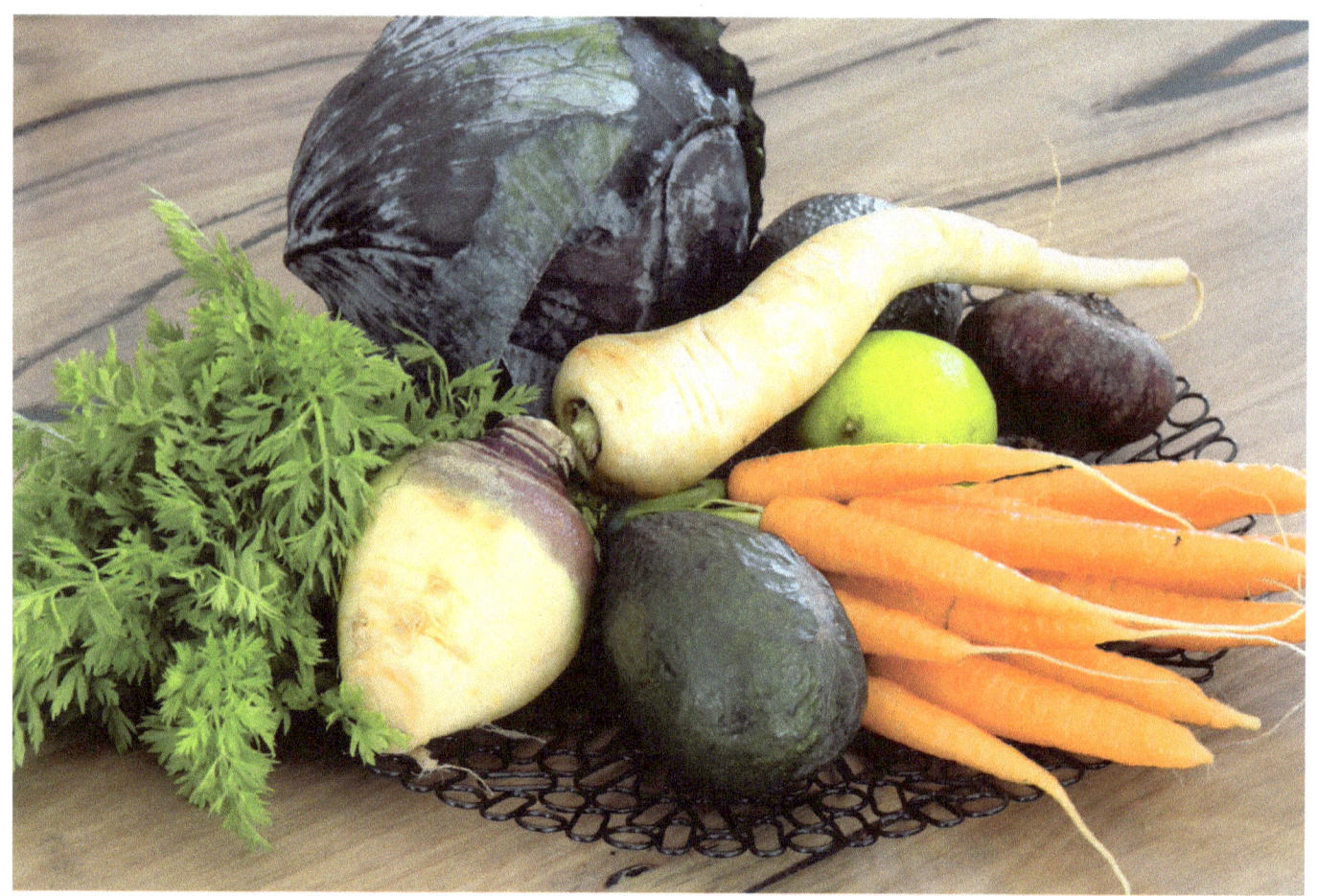

WHAT IS A PALEO LIFESTYLE?

Paleo is a lifestyle where you are eating whole, real, natural foods and removing processed foods and additives. It is going back to what our ancestors would have eaten; not the highly processed, gluten and grain based foods and refined sugars that have only been recently introduced into our diets. One of the main goals is to remove foods that cause inflammation in the body, which in turn cause illness and disease.

A quick look at the basics of the Paleo Diet:

WHAT YOU CAN EAT	WHAT TO AVOID
Meat, Fish and Seafood	Legumes (peanuts, lentils, kidney beans, etc.)
Poultry and Eggs	Grains (Wheat, barley, oats, rye, corn, rice)
Fruit and Vegetables	Dairy
Fermented Foods	Hydrogenated oils (canola, soybean, margarine, corn, safflower)
Natural Oils (coconut oil, ghee, lard, nut oils, olive and avocado)	Processed foods and refined sugar
Nuts and Seeds	Soy

Neurosurgeon, Dr David Perlmutter's book "Grain Brain" and Dr William Davis' book "Wheat Belly" are brilliant reads, giving an insight into what illness' can be reversed or improved by eliminating grains from our diet.

In the last few years many nutritionists, doctors, researchers and health experts have realized that our dietary guidelines must change for our societies' health to improve. The solution is to go back to ancient times and eat like our ancestors. There are many stories now of people recovering from illnesses that they have had for many years; and I'm one of them.

Although I do not endorse the many references incorporating evolution, I knew in my heart that this way of eating was nourishing and starting to heal my body. So whether you believe we are designed by God or evolved, don't over look the health benefits of the Paleo lifestyle.

I have recommended several books below on the subject, and while each author may have their own slant on the ancestral diet, one thing is in common, we need to remove grains, refined sugars, legumes, vegetable oils and food chemicals from our diets.

Here are a few great books that expand upon and help in understanding the Paleo lifestyle:

'Eat The Yolks' by Liz Wolfe

'The Paleo Answer' by Lauren Cordain

'Primal Body, Primal Mind' by Nora Gedgaudas

'The Paleo Solution' by Robb Wolf

A website that is also a great place to start is paleohacks.com.

If we look back in history to only 120 years ago, nothing came in bags, boxes or premade mixes. What people ate was picked straight from the garden and cooked fresh. Wheat is not the same as it was many years ago, as it has been modified to stop pests from eating it, yet we eat it too - pesticides and all. If it is killing the bugs what is it doing to our bodies and our children's? If you are finding all of this a bit daunting, just start by changing your diet one step at a time. The first and most damaging foods are wheat and sugar. Wheat contains Phytic Acid, a mineral blocker that prevents absorption of calcium, magnesium, iron, copper and zinc. Wheat is a common culprit for bloating, diarrhea, constipation, skin rashes, Irritable Bowel Syndrome, Leaky Gut, Celiac disease, migraines and the list goes on. Research by Dr Robert Lustig, an expert on childhood obesity from the University of California, states:

"Sugar is toxic and a poison. Your liver has no choice but to turn the energy into liver fat and that liver fat causes diseases".

This is something I had experienced first hand. Carbs are not created equal. I do not think fruit and vegetables should be in the same group as grains, processed sugars, lollies and bags of crisps but they are all carbohydrates. It was tough for me to give up bread and pasta but just because we like it or we have always eaten it doesn't mean it is good for us.

I believe we all have a responsibility to look after our bodies. I struggled when I discovered that the foods I ate had made me ill. It had happened due to my choices but I did not know any better at the time. I believed the ads on TV and the "natural" or "low fat" labels on the food packaging. However, once you are given the correct information you then need to act on it and therefore, I urge you to investigate further. The internet is an amazing tool and can assist with your start on a road to a healthier you. I have given you a start with my recipes but now you need to do some of your own work. It is not going to be easy but it is certainly going to be worth it. Something else to look forward to; you can not help but lose weight when gluten and grains are removed from your diet.

SO, LETS SEE WHAT YOU WILL BE EATING

'Your Paleo meal plate should consist of: ⅔ vegetables and salad, ⅓ protein (meat or eggs) and include some healthy fats (like avocado or olive oil as a dressing for your vegetables). A glass of filtered water or bone broth.'

MEAT, POULTRY, EGGS AND SEAFOOD

As part of a grain free diet, you also need to look at what the protein you are eating has been fed. Look for grass-fed meat, free-range chickens and free-range eggs. What we eat affects our health, so what these animals eat will surely affect their health. Do you want to eat unhealthy food? They were created to eat grass not to be fattened up quickly with grains. Make sure you check with your butcher before making your purchases to ensure you get 100% grass-fed.

All processed meats ladened with chemicals, additives and sugar are off the menu. However, you can find nitrate free, organic choices for sausages, cold cuts, bacon etc. The best place to source these is Gourmet Delicatessens.

When purchasing seafood opt for wild caught fish, not farmed. Salmon is one of the best choices as it contains good amounts of omega 3 fatty acids. When purchasing canned fish, look for "pole and line caught" on the label. You will have many choices of white fish to choose from, in addition; prawns, scallops, crab, mussels, oysters, and my favourite crayfish (lobster).

FRUIT AND VEGETABLES

In season organic or pesticide-free fruits and vegetables are the best choice. If that is not possible, look at purchasing from a local Farmers Market. Don't stress if it is not always affordable or available, I've purchased a good fruit and veg wash (Enviro Clean) to help remove the chemicals, waxes and pesticides from the outer skins of my produce.

Some crops absorb more pesticides than others. To help you know and be aware, you can search online or download an app called "The Dirty Dozen".

Fresh produce is essential for good health but there are a few exceptions: white potatoes, sweet corn (which is not a vegetable it is a grain) and legumes. Avoid canned fruit in syrups and limit your quantities of dried fruits, as they contain large amounts of concentrated sugars. The biggest concern with dried fruit is the sulfur that is used to preserve them, so choose organic. If you are trying to lose weight, the best option is to avoid very high sugar fruits such as, grapes, bananas, mango and pineapple for the time being. Any of the berries or an apple would be a better choice.

Fermented foods are one of the best things you can do for your health. They keep our digestive system healthy, in turn our immune system will be strong.

OILS AND FATS

Healthy fats are essential for brain function and to transport vitamins and minerals throughout our bodies. Stay away from the saturated fats in processed foods. The good saturated fats to consume are from grass-fed meats, eggs, seafood and coconut. Not all saturated fats are created equal.

The most nutritious fats to cook with are; coconut oil, ghee-clarified butter (ghee is pure butter fat and has had the milk solids removed), avocado oil, tallow, or lard. Oils that you need to avoid heating to high temperatures are olive oil and macadamia oil but these may be used for baking at lower temperatures. They are also delicious drizzled over salads and vegetables.

Flaxseed and hemp oils must not be heated. They are great oils to add to smoothies or to use for salad dressings. Highly processed oils derived from seeds and grains (corn, soybean, canola, vegetable etc.) are highly inflammatory to the body and are believed to contribute to many illnesses. When purchasing oils ensure they come in dark bottles, this helps to keep them fresher and prevent oxidization.

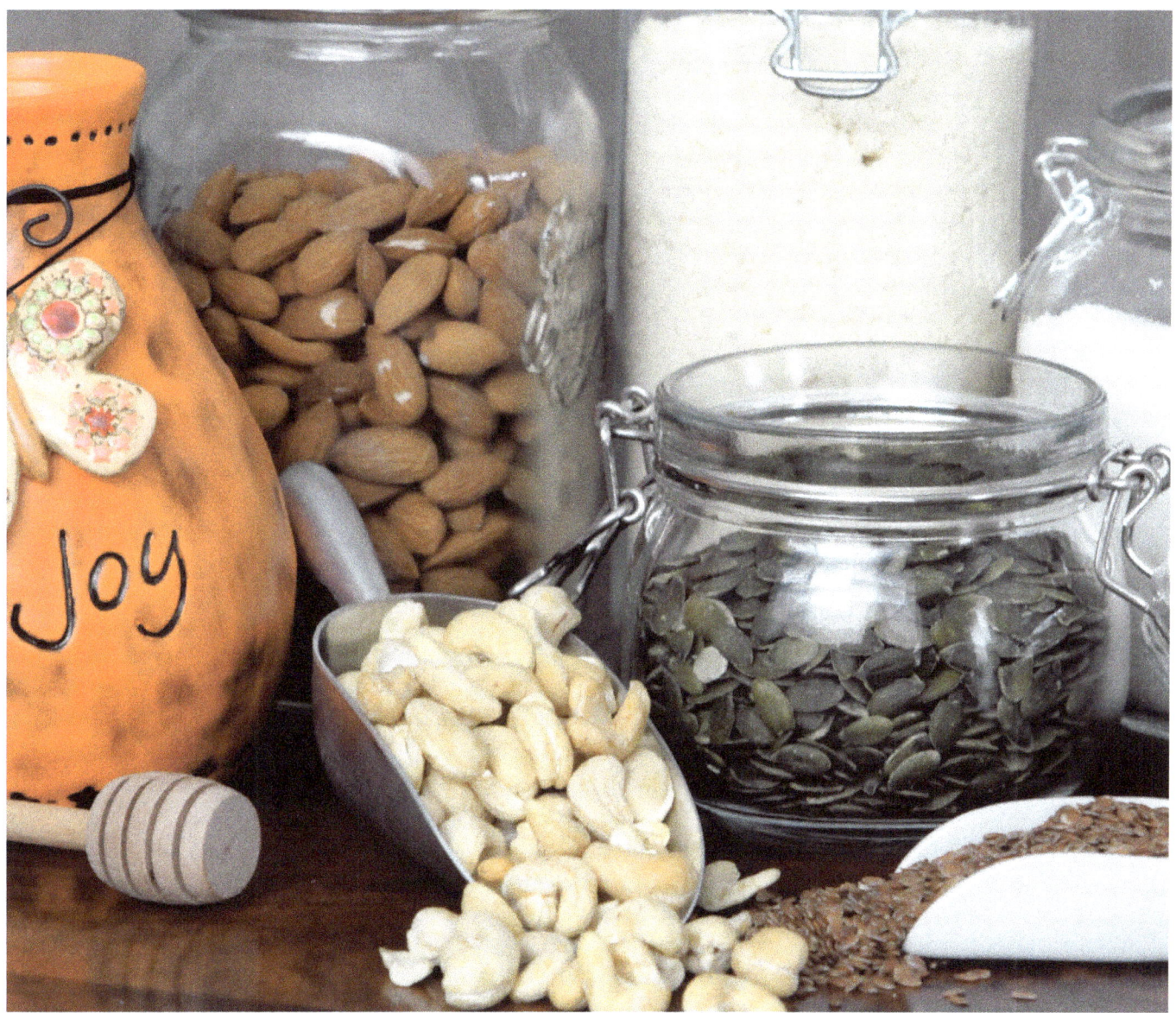

NUTS AND SEEDS

Nuts and seeds are a great protein snack. Eat them raw but in moderation. Stay away from store bought roasted nuts that have been cooked in canola, sunflower or similar vegetable oils. If you don't like them raw, try dry roasting them. They can also be used to garnish your salads. The best thing of all however, is that they make wonderful nut meals/flours for grain-free baking. You will find recipes in this book for delicious nut and seed butters. Where possible, it is best to soak nuts before using to assist with digestion.

OTHER INGREDIENTS IN MY PALEO KITCHEN

ARROWROOT FLOUR

Arrowroot (Maranta arundinacea) is a large perennial herb; the roots are cultivated for its starch properties. Combining arrowroot with nut meals and coconut flour helps create a lighter texture for your baking and helps do the job of holding the ingredients together in the absence of gluten. It's a perfect thickener for stews and doesn't have any noticeable smell or taste (add at the end of your cooking time). Arrowroot has many health benefits and is useful for those suffering with digestive issues and sensitivities, as it's gentle on the gut and has healing properties. It's also used as a nutritional food for infants and for people recovering from illness. Arrowroot contains protein and provides good amounts of folate (B Vitamins), potassium, copper, iron, calcium ash and fibre. Purchase organic if possible and I find online or from a health food store is best, if purchasing from a supermarket it can contain preservatives and can also contain tapioca. Tapioca can be used in place of arrowroot in baked goods but I wouldn't recommend it as a thickener for stews or fruit dishes. Tapioca flour is made from the dried roots of the cassava plant. (When substituting arrowroot for cornflour to thicken a dish, 2 teaspoons arrowroot = 1 tablespoon cornflour/starch).

BAKING SODA

Also known as Bicarbonate Soda is used as a rising agent in baking, it contains no gluten or grains. Baking Soda/bicarb is concentrated, ¼ teaspoon of baking soda = 1 teaspoon of baking powder.

BAKING POWDER

Baking Powder is also a rising agent. If substituting for baking soda you will need 4 times the quantity. Ensure you purchase a gluten free, no aluminum brand. Alternatively, you can make your own baking powder; 1 teaspoon of baking powder is equal to ¼ teaspoon of baking soda and add ½ teaspoon of cream of tartar. Note, that they should only be combined when preparing your recipe. Store bought baking powder may also contain corn starch or similar as a filler and anti-caking agent, so making your own is a better option.

BROTHS AND STOCKS

Making home-made broth is a great way to heal Leaky Gut and bring minerals and nutrients into your diet. If purchasing store bought stocks, read your labels as many companies have changed the name of MSG to yeast extract. Organic or free-range brands are available. I keep one on hand for emergencies, but I have gotten into the habit of keeping our chicken bones and making broth in my slow cooker. The recipe for this is on page 295. I keep ice block trays filled with broth in the freezer ready for when just a small amount is required for a recipe.

CACAO POWDER

Raw cacao powder is not the same as cocoa powder, which has been heated and processed; it is raw and unsweetened. It has a stronger flavour and you would use less than cocoa powder. It is so good for you; high in dietary fibre, iron and is a good source of magnesium and antioxidants.

CHIA SEEDS

These little seeds absorb 9-12 times their weight in water and are great to add as a thickener to sauces and fruit spreads. They can also be used as an egg replacement in muffins and cakes (1 tablespoon chia seeds mixed with 3 tablespoons of water). There are many health benefits of chia. It is the richest plant source of Omega 3, dietary fibre and protein. Chia seeds are also packed with a variety of vitamins and minerals, antioxidants, amino acids and fatty acids.

CHOCOLATE

In some of my recipes I have used Paleo approved dark chocolate chips, they are dairy, soy, nut and gluten free. My favourite brand is 'Chef's Choice' organic drops (70% cacao), they can be purchase from health stores or online.

CINNAMON POWDER

I am sure you will notice as you read my recipes that cinnamon appears quite frequently. It lends itself to savoury and sweet dishes. The best cinnamon to use is Ceylon (Verum). It has huge health benefits in regulating blood sugar levels. Cinnamon has antifungal properties and candida (yeast overgrowth) cannot live in a cinnamon environment. Added to food it inhibits bacterial growth, making it a natural food preservative and these are just a few of the benefits.

COCONUT

In all my recipes, I use unsweetened desiccated coconut, unless I have stated otherwise. Use organic coconut, which does not contain preservatives (sulphur).

COCONUT AMINOS

A great soy free alternative to soy sauce and tamari. It comes from the sap of the coconut tree and has a sweeter flavour than soy sauce and is not as salty. Coconut aminos can be purchased from health food stores or online.

COCONUT BUTTER

Coconut butter is delicious added to smoothies or just eaten out of the jar when a sweet treat is needed. It is so easy to make yourself, saving you lots of money. It can be warmed and mixed into slices and bars to give a rich coconut flavour. An added benefit is that it does not melt as easy as coconut oil and stays firmer in recipes.

COCONUT FLOUR

This flour is made by drying and grinding the meat of a coconut to a fine texture. Coconut flour is an excellent source of dietary fiber and protein. It is another great grain-free alternative for baking but does require a larger amount of liquid than normal when baking.

COCONUT MILK AND CREAM

I use this extensively throughout my book; from soups to dinners to desserts and cakes. I think it is the best dairy-free alternative. It gives so much flavour and creaminess to a wide variety of dishes. See coconut milk recipe on page 299. If purchasing in the can read your labels, even some organic brands contain gums and thickeners, choose full-fat not low-fat varieties. I use Ayam Coconut Milk and Cream (the cans are BPA free).

COCONUT WATER

This is the liquid found inside young coconuts. It is packed with electrolytes, excellent for after exercise. Coconut water contains potassium, calcium and magnesium and is also a natural hydrator. I use it in my smoothies and have added it to a few of my recipes. You can find it in health food stores and supermarkets. Ensure you read the label carefully as some contain preservatives and/or sugar and may not be 100% coconut water.

FISH SAUCE

Just a little of this sauce will make a big difference to a recipe. Read your label when purchasing, as you just want fish and salt, no preservatives or sugar added.

FLAXSEED MEAL

Flaxseed meal is finely ground linseed. I prefer to use the golden flaxseed variety, as the colour isn't as dark when using it in recipes as a replacement for flours. It is also a great egg substitute when mixed with water. Flaxseed is very low in carbohydrates, making it ideal for people who limit their intake of starches. It is rich in Omega-3 fatty acids, which is the key force against inflammation in our bodies. Flaxseed must be stored in the fridge.

GELATIN

Ensure you use unflavoured gelatin. 'Great Lakes' is a brand I use which is made from Kosher grass-fed beef. When using gelatin to thicken desserts, use the red carton. The green carton (which is cold water soluble and does not thicken) I use to add to smoothies and drinks. Gelatin is pure collagen protein, which is good for bone and joint care. It is also excellent for skin, hair and nails (helps the wrinkles from the inside).

HERBS, SPICES AND SEASONINGS

They bring flavour and life to your food. When I use fresh herbs they come from my garden but are available from any supermarket. I purchase organic dried herbs online from iherb.com. I also use an organic herbed sea-salt called Herbamare, which can be bought at any supermarket or health food store.

NUT MEALS/FLOURS

The most favoured in my kitchen is almond meal. It is finely ground blanched almonds and in some countries, it is call almond flour. It has a slightly sweet flavour so you don't have to add as much sweetener when baking with it. All kinds of nuts can be ground down to make a meal and are excellent for raw cheesecake or pie bases. I shop in bulk and online where possible in order to save money. Nut meal/flour, nuts and seeds are all best stored in airtight containers in the fridge or freezer to prevent them going rancid.

NUTRITIONAL YEAST FLAKES

Also known as Savoury Yeast Flakes. It is a fermented and deactivated yeast, which means it isn't going to grow (and has nothing to do with brewer's yeast or bakers' yeast). It has a creamy cheesy flavour and I've used it in a few recipes to create a cheese flavour. Vegans use it as a condiment and a cheese substitute, and to also add additional protein and vitamins to their diet (it's a complete protein). Nutritional yeast flakes are free from sugar, dairy, grains, and gluten. Do not confuse it with yeast extract (MSG). Purchase from health food stores.

PROBIOTICS

I use 'Changing Habits' brand of fermented raw food probiotics to add to my smoothies. I also use a very good quality dairy free probiotic capsule (Acidophilus) to make Cashew 'Cheeze'.

SEA SALT

Organic unbleached, unrefined Celtic sea salt or Himalayan pink salt is my salt of choice as these contain healthy minerals that our body needs. Table salt has been bleached, refined and processed leaving minimal health benefits. If you choose to use table salt, reduce the quantity in my recipes.

SWEETENERS

I use natural unrefined sweeteners in my recipes but use them in moderation and only for treats. I have reduced the amount of sweetness in each recipe to the lowest possible without compromising taste. Feel free to adjust to your liking. Honey is the most common sweetener in my recipes. It is best to buy local unprocessed honey, as it has wonderful health benefits and can help with allergies. Generally, honey sold in supermarkets has been processed. Medjool Dates are plump and moist and high in fibre they give a lovely caramel flavoured sweetness to recipes. Organic 100% maple syrup is a natural food sweetener (not flavoured maple syrup). Coconut sugar is produced from the sap of the flower bud of the coconut palm tree. I use it when a dry sweetener is required.

During your first 6 weeks of your new Paleo lifestyle, I recommend removing even natural sweeteners from your diet while your body eliminates toxins and addiction to sugar. I have cookies and desserts in my book made from whole food ingredients with natural sugars but please don't overindulge. Use as a treat only for special occasions and to take to friends so you don't feel left out.

TAHINI

This is a smooth and creamy paste made from ground sesame seeds. I use it to make dips and salad dressings.

TOMATO PRODUCTS

Use fresh where possible or organic tomato passata/puree in glass containers. Tomatoes are acidic which increases the rate at which BPA enters food and this can be a concern with canned tomato products. If canned tomatoes are required make sure you purchase in a BPA free can.

VANILLA AND ALMOND EXTRACTS

Vanilla makes a big difference to the flavour of a recipe, I recommend keeping to the quantities I have stated in a recipe. Use an organic vanilla extract (not an essence) or powder. I like Madagascar pure vanilla extract manufactured by 'Simply Organic'. I have also used organic almond extract in a few recipes. The best quality and price I have found is manufactured by 'Frontier Natural Flavors'. I purchase both online.

VINEGARS

Apple cider vinegar is used many times in my recipes due to its health benefits. When purchasing, look for raw unfiltered apple cider vinegar 'with the mother' it has a cloudy appearance. For salads, I like balsamic vinegar and you will find organic white and red wine vinegars in a few recipes. Coconut vinegar is wonderful over salads with its slight sweet taste. Avoid malt vinegars as they are made from barley and contain gluten.

WORCESTERSHIRE SAUCE

My choice in Worcestershire sauce is the 'Melrose' organic brand. This sauce adds a great savoury flavour to meat dishes. Regular brands contain gluten and most have MSG, colours and flavours.

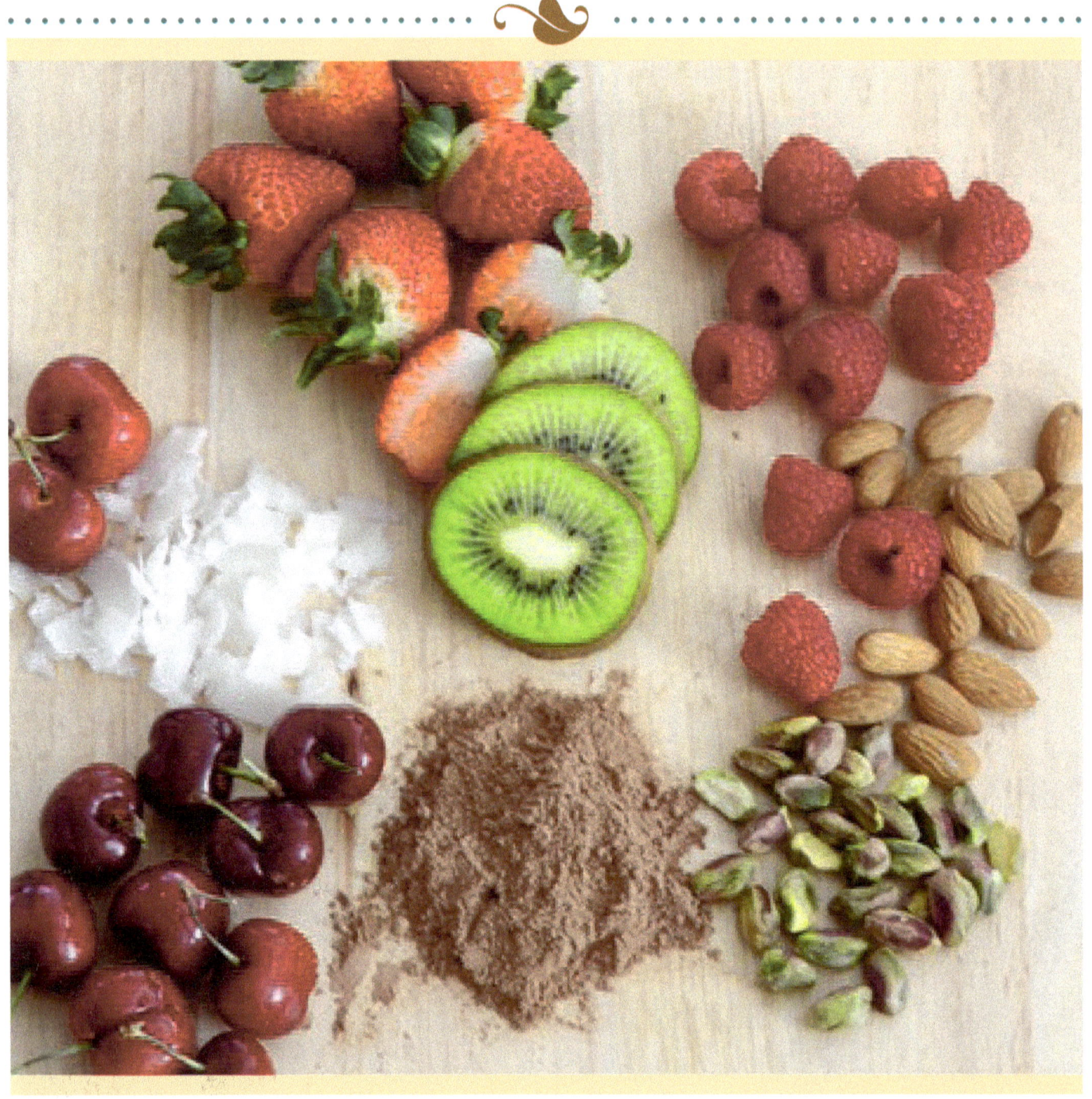

WHERE CAN I PURCHASE MY INGREDIENTS?

Supermarkets, health food or organic stores stock much of the ingredients listed in this book. I tend to purchase a lot online from iherb.com, due to the variety and huge savings. I also purchase locally from specialty stores that provide baking goods in either bulk or weigh and pay.

TIPS FOR SUCCESSFUL BAKING:

- When using my recipes I recommend having all your ingredients out and prepared before starting. Follow my recipe in its entirety. Once you have cooked a recipe and tested my flavours and textures, then go ahead and experiment and adjust to your preferences.

- When measuring flours and other ingredients, I have used a level cup or spoon. Use the back of a knife to smooth over the top. When using coconut flour, ensure you measure exactly, as even the slightest difference may not get the results desired. It is a very fibrous flour and absorbs a lot more liquid than other flours.

- Australian metric measurements have been used in the recipes and I have also given imperial options for many of them. I have tried to make the measuring as uncomplicated as possible.

- If you use a different size baking tin, take note that baking times will vary.

- I have calculated cooking times using a fan-forced oven and centre rack.

- I have used large eggs from a 700g carton.

- Wherever possible, I used organic ingredients.

- The main tools I use in my kitchen consists of; a slow cooker, good quality enamel pots and non toxic frying pans, spiral slicer, food processor and Vitamix blender. Using a food processor when baking with almond meal and coconut flour will give you an aerated and finer texture.

HOW CAN I SUCCEED?

- Get rid of all the junk food. If it is in the house it's too easy to be tempted. Give it away.

- Don't eat out at restaurants until you can resist temptation. Give yourself time to adjust to your new eating lifestyle so you can make the right choices.

- If you are invited to a dinner party, ask if you can contribute. This will always ensure you have a Paleo option.

- Do not stress, make it simple and just eat real food.

- Cook extra food at dinner so you have lunch for the next day.

- Get plenty of sleep and moderate exercise.

- When shopping buy foods from the outer aisles where you find the fruit, vegetables and meat. Don't enter the aisles where the packaged, processed foods are and you can't be tempted. Once you have studied your food labels, write down the brands that fit into your Paleo lifestyle. This way, when shopping, you can go straight to them. It will save time and also keep you away from the other tempting aisles.

- My best advice is to read and research to help yourself make good choices. Take your time, as this will ensure that the changes will be permanent and sustainable. I want this to work for you like it did for me.

BREAKFAST

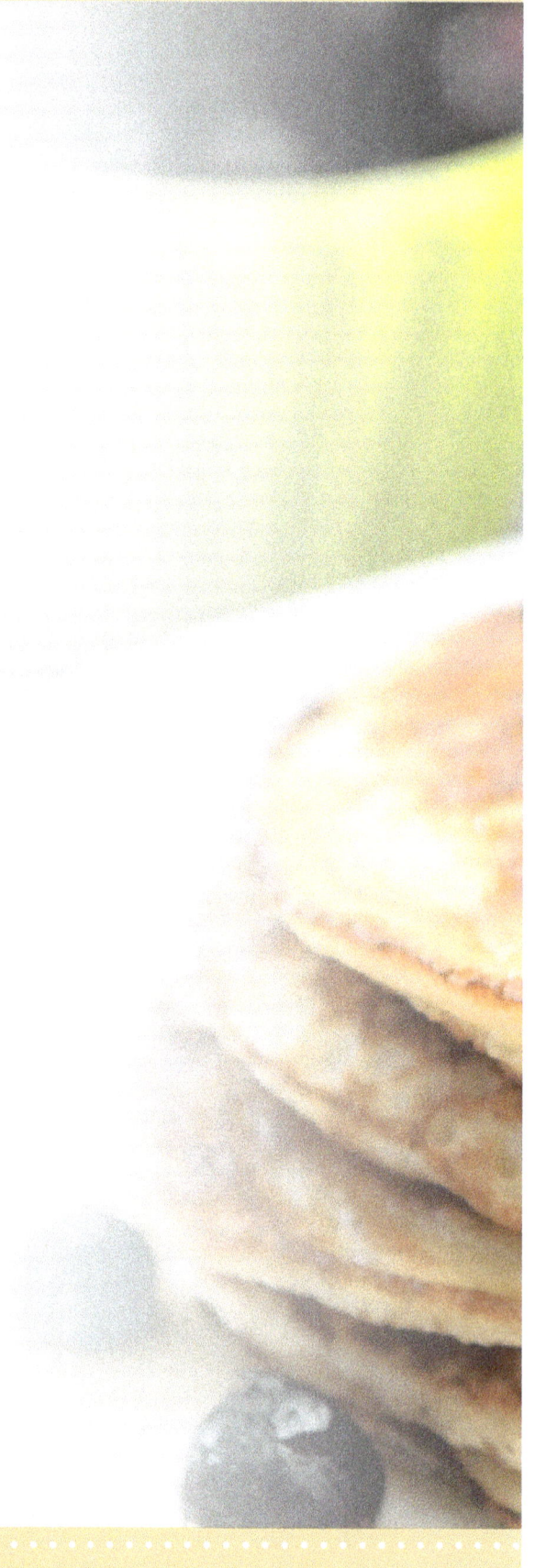

Bircher Style Muesli 19

"Granola Cereal" Grain free 20

Muesli Breakfast Slice 23

Green Banana Smoothie 24

Blueberry Smoothie 25

Chocolate Coconut Smoothie 26

Pancakes 29

Breakfast Sausages 31

Egg Burrito with leftovers 33

English Muffins with Egg and Avocado 34

Greens Eggs and Ham Muffins 37

Sweet Potato Hash Browns 38

Sweet Potato & Onion Hash Browns 41

Vegetable and Bacon Slice 42

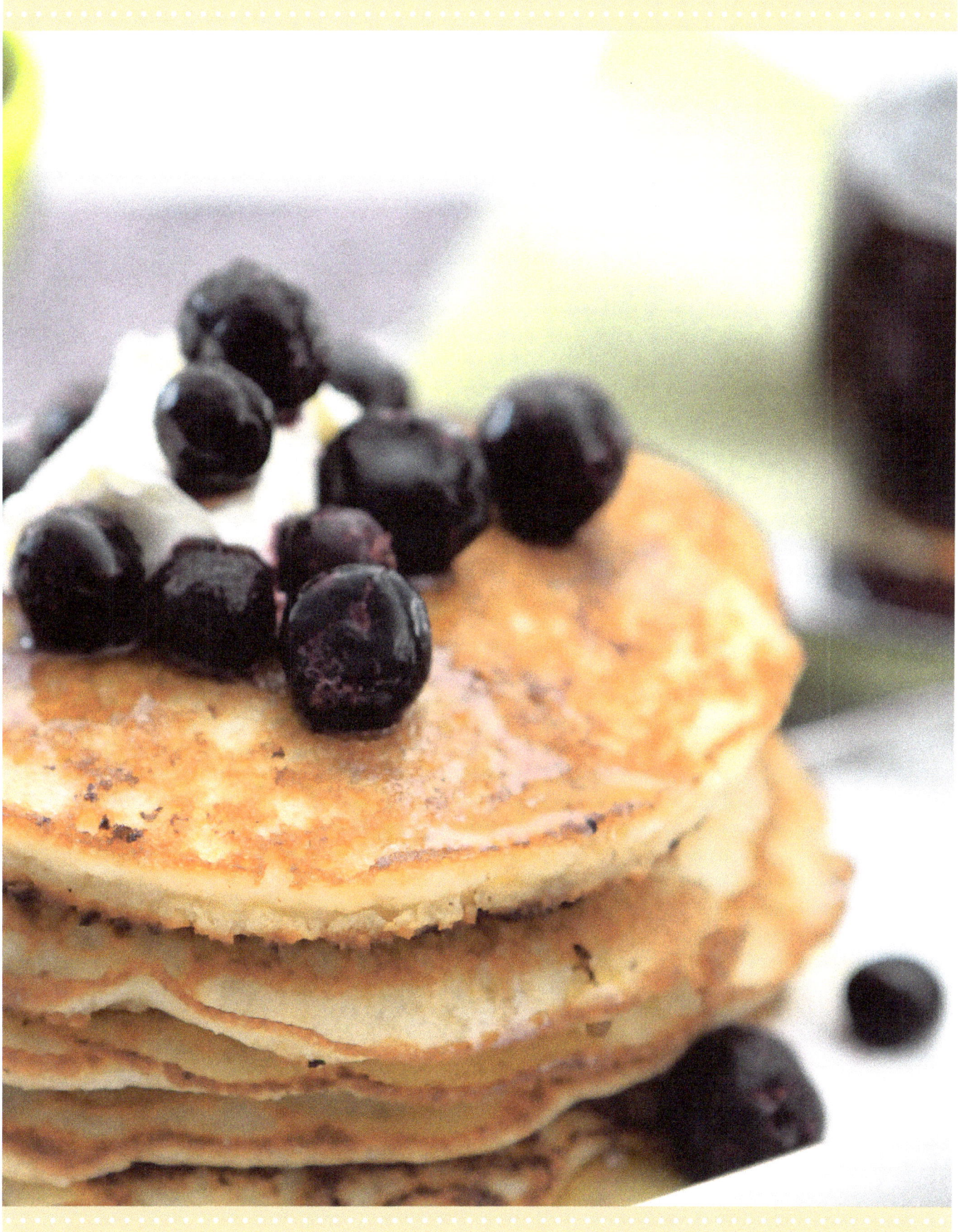

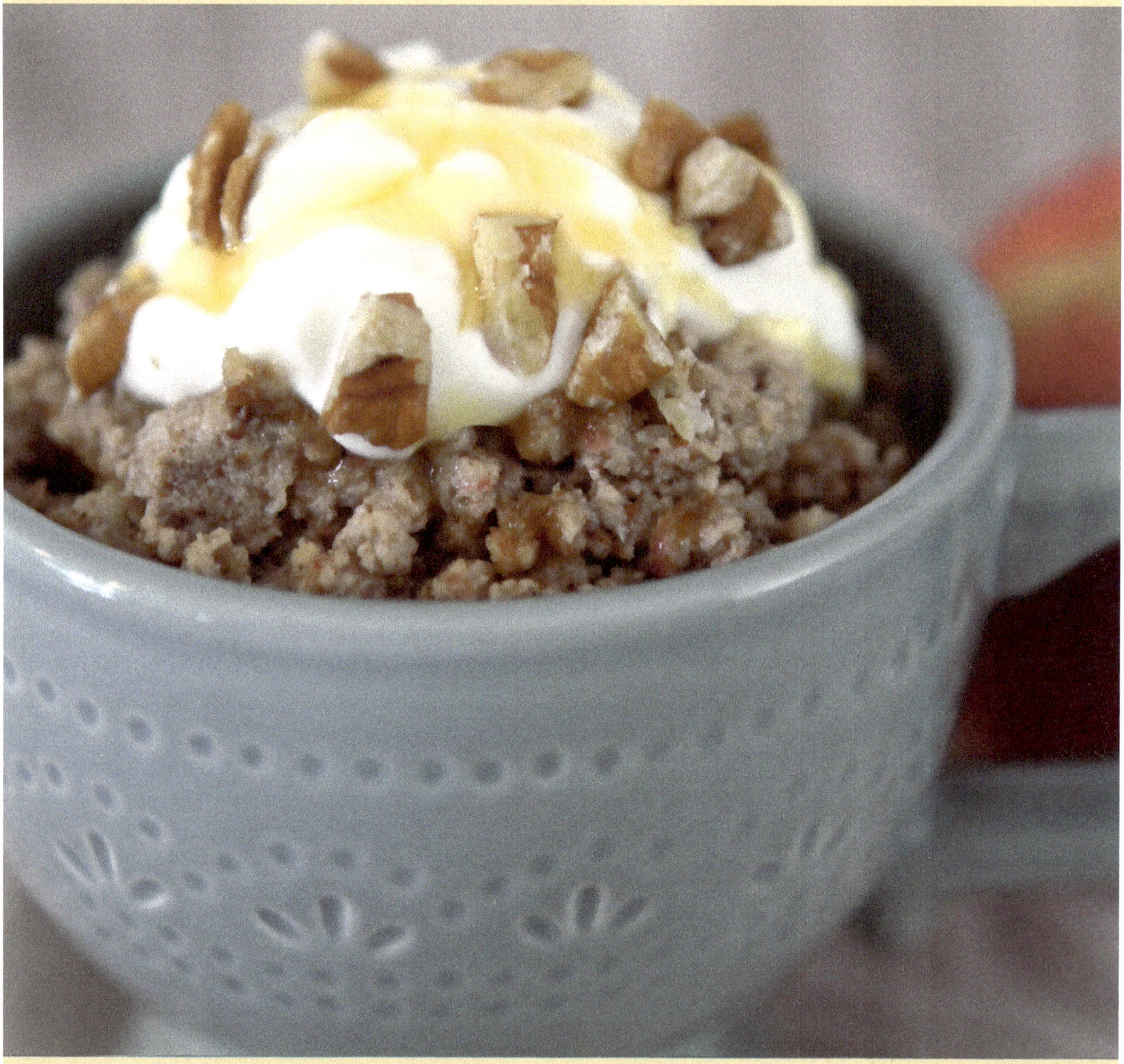

18 | BREAKFAST

Bircher Style Muesli

I like how the apple makes this muesli or porridge, whatever you wish to call it, taste so fresh and sweet. Normally oats are used and soaked overnight in milk to soften them, fruit and nuts are added in the morning. I'm using a mix of nuts and seeds. You will be surprised how filling this breakfast is.

Prep time: 10 minutes plus soaking time Cooking time: none Serves: 2 or 1 large

Ingredients:

- 2 Tbsp pecans
- 2 Tbsp almonds
- 2 tsp sunflower seeds
- 2 tsp pumpkin seeds
- 2 Tbsp desiccated coconut
- 2 medjool dates, pitted
- 1 small apple, cut into small chunks
- ¾ tsp ground cinnamon
- Squeeze of lemon juice
- Pinch of fine sea salt
- 2-3 Tbsp coconut yoghurt
- Drizzle of honey, optional

Method:

The night before, soak the nuts, sunflower and pumpkin seeds in a large cup, and fill to the top with water to soak overnight. The nuts and seeds will soak up quite a bit of water. You will need to have at least 6cm(2.5ins) of water above the nuts. In the morning using a metal sieve, drain off the soaking water and rinse nuts and seeds with fresh water, and drain.

Place nuts and seeds in a blender or food processor and pulse a few times until they are broken up. Add coconut, dates, apple (leave skin on), cinnamon, lemon juice and salt. Process to break up the apple and dates. If using a blender you will need to use the tamper to help push food onto the blades.

Serve muesli in a bowl or cup, add a dollop or two of coconut yoghurt, and a drizzle of honey and mix through.

"Granola Cereal" Grain free

This recipe makes 10 cups. If stored in an airtight container it will keep for up to 2 months. You can halve the recipe amounts but it's useful to have on hand. Excellent as a snack or treat, place 3 tablespoons in a bowl, top with chopped strawberries and a dollop of cream or yoghurt. It is also handy if a dessert is needed quickly, just add 3-4 cups to a food processor with ¼-⅓ cup of melted coconut oil. Whizz until it all comes together, press into the base of a pie dish and top with a raw cheesecake or pie filling. You can also sprinkle it on top of a bowl of stewed cinnamon apples to make your own individual serve of apple crumble.

Prep time: 15 minutes plus soaking time
Makes: 10 cups Cooking time: 1 hour 15 minutes

Ingredients:

- 1 cup almonds
- 1 cup macadamia nuts
- 1 cup pecans
- 1 cup pumpkin seeds
- Filtered water for soaking
- 1 cup/10 fresh medjool dates, pitted
- 1½ cups desiccated coconut
- 2 tsp vanilla powder or 1 Tbsp vanilla extract
- 1 tsp ground cinnamon
- ½ tsp fine sea salt

Method:

Place nuts and pumpkin seeds in a large bowl, cover with filtered water. Allow 8cm(3ins) of water above the nuts and soak overnight. Place dates in a separate bowl. Cover with 1 cup of water and soak overnight.

The next day place the dates with soaking water in a food processor. Puree until smooth.

Preheat oven to 120c/250f. Line 2 large baking trays with baking paper.

Using a fine metal strainer, drain the nuts and seeds. Rinse well until water is clear, drain well, shake out excess water.

Add nuts, seeds, coconut, vanilla, cinnamon and salt to date paste and pulse briefly to mix. Try to keep the nuts coarsely chopped. Transfer mixture onto the lined baking trays and spread out evenly.

Bake for approximately 1 hour 15 mins-1 hour 25 mins or until golden and dry, watch it doesn't burn. Leave to cool on trays. Store in an airtight container.

To this basic mixture you can add chopped dried fruit or toasted coconut flakes. Serve with your choice of dairy free milk and yoghurt for breakfast.

BREAKFAST | 21

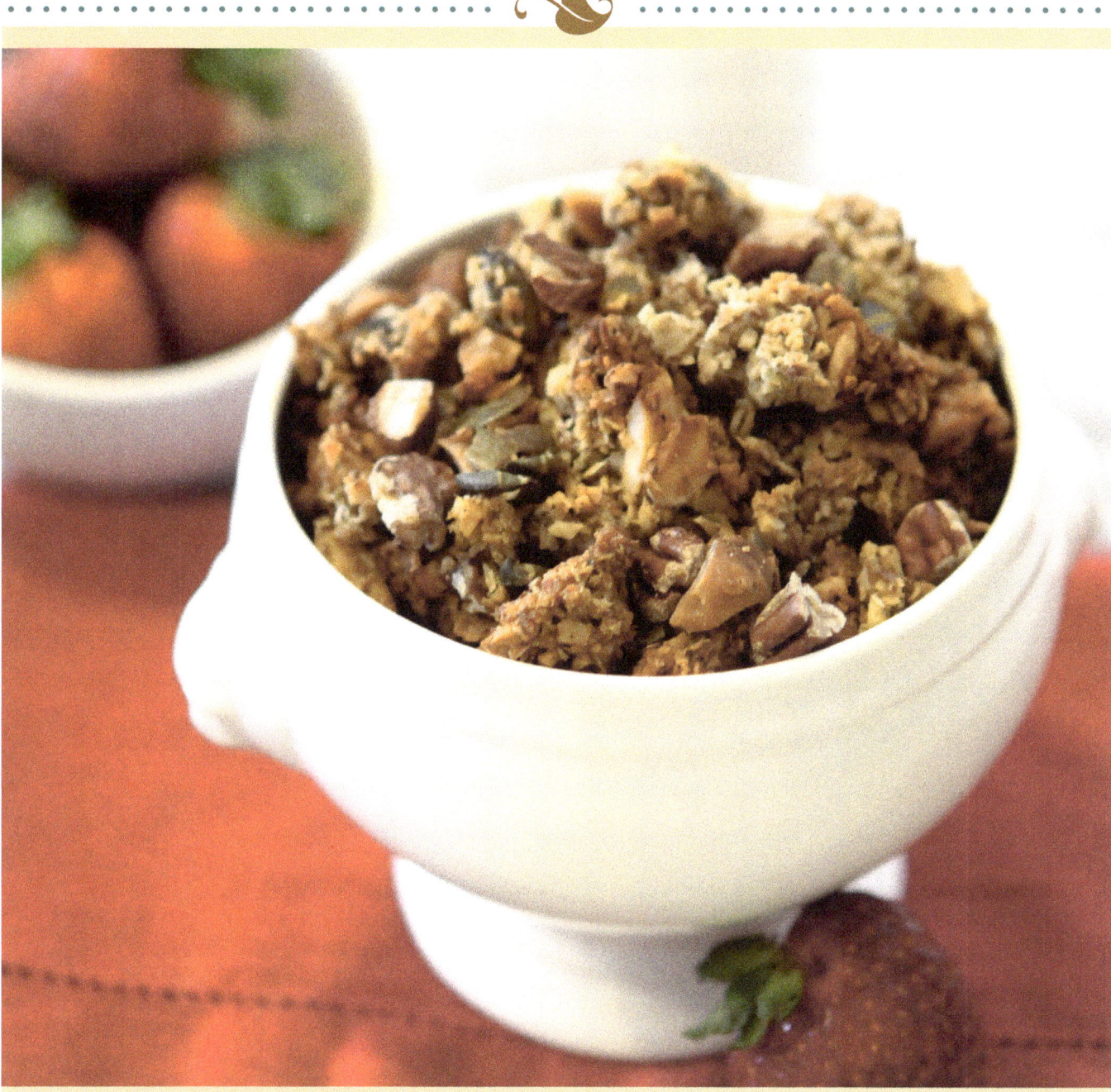

22 | BREAKFAST

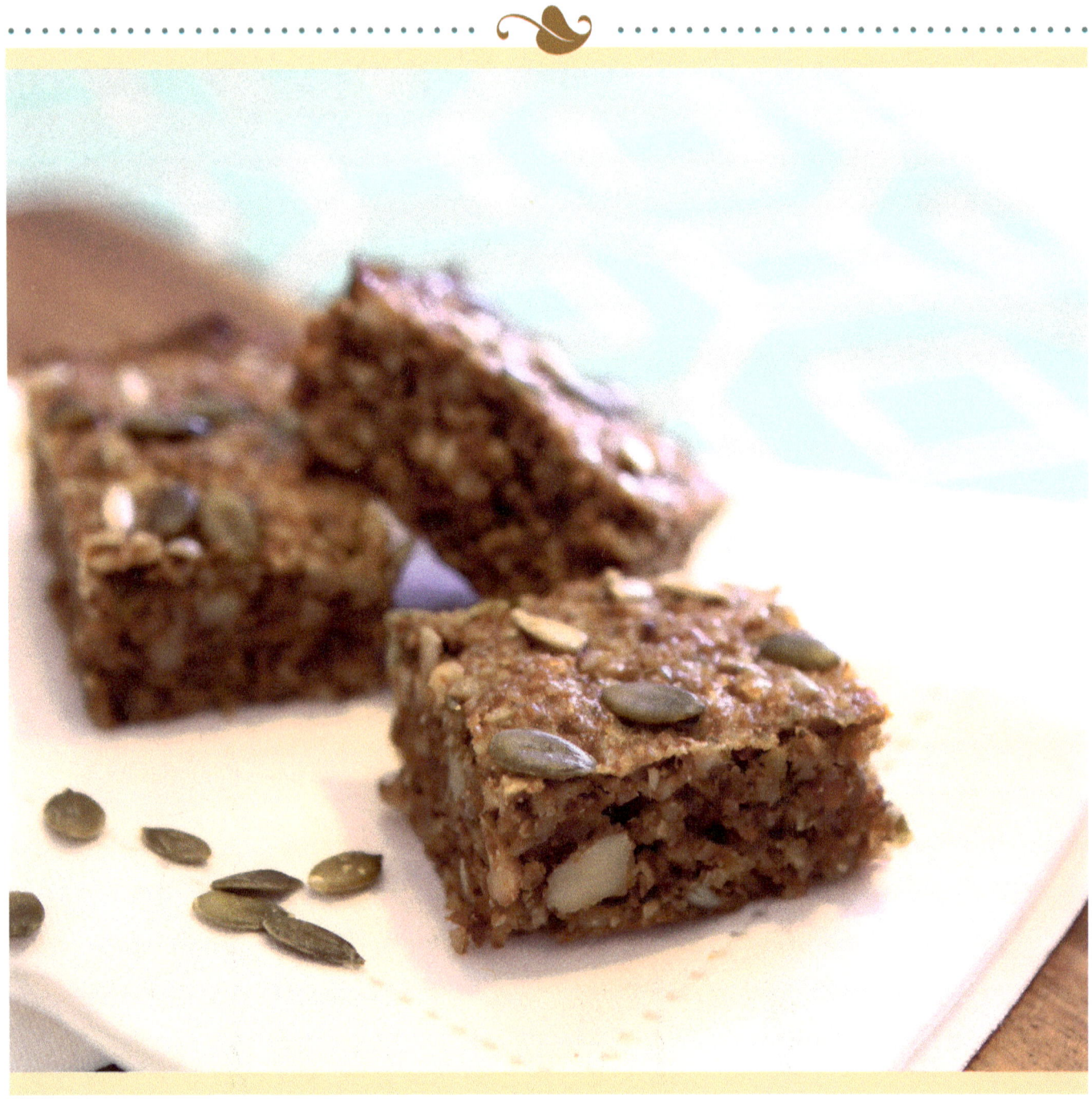

Muesli Breakfast Slice

These are great for breakfast on the run or for people who can't handle eating too early. Just pack and take with you. I have chosen an assortment of nuts and seeds to provide a wider spectrum of vitamins, minerals and protein to keep you going throughout the morning.

Prep time: 15 minutes   Cooking time: 20 minutes   Makes: 15

Ingredients:

- ¾ cup almonds
- ½ cup macadamia nuts
- ½ cup walnuts
- ⅓ cup pumpkin seeds
- ⅓ cup sunflower seeds
- ⅓ cup flaxseed meal
- 8 medjool dates, pitted
- ¼ cup honey
- ¼ cup coconut oil, melted
- 3 large eggs
- ½ tsp ground cinnamon
- 2 tsp vanilla extract
- ½ tsp fine sea salt
- 2 tsp each of pumpkin and sunflower seeds for top

Method:

Preheat oven to 160c/320f. Line and grease a 27x17cm(10.5x6.5ins) slice tin with baking paper.

Add to a food processor, almonds, macadamia nuts, walnuts, pumpkin and sunflower seeds. Pulse to just break up the nuts and seeds.

Then add the remaining ingredients, except for the seeds to go on top. Pulse until combined but pieces of nuts should still be seen.

Press mixture into prepared slice tin. Flatten and smooth top, then sprinkle with the extra few teaspoons of seeds and lightly press into mixture.

Bake for 20 minutes or until firm to touch and lightly browning. The inside will be soft and chewy. Let cool in tin, then cut into bars.

Store in an airtight container. They will keep fresh for up to 7 days or they can be frozen.

Green Banana Smoothie

My husband and I regularly have a smoothie for breakfast. It's a great way to fuel your body for that busy day ahead. We include all the additions listed below. It's like getting as much as possible at once and disguising it in a smoothie. I also try for extra Omega 3, because most of our diets are out of balance with way too much Omega 6 and 9. Chia seeds, hemp and flaxseed oils will give a boost of Omega 3.

Prep time: 10 minutes Cooking time: none Serves: 2 large or 3 small glasses

Ingredients:

- 1 banana
- 1 small apple
- 1 stick celery
- 2-3 kale leaves, stalks removed or 2 cups baby spinach
- Small handful of fresh parsley
- 2 Tbsp chia seeds
- 2 medjool dates, pitted
- 2 Tbsp hemp oil or flaxseed oil
- 1 Tbsp raw honey
- 1 Tbsp coconut butter, optional
- 2 tsp spirulina powder or a green superfood blend
- 2 cups of liquid, I use one of coconut water and one of filtered water or use nut milk
- Cinnamon to taste
- 2 cups ice cubes

Method:

Add all the above ingredients into a high speed blender. Start on variable speed, then turn to high. Blend until smooth. Be patient it's nicer drinking it smooth and creamy without bits in it. Drink immediately, as the chia seeds thicken the smoothie.

Additional options to boost your immune system and increase protein and antioxidants are:

1 Tbsp colloidal minerals, 1-2 tsp raw probiotic powder (immune & gut health), heaped Tbsp organic vanilla pea protein powder or gelatin, 1 Tbsp acai powder (antioxidant), 1 tsp camu powder (vitamin C), 2 eggs (protein); you can't taste them so don't cringe.

Tip: To change things up a little, add some mango or substitute fresh pineapple for the banana and apple, cucumber for celery. Add 1-2 sprigs of fresh mint leaves in place of parsley and some fresh young coconut meat.

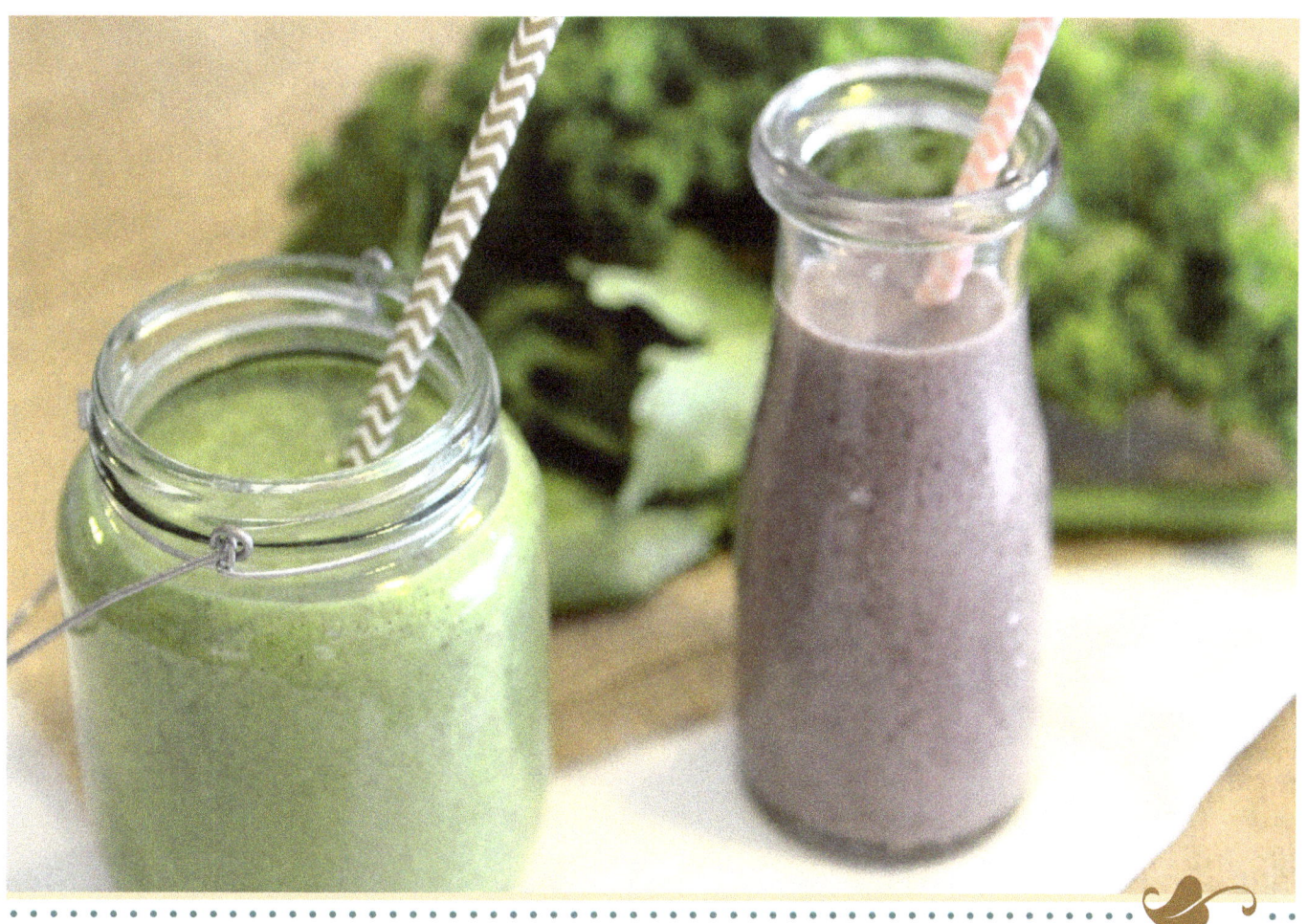

Blueberry Smoothie

Prep time: 10 minutes Cooking time: none Serves: 2 large or 3 small glasses

Ingredients:

- 1 cup frozen blueberries
- 1 banana
- 1 small apple
- 1 stick celery
- 2 Tbsp chia seeds
- 2 medjool dates, pitted
- 2 Tbsp hemp oil or flaxseed oil
- 1 Tbsp raw honey
- 1 Tbsp coconut butter, optional
- 2 cups of liquid, I use one of coconut water and one of filtered water or use a nut milk
- 1 tsp vanilla extract
- 1-1½ cups ice cubes

Method:

Add all the above ingredients into a high speed blender, start on variable speed, then turn to high. Blend until smooth. Be patient, it's nicer drinking it smooth and creamy without bits in it. Drink immediately.

See additional options to boost your immune system, protein and antioxidants on page 24.

Chocolate Coconut Smoothie

Now here is a treat for you and the kids for breakfast. Raw cacao will give you fiber, it's heart-healthy and is beneficial in helping blood glucose levels. I'm sneaking in some powdered greens but you can't tell with all that chocolate! Enjoy this healthy treat! "It's just like a chocolate thick shake".

Prep time: 10 minutes Cooking time: none Serves: 2

Ingredients:

- 1 small banana
- 2 Tbsp chia seeds
- 2 medjool dates, pitted
- 2 Tbsp coconut butter
- 2 Tbsp almond butter/spread or tahini
- 2 Tbsp raw cacao powder
- 2 Tbsp hemp oil or flaxseed oil
- 1½ tsp spirulina or a green superfood blend
- 1 cup coconut milk
- 1¼ cups filtered water or coconut water
- 2 cups ice cubes

Method:

Put all the above ingredients into a high speed blender, start on variable speed, then turn to high. Blend until smooth. Drink immediately.

Additional options you can include to boost your immune system and increase protein and antioxidants: 1 Tbsp colloidal minerals, 1-2 tsp raw probiotic powder (immune & gut health), 1 Tbsp acai powder (antioxidant), ½-1 tsp camu powder (vitamin C), 2 eggs (protein).

BREAKFAST | 27

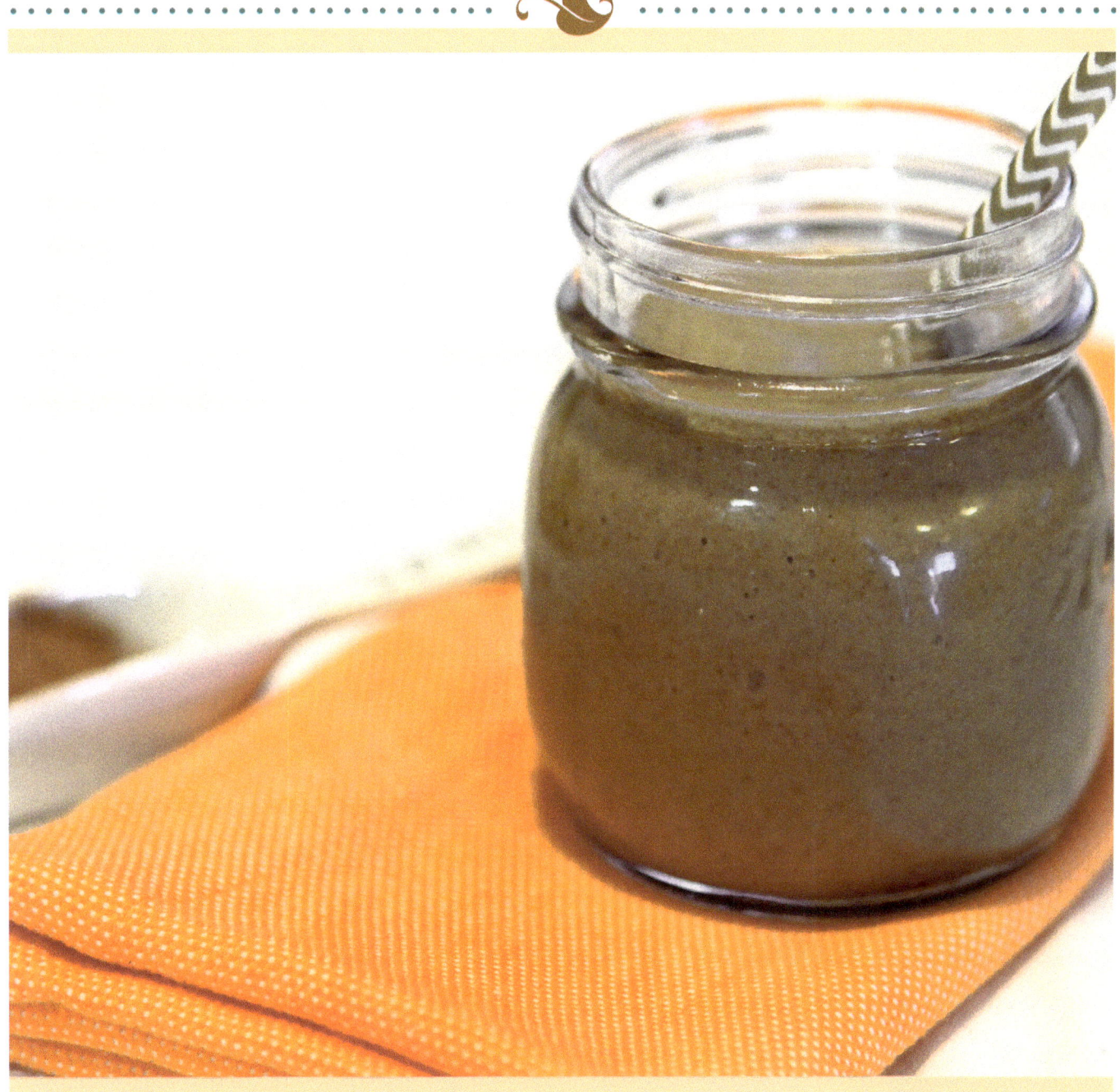

28 | BREAKFAST

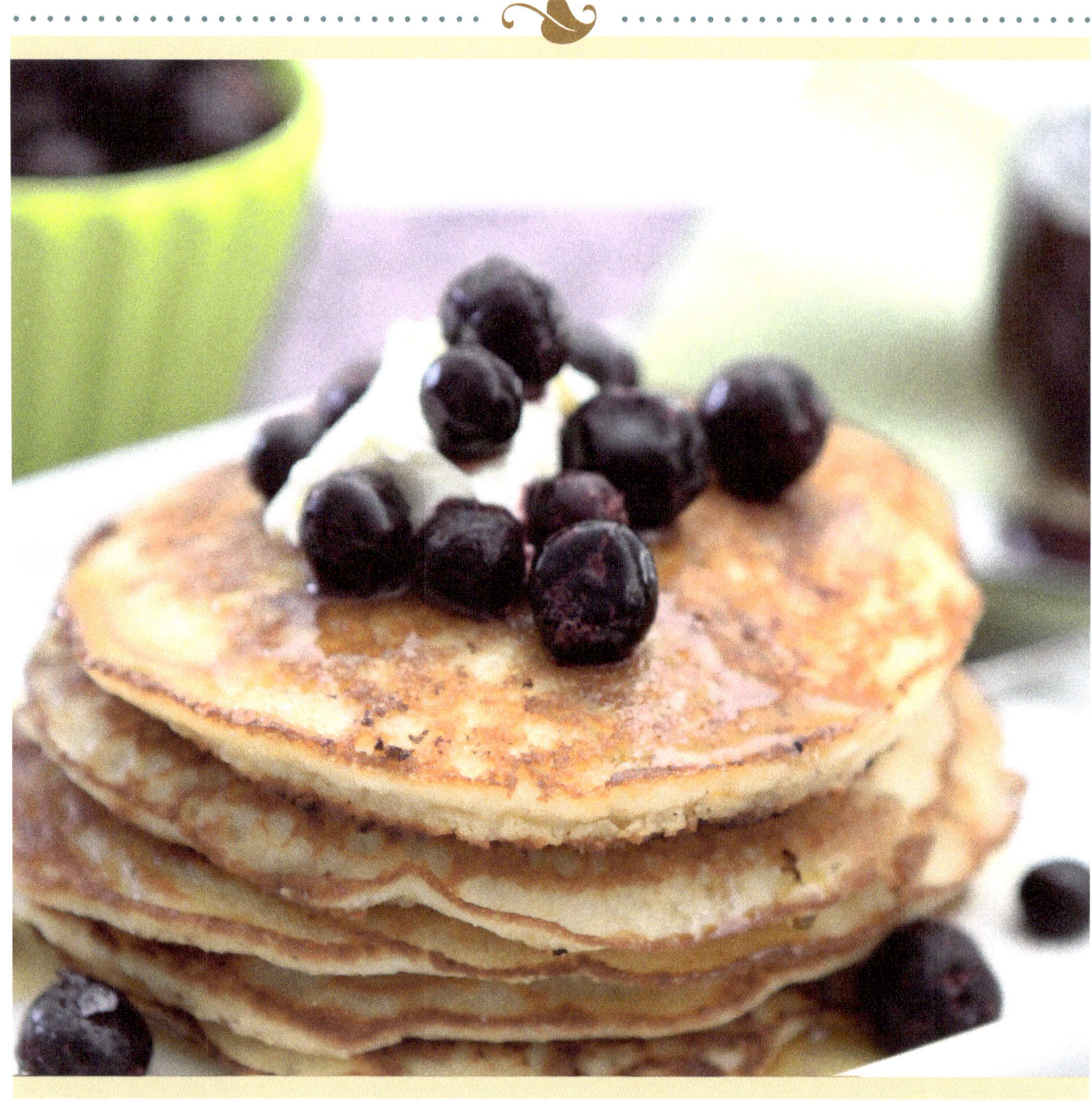

Pancakes

For a grain free pancake, these are super light and fluffy. It is achieved by separating the eggs and adding a small amount of arrowroot flour.

Prep time: 12 minutes Cooking time: 15 minutes Makes: 12

Ingredients:

- 3 large eggs, separated
- 1 cup almond or cashew milk, or milk of your choice
- 1 Tbsp 100% maple syrup
- 2 tsp vanilla extract
- 1¾ cups almond meal/flour
- 3 Tbsp arrowroot flour
- ½ tsp baking soda
- Ghee for frying

Method:

Beat egg whites until stiff peaks form and set aside.

In a large bowl beat egg yolks, milk, maple syrup and vanilla.

Add to the wet ingredients, almond meal, arrowroot flour and baking soda. Beat to blend.

Using a spatula, fold half the beaten egg whites into the batter, then fold in the remaining egg whites. Add additional milk if consistency is too thick.

Heat a large nonstick frying pan on medium heat. Smear a coat of ghee over the pan.

Pour a ¼ cup of mixture into the pan for each pancake. Cook 2 or more at a time. Cook for 3-4 minutes on first side. Flip over and cook for approximately 2 minutes or until cooked through.

Transfer to a plate and keep warm. Repeat with remaining batter, greasing pan with ghee between batches.

Serve with 100% maple syrup, coconut cream or yoghurt and fruit.

For variety, add cinnamon to the batter.

30 | BREAKFAST

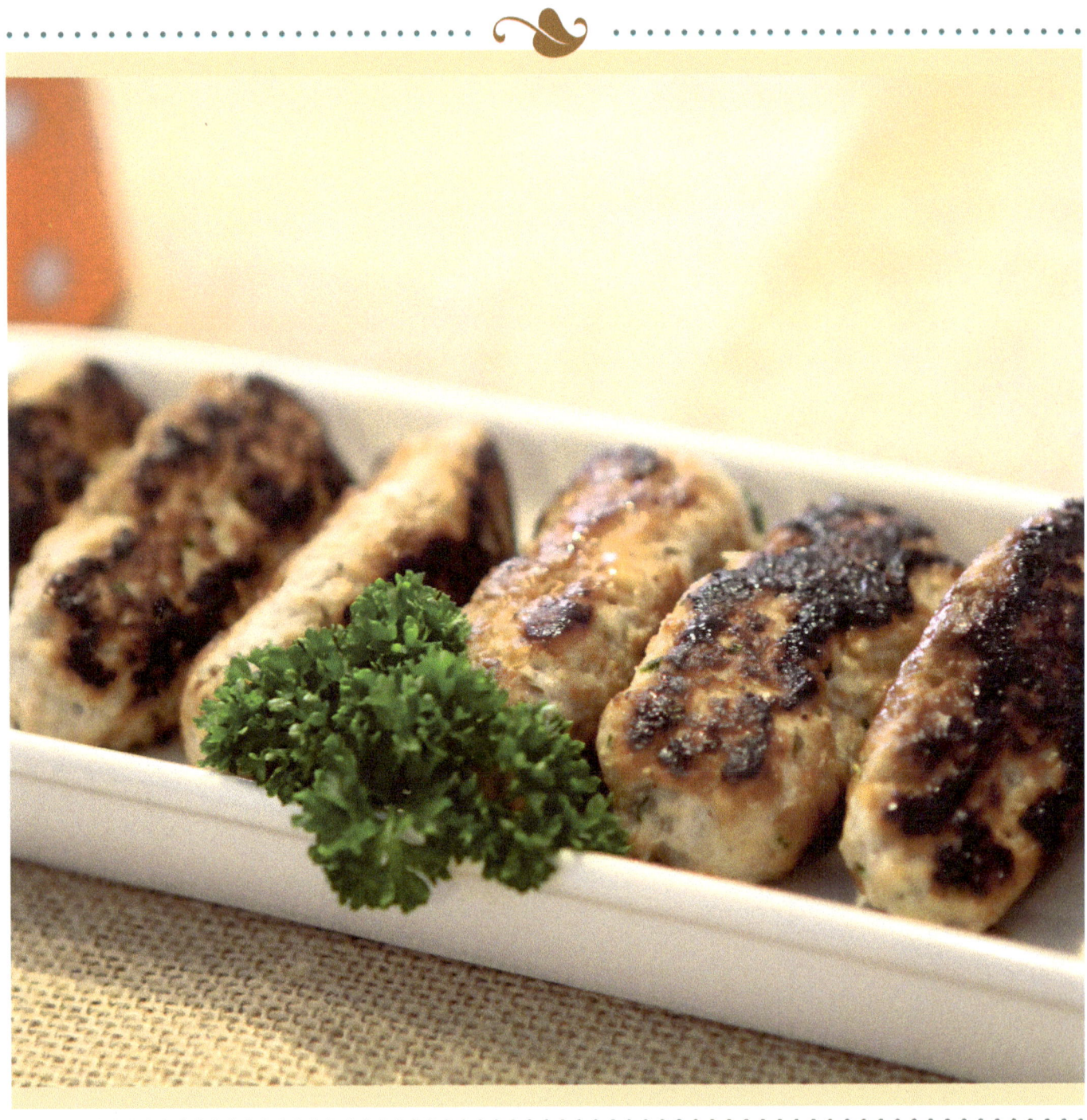

Breakfast Sausages

As the ingredients of commercially made sausages are always a mystery, I thought we had better have ones that we know exactly what is in them. To make a hearty breakfast, these sausages can be served with fried eggs, tomato and mushrooms. Plan ahead and make extra to freeze and have on hand for breakfast or lunch, they are excellent cold in a packed lunch.

Prep time: 10 minutes Cooking time: 8 minutes Makes: 12 small sausages

Ingredients:

- 1 small onion, chopped in quarters
- 500g/1 lb minced pork or meat of your choice
- 2 Tbsp fresh parsley leaves
- 2 tsp maple syrup or honey
- ¾ tsp sea salt
- ½ tsp ground cinnamon
- ¼ tsp dried thyme leaves
- ¼ tsp nutmeg
- ¼ tsp black pepper
- Coconut oil for cooking

Method:

To a food processor add the onion and pulse a couple of times until it's roughly minced. Add pork and remaining ingredients. Blend until well combined. You can also mix by hand if you prefer but mince or grate the onion first. I just like the texture that comes from using the food processor.

Heat a frying pan over medium-high heat and melt coconut oil. Scoop out 2 rounded tablespoons of mixture into your hand and mold to make a sausage shape, approximately 10cm/4ins long.

Fry the sausages until cooked through, turning as they cook to brown on all sides, approximately 8 minutes in total. When cooked, place on paper towels to drain.

For freezing, make up and form your uncooked sausages and lay them on a paper-lined tray. Place the tray in freezer and when sausages are frozen, remove to a sealed container and return to store in the freezer.

For a speedy breakfast, add the frozen sausages to a frying pan on medium heat, add oil and cook covered for a few minutes to help thaw, then uncover and turn the heat up, brown on all sides, serve when cooked through.

32 | BREAKFAST

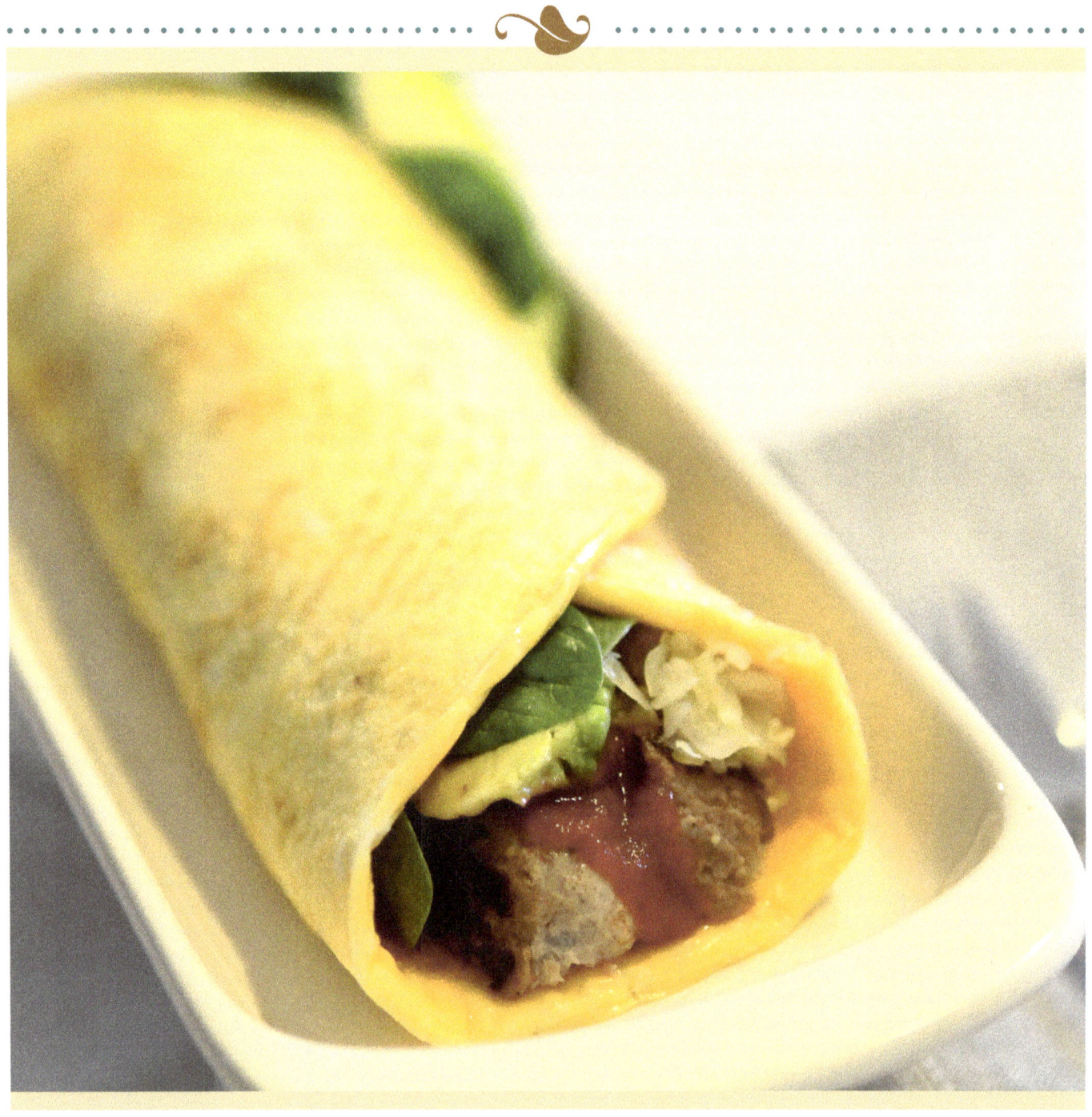

Egg Burrito
with leftovers

This is a thin plain omelet used to hold your food together and given a fancy name. Using leftovers in your breakfast burrito is a good way to not waste food. The kids will think it's fun! I'm sure you will find many uses for this egg burrito!

Prep time: 10 minutes   Cooking time: 7 minutes   Serves: 1 large

Ingredients:

- 1 serve of leftover meat dish, casserole, meatballs, sausage or vegetables, heated
- 3 eggs
- 2 tsp filtered water
- ½-1 tsp ghee or coconut oil
- Sea salt and pepper to taste
- Your favourite paleo sauce
- Optional: sliced avocado, sauerkraut, sliced tomatoes, sautéed mushrooms

Method:

Heat up leftovers and slice up any additional items to go inside your burrito.

Whisk eggs and water in a small bowl.

Heat ghee or coconut oil in a large nonstick frying pan 28 or 30cm(11ins) over low heat. Pour eggs into pan, move your pan a little to spread egg out in a thin even layer.

Cook eggs on low for 3-4 minutes, then gradually turn up to medium to finish cooking eggs, it will take approximately 7-8 minutes to cook. Don't turn the egg over.

When cooked, carefully slide your burrito onto a plate. Place your leftover meat or vegetables and any additions you fancy onto your egg burrito. Add salt, pepper and sauce if required. Roll up and serve.

You can use 2 eggs and 1 tsp water if you would prefer a smaller serve, and reduce the size of the pan.

English Muffins
with Egg and Avocado

So quick and easy, just throw everything into a blender. After baking you just need to toast the muffins in a frying pan to make them look like an English Muffin. For a nut free version, substitute sunflower meal for the almond meal.

Prep time: 5 minutes Cooking time: 25 minutes Makes: 2 whole or 4 halves

Ingredients:

- ⅓ cup almond meal/flour
- 1 Tbsp golden flaxseed meal
- 1 tsp gluten free baking powder
- ⅓ tsp sea salt
- 2 large eggs
- 3 Tbsp full fat coconut milk
- 2 tsp macadamia oil, plus extra for coating ramekins
- Ghee for frying
- Muffin fillings, 2 fried eggs and sliced avocado

Method:

Preheat oven to 180c/350f. Grease two 9cm (3.5in) ramekins with the extra macadamia oil.

To a blender add, almond meal, flaxseed, baking powder, salt, eggs, coconut milk and 2 teaspoons of macadamia oil. Blend on variable speed then switch to high for one or two seconds.

Divide batter between the ramekins and bake for 18-20 minutes or until tops are firm to touch and are starting to brown.

Remove from oven and let cool for 10 minutes. Using a knife, run around the sides to loosen the muffins and remove. Use a serrated bread knife to slice in half.

Toast in a frying pan with a small amount of melted ghee. Use an egg slice or spatula to press down on the muffins to lightly brown. Flip to cook on both sides, this will make it look like an English muffin.

Eat straight away, topped with an egg and avocado slices, add your favourite sauce. Your children may like them topped with almond or sunflower butter or homemade jam.

Double or triple recipe for larger quantities.

To freeze, place baking paper between cooled fried muffins and seal in a freezer safe container. After thawing, just pop into a toaster or into a fry pan again and they are ready to eat.

BREAKFAST | 35

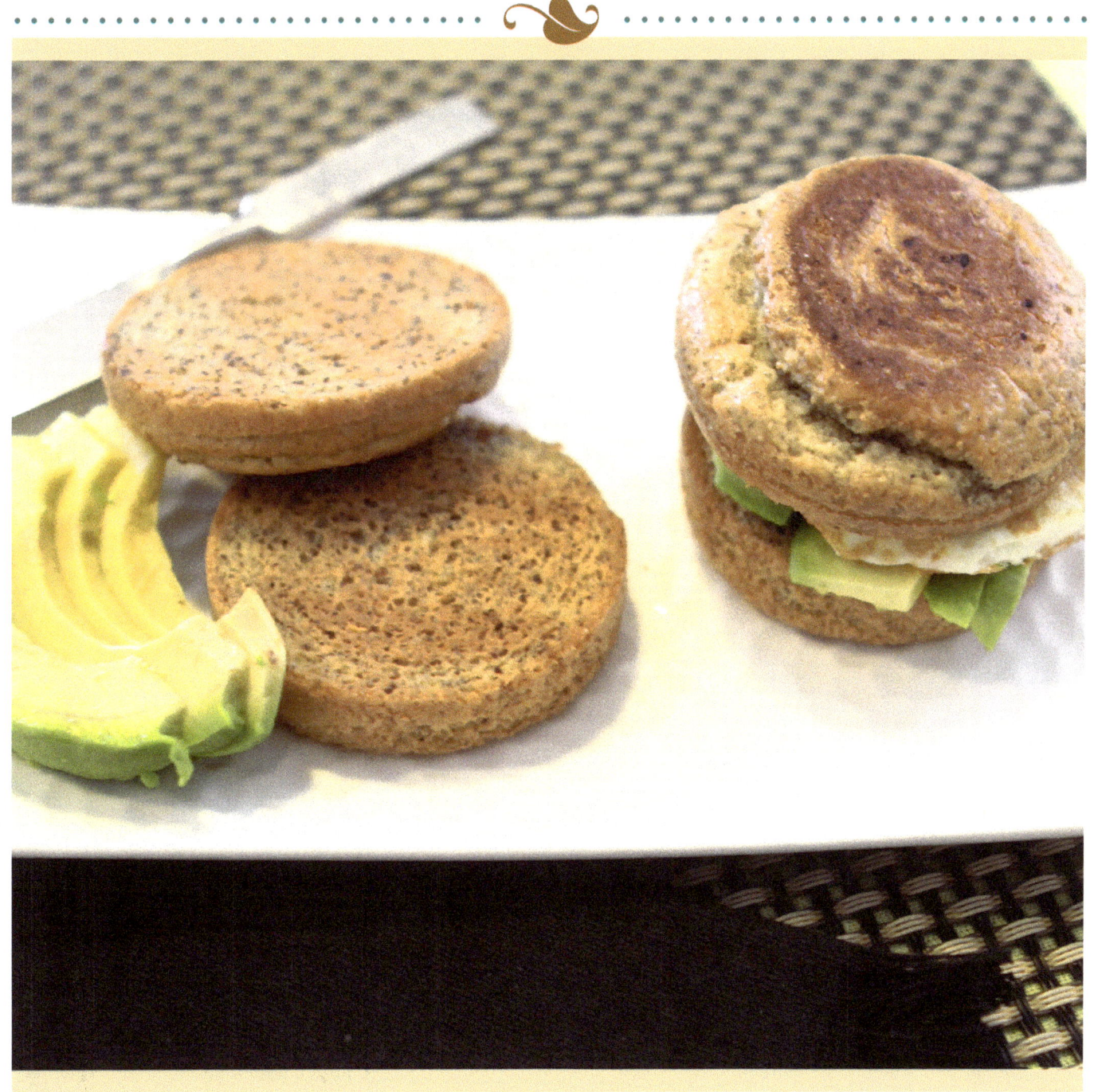

36 | BREAKFAST

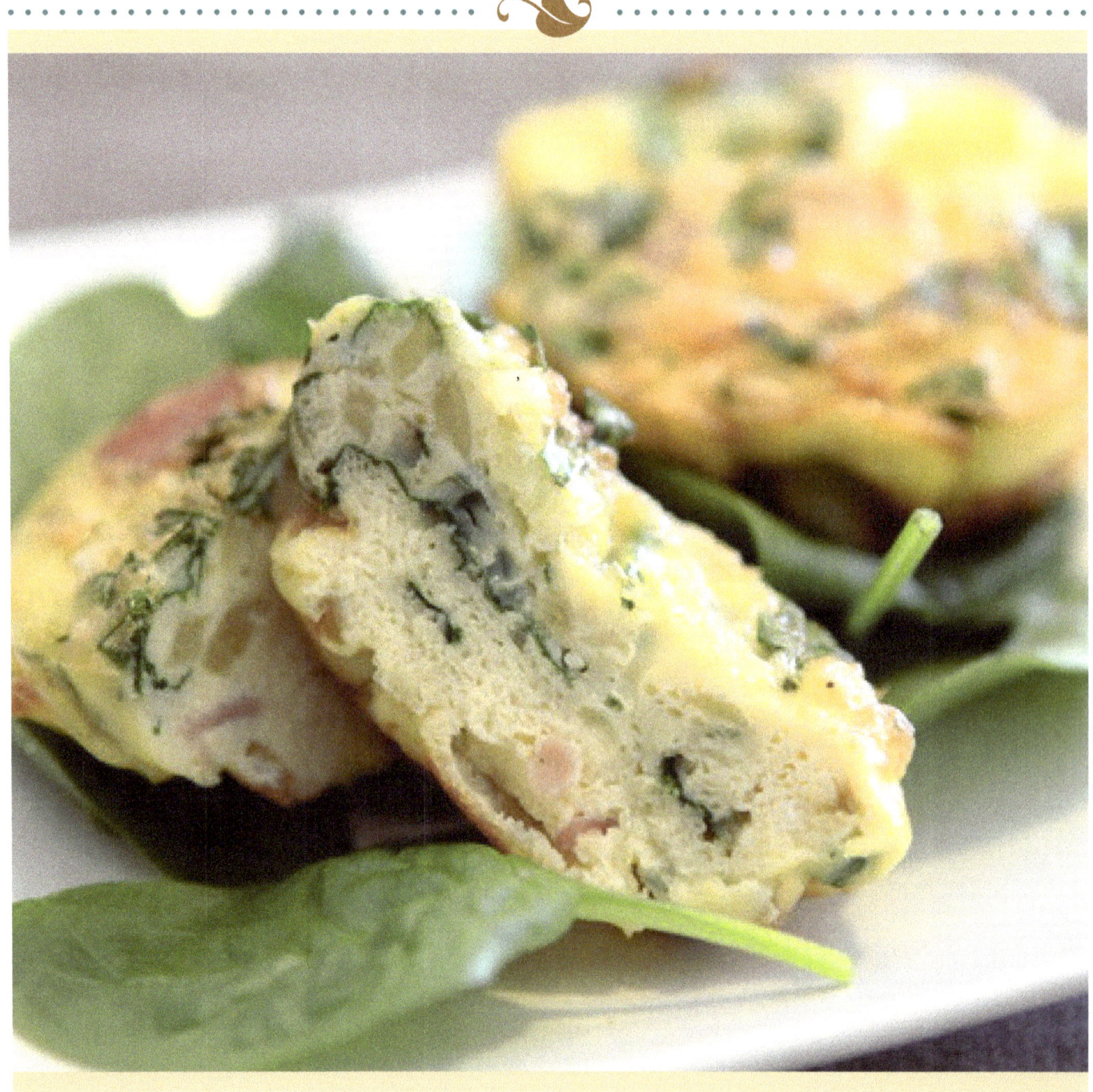

Greens Eggs and Ham Muffins

I am hoping your children or grandchildren will love these. The name of my recipe was inspired by Dr Seuss' book Green Eggs and Ham. You could also add diced green capsicum, instead of spinach. I think they would work well for school lunches too.

Prep time: 12 minutes Cooking time: 20 minutes Makes: 10

Ingredients:

- 8 large eggs
- 4-5/120g ham slices, diced (nitrate free)
- 1 small onion, finely diced
- 1 cup baby spinach, finely chopped
- ½ cup mature cheese grated or
    - 3 Tbsp Nutritional Yeast Flakes for dairy free
- 3 Tbsp coconut milk
- ⅓ tsp fine sea salt
- ¼ tsp ground nutmeg, optional
- ⅛ tsp ground black pepper

Method:

Preheat oven to 170c/340f and line a muffin tin with paper liners. I use café style liners; there's no sticking and the muffins pop right out.

Beat eggs in a large bowl. Add ham, onion, spinach, cheese or Nutritional Yeast Flakes, coconut milk or milk of choice and seasonings. Mix well to combine.

Spoon mixture into prepared muffin cups.

Bake for 20-25 minutes or until muffins are set in the middle.

Sweet Potato Hash Browns

I love cinnamon with sweet potato but not all people like sweet flavours for breakfast. (As I was reminded by my savoury loving husband.) So we have two varieties now. Hope you enjoy one or both of my hash brown recipes.

Prep time: 10 minutes Cooking time: 12 minutes Makes: 7

Ingredients:

- 2 large eggs, beaten
- 2 Tbsp coconut flour
- 1 tsp cinnamon
- ½ tsp fine sea salt
- 1 medium/500g sweet potato, peeled and grated
- Coconut oil for cooking

Method:

To a large bowl add, eggs and whisk. Add coconut flour, cinnamon and salt. Mix well.

Remove excess water from the grated sweet potatoes by pressing between sheets of paper towels.

Add the sweet potato to the egg mixture. Combine well, (I find a fork is best to mix with or your hands.)

Heat a large frying pan over medium-high heat. Add coconut oil. Be generous with the oil, as the hash browns will cook and stay together better and be nice and crunchy.

Spoon the mixture into the frying pan. Shape and flatten with a fork to make approximately 9-10cm(4in) rounds. Add additional oil between batches if required. Cook for approximately 3-4 minutes on each side. (I use a big 32cm frying pan and fit 4 in at a time.) Serve immediately so they keep their crunch.

Serve with lightly fried spinach, bacon and eggs. I love a little sour cream with my hash browns. (Dairy free sour cream recipe on page 302).

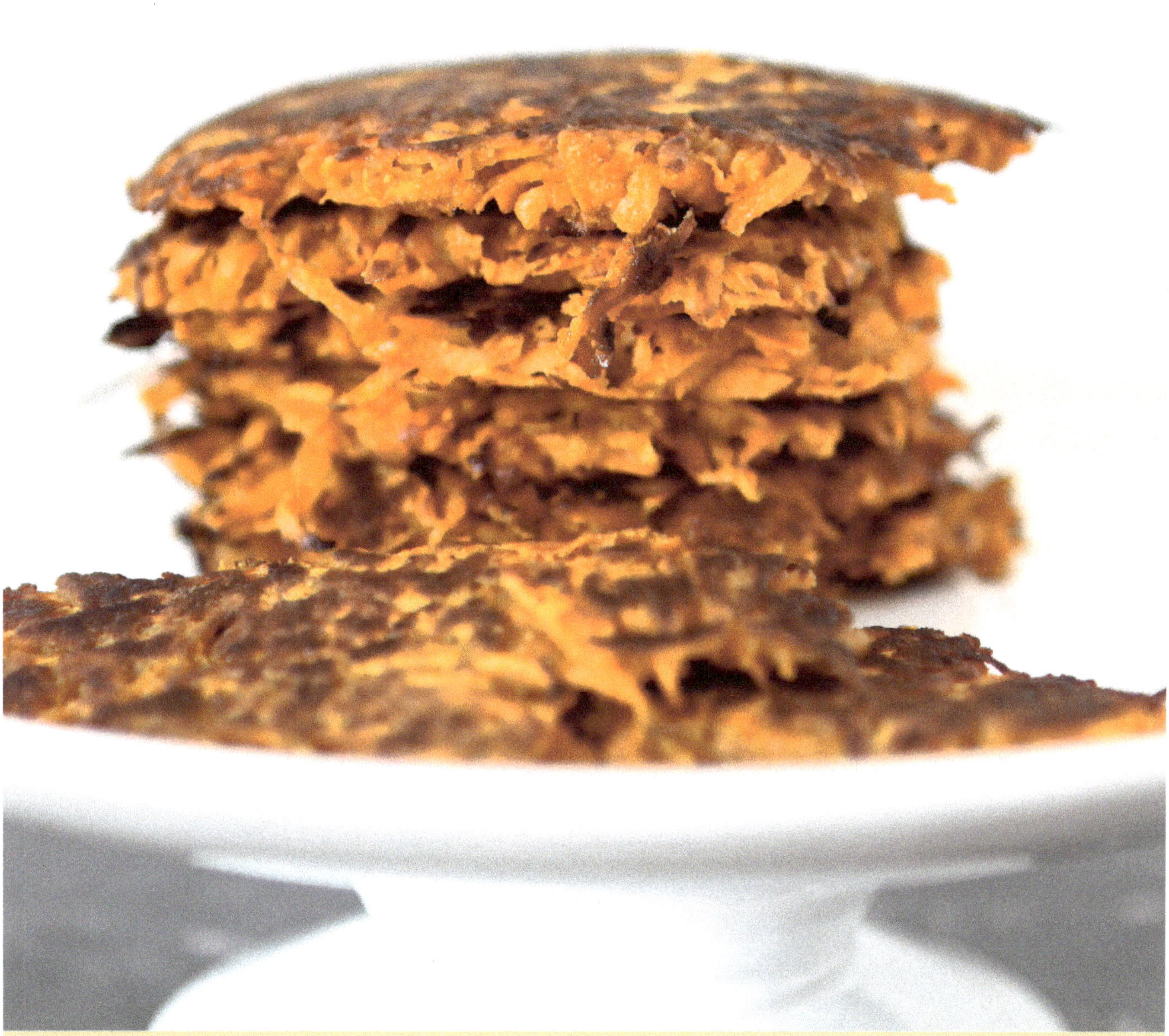

BREAKFAST | 39

40 | BREAKFAST

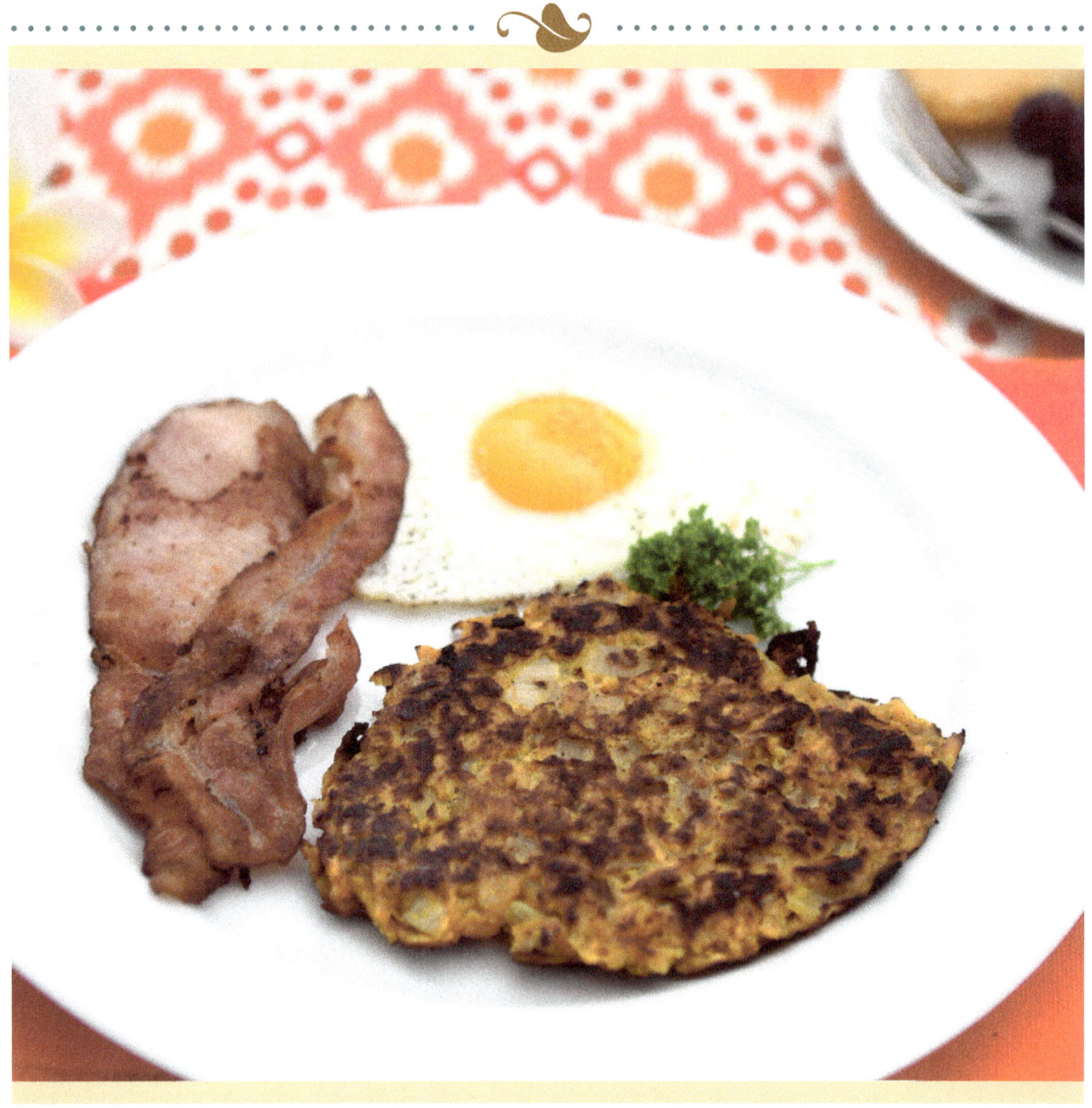

Sweet Potato & Onion Hash Browns

Savoury version of sweet potato hash browns, to please all family members. Serve with bacon and eggs.

Prep time: 15 minutes   Cooking time: 12 minutes   Makes: 7

Ingredients:

- 2 large eggs, beaten
- 2 Tbsp coconut flour
- ½ onion, finely diced
- ¾ tsp garlic, minced
- 1 tsp fine sea salt
- ¼ tsp pepper
- 1 medium/500g sweet potato, peeled and grated
- Coconut oil for cooking

Method:

To a large bowl add, eggs and whisk. Add coconut flour, onion, garlic, salt and pepper. Mix to combine.

Remove excess water from the grated sweet potatoes by pressing between sheets of paper towels.

Mix in the sweet potato. Combine well. (I find a fork is best to mix with).

Heat a large frying pan over medium-high heat. Add coconut oil, be generous, it will help the hash browns to stay together and turn out nice and crunchy.

Spoon the mixture into the frying pan. Shape and flatten with a fork to make 9cm(3.5in) rounds. Add extra oil between batches when required.

Cook for approximately 3-4 minutes on each side. I use a big 32cm frying pan and fit 4 in at a time. Serve immediately so they keep their crunch.

Vegetable and Bacon Slice

Since removing potatoes from my life, I've fallen in love with swede. So I couldn't help adding some to this slice. Swede is very high in dietary fibre and good source of magnesium, niacin, phosphorus, potassium, vitamins B6 and C, zinc and so much more. It's always hard changing habits but who said you can't eat vegetables for breakfast? To save time, make the night before and just warm in the morning for breakfast. This slice also makes a great dish for a weekend brunch.

Prep time: 25 minutes Cooking time: 50 minutes Serves: 6

Ingredients:

- 3 full rashes of bacon, chopped (nitrate free)
- 1 onion, diced
- 2 tsp garlic, minced
- 1 large swede, grated
- 1 large carrot, grated
- ½ medium zucchini, grated with skin on
- 2 cups firmly packed baby spinach, finely sliced
- 1 Tbsp chopped fresh parsley or 1½ tsp dried
- 3 Tbsp coconut flour
- ¼ cup Nutritional Yeast Flakes or ¾ cup matured cheese grated
- ¾ tsp fine sea salt
- ¼ tsp ground black pepper or to taste
- 5 large eggs, beaten
- ½ cup coconut milk, or milk of choice

Method:

Preheat oven to 180c/350f. Grease an oven-proof dish (I use a 24cm square dish), with ghee or coconut oil.

Heat a frying pan over medium heat. Add bacon, onion and garlic. Cook for 5 minutes until onions are soft. If not enough fat is left from the bacon, add a little ghee. Set aside.

Grate swede, carrot and zucchini, place between paper towels or tea towels. Press to squeeze out excess liquid.

To a large bowl add, grated vegetables, onion mixture, sliced spinach, parsley, coconut flour, Nutritional Yeast Flakes, salt and pepper. Mix well to combine.

Whisk eggs and coconut milk together. Add to vegetable mixture and stir well to combine. Spoon into prepared dish, smooth top with a spatula.

Bake for 45-50 minutes, or until liquid has absorbed and top is set. Cut into squares to serve warm or cold.

BREAKFAST | 43

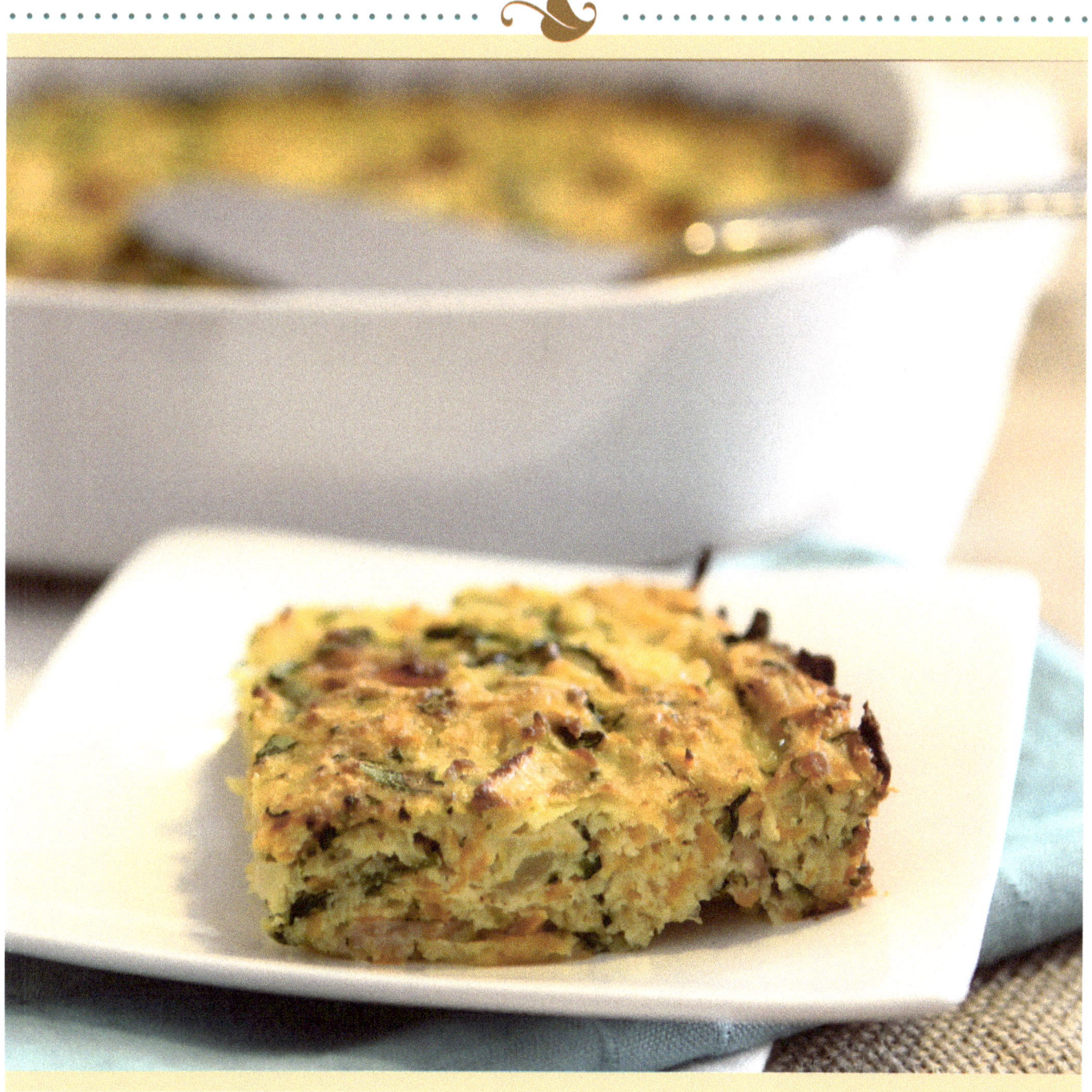

SOUPS

Cream of Asparagus Soup 47

Cream of Broccoli Soup 48

Cream of Cauliflower Soup 51

"Potato" and Leek Soup 52

Pumpkin Soup 55

Taco Soup 56

Sweet Potato and Vegetable Soup 59

Seafood Chowder 60

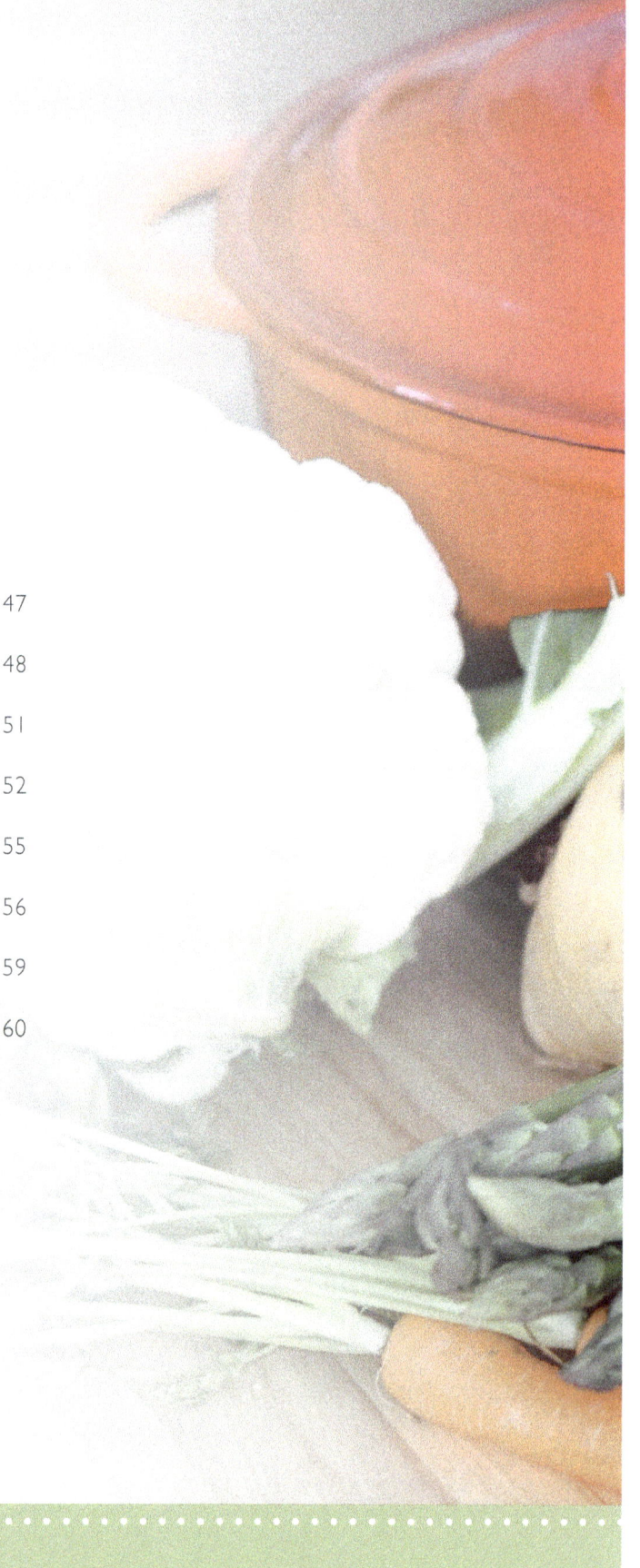

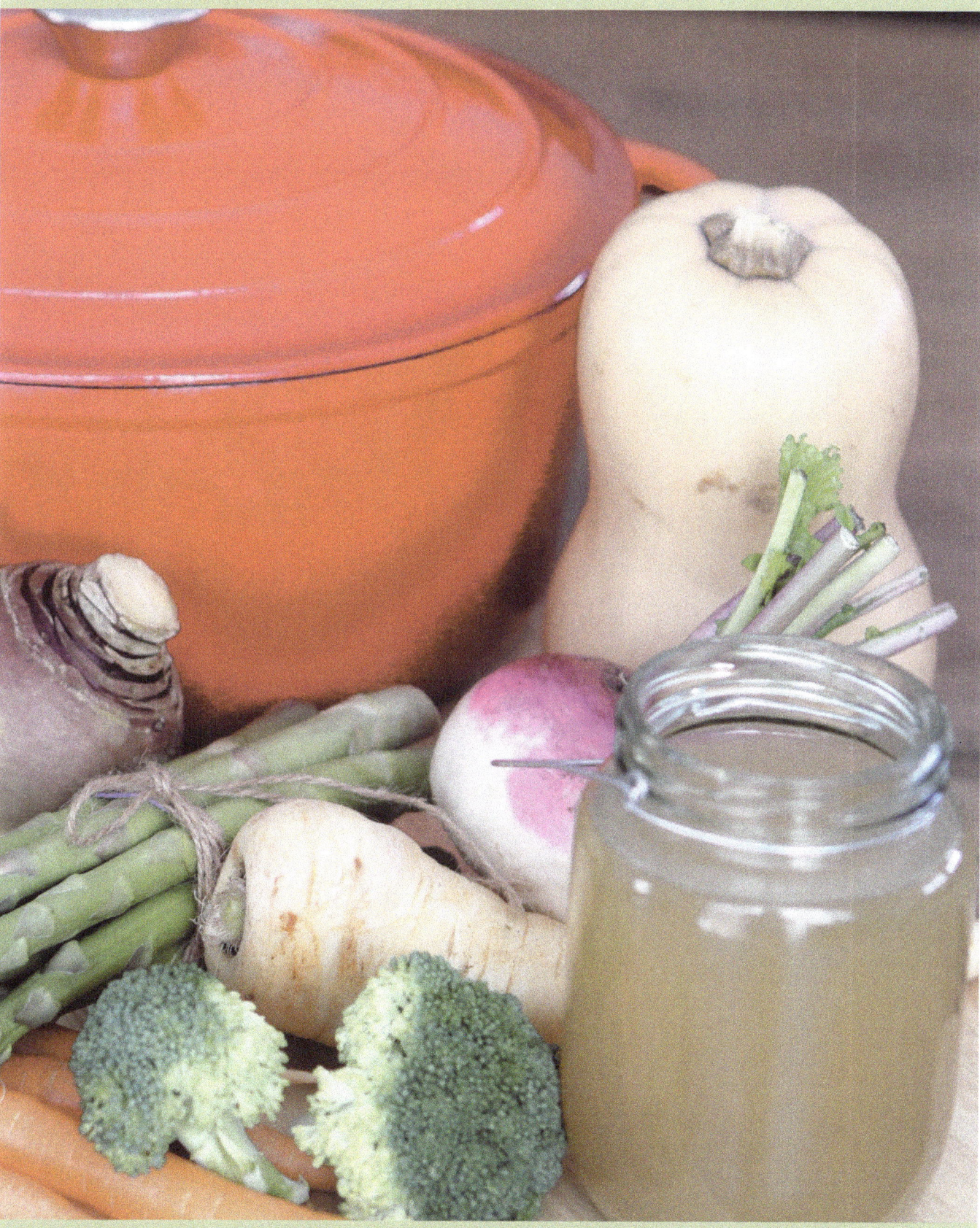

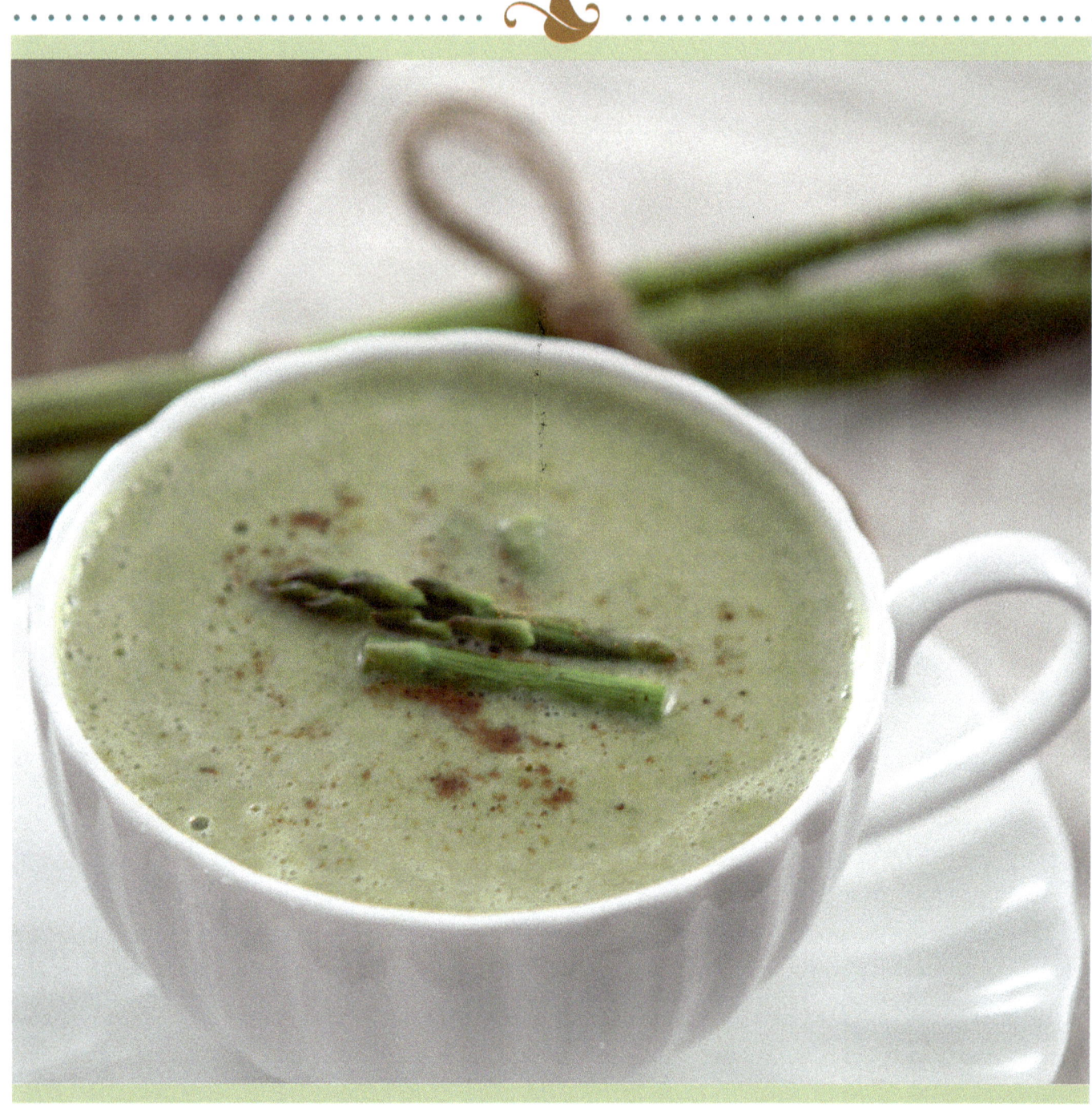

Cream of Asparagus Soup

This is a lovely quick and simple soup to make. There are huge health benefits. Asparagus is one of the healthiest vegetables. Loads of nutrients: folate, vitamins A, C, E, K and chromium. High levels of antioxidants and a good source of prebiotics. I've added a little spinach to help give a nice shade of green to the soup.

Prep time: 10 minutes Cooking time: 30 minutes Serves: 4

Ingredients:

- 1½ Tbsp coconut oil or ghee
- 500g/2½ bunches asparagus, cut into 2.5cm (1in) pieces
- 3 stalks celery, chopped
- 1 large onion, diced
- 3 tsp garlic, minced
- 1½ tsp coarse sea salt, divided
- 1L/4 cups chicken broth/stock
- ⅓ tsp ground pepper or to taste
- ⅓–½ tsp ground nutmeg, plus extra to sprinkle when serving
- 1 cup firmly packed baby spinach
- 1 cup canned coconut cream or cashew cream (recipe below)

Method:

Heat a large pot on medium heat, melt the coconut oil. Add cut asparagus, celery, onion, garlic and ½ teaspoon sea salt. Cook for 10 minutes or until vegetables have started to soften. The salt will help moisture come out of the vegetables and prevent browning.

Add broth/stock, remaining sea salt, pepper and nutmeg to pot, cover and bring to a boil. Reduce and simmer for 15 minutes covered. Add spinach, coconut cream or cashew cream and cook uncovered for a further 5 minutes.

Transfer to a high-speed blender and blend well. Make sure asparagus and celery are fully blended and smooth, as they are very fibrous vegetables. Adjust seasoning if required.

Serve garnished with a sprinkling of nutmeg and cut pieces of steamed asparagus.

CASHEW CREAM:

Soak 1 cup of raw cashews with a pinch of sea salt in filtered water for 1 hour. Drain and rinse well. Add to a high-speed blender with enough filtered water to just cover the nuts. Blend on high for several minutes until very smooth. You may need to use a tamper to push the nuts onto the blade. (Cashew Cream can be used to replace any type of cream in a recipe).

Cream of Broccoli Soup

When my sons were schoolboys, they loved coming home to warm Broccoli soup on the stove in winter. This old favourite only under went two changes to make it Paleo, swapping canned evaporated milk with coconut milk and potato with swede. Tastes even yummier! Don't discard the broccoli stalks, all that goodness will be blended into the soup and it helps to bulk it up.

Prep time: 15 minutes Cooking time: 40 minutes Serves: 4-6

Ingredients:

- 1½ Tbsp coconut oil
- 2 onions, diced
- 3 tsp garlic, minced
- 1 swede, peeled and diced finely
- 1.5L/6 cups chicken broth/stock
- 2 bunches broccoli, chopped (use stalks)
- 1 cup coconut milk or more if you like it creamier
- 1 tsp coarse sea salt and pepper to taste (be generous)

Method:

Heat a large soup pot on low-medium heat, melt coconut oil. Add onion, garlic and swede. Cook for 5 minutes, don't allow to brown.

Add broth/stock to pot and bring to a boil, reduce and simmer for 15 minutes.

Add broccoli, cook a further 15-20 minutes or until vegetables have softened enough to blend. Add to the pot, coconut milk, salt and pepper to taste.

Transfer to a blender and blend in batches until smooth.

Serve with coconut milk or cream drizzled over the top. Run a toothpick through the cream if you would like to make a pattern.

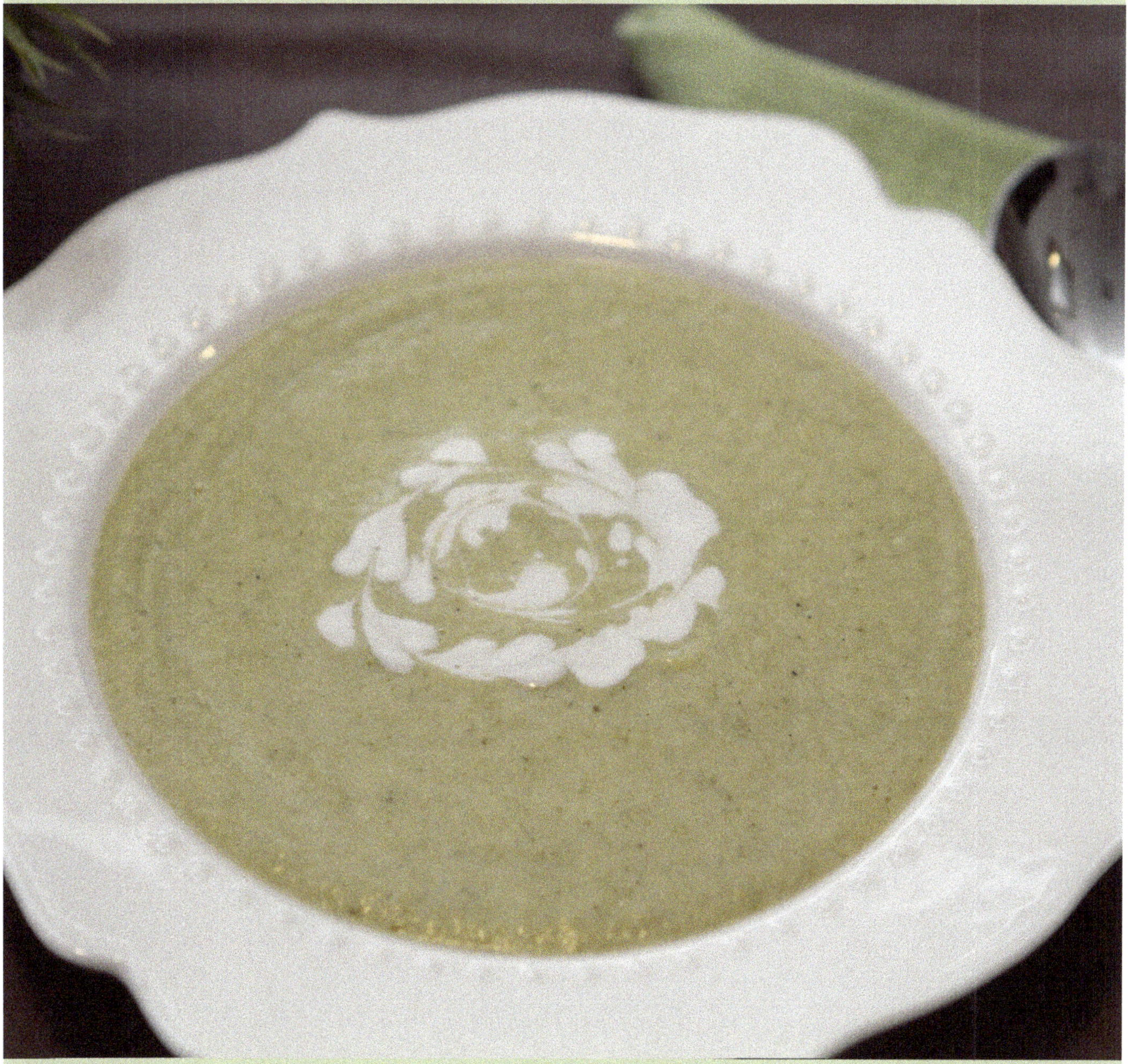

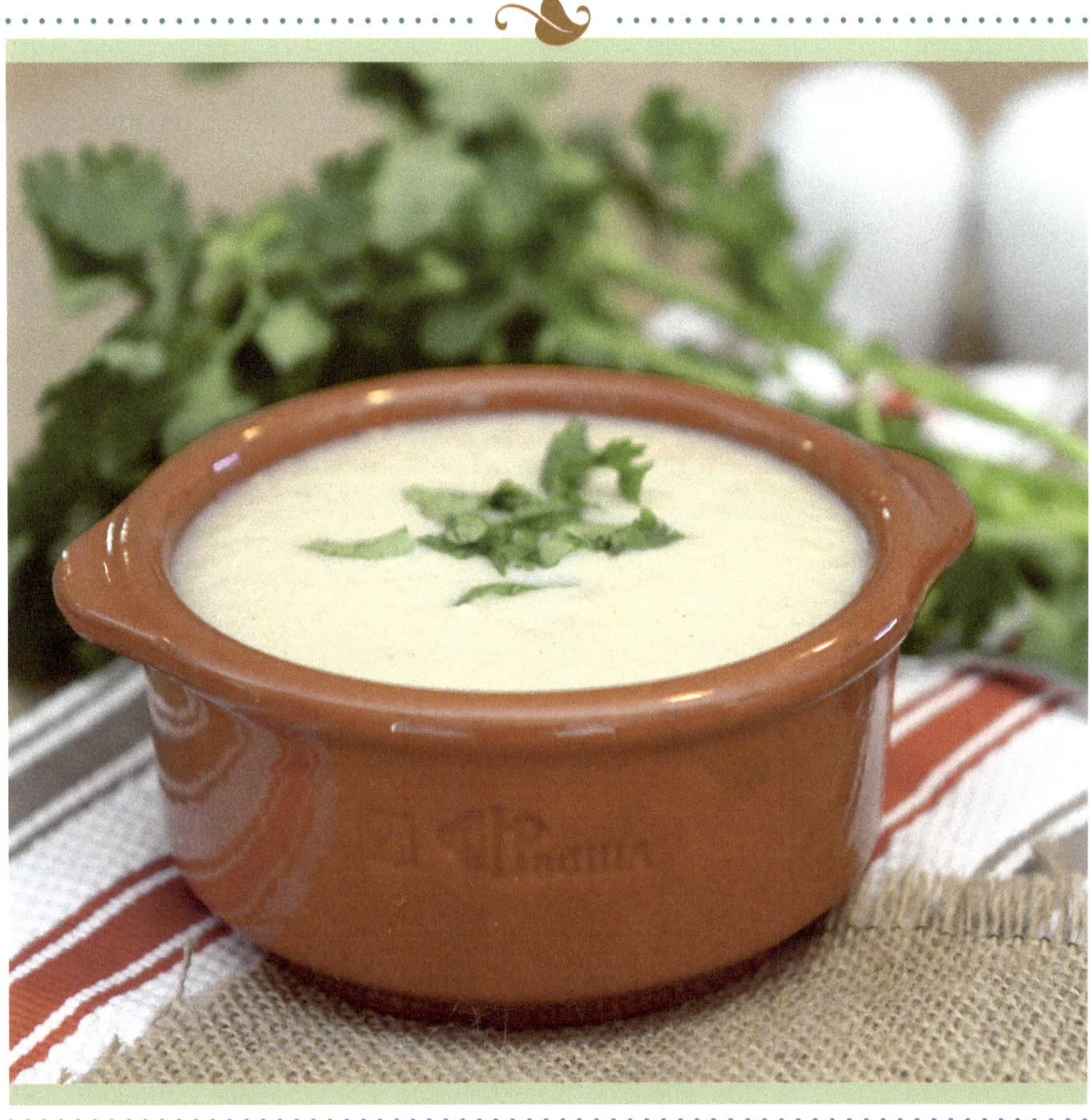

Cream of Cauliflower Soup

I hope you like cauliflower. I have a new appreciation for it since going Paleo. Cauliflower has the ability to give a lovely creamy texture, which makes for a delicious soup. For the chili lovers, add ¼ - ½ teaspoon of chili to spice it up.

Prep time: 10 minutes   Cooking time: 35 minutes   Serves: 4

Ingredients:

- 1 Tbsp coconut oil
- 2 medium onions, diced
- 2 tsp garlic, minced
- 2 tsp ground coriander
- 2 tsp ground cumin
- 1 large cauliflower, chopped in chunks (use stalks)
- 1.5L/6 cups chicken or vegetable broth/stock
- ½ cup coconut milk or almond milk
- Sea salt and pepper to taste (be generous)
- Chopped fresh coriander to garnish

Method:

Heat a large soup pot on medium heat and melt the coconut oil. Add onions and garlic, cook for 3 minutes or until transparent. Add coriander and cumin, cook stirring for 1 minute or until the spices are fragrant.

Add cauliflower and broth/stock, cover and bring to a boil. Reduce heat to low, simmer for 20 minutes until cauliflower is tender.

Add coconut milk or almond milk and season with salt and pepper. Let warm through. Transfer to a blender, blend in batches until smooth.

Serve with a sprinkling of chopped fresh coriander.

"Potato" and Leek Soup

I have used swede and cauliflower in place of white starchy potatoes. My family was so surprised that it tasted even better than my old potato and leek recipe. It is so much healthier to use home made chicken broth, see recipe on page 295. For a treat, fry up diced bacon and serve with fresh chopped parsley sprinkled over your soup.

Prep time: 15 minutes Cooking time: 45 minutes Serves: 4-6

Ingredients:

- 1½ Tbsp coconut oil
- 2 large leeks, sliced
- 2 tsp garlic, minced
- ½ tsp ground cinnamon
- ½ tsp ground nutmeg
- 3 swedes, chopped into chunks
- 1.5L/6 cups chicken broth/stock
- ½ head cauliflower
- 1 tsp coarse sea salt
- ¼ tsp pepper or to taste
- 1 cup coconut milk

Method:

In a large soup pot over medium heat, melt coconut oil. Add leeks and garlic, sauté until softened but not brown.

Add cinnamon and nutmeg, cook for 30 seconds or until fragrant. Add swede and broth/stock and bring to the boil and cook for 15 minutes. Add cauliflower, salt and pepper. Simmer for a further 15-20 minutes or until vegetables have softened.

Check seasonings and adjust to your liking. Add coconut milk and stir.

Transfer soup to a blender, work in batches until all the soup is blended and smooth.

If you find the soup a bit too thick, add a little more stock.

SOUPS | 53

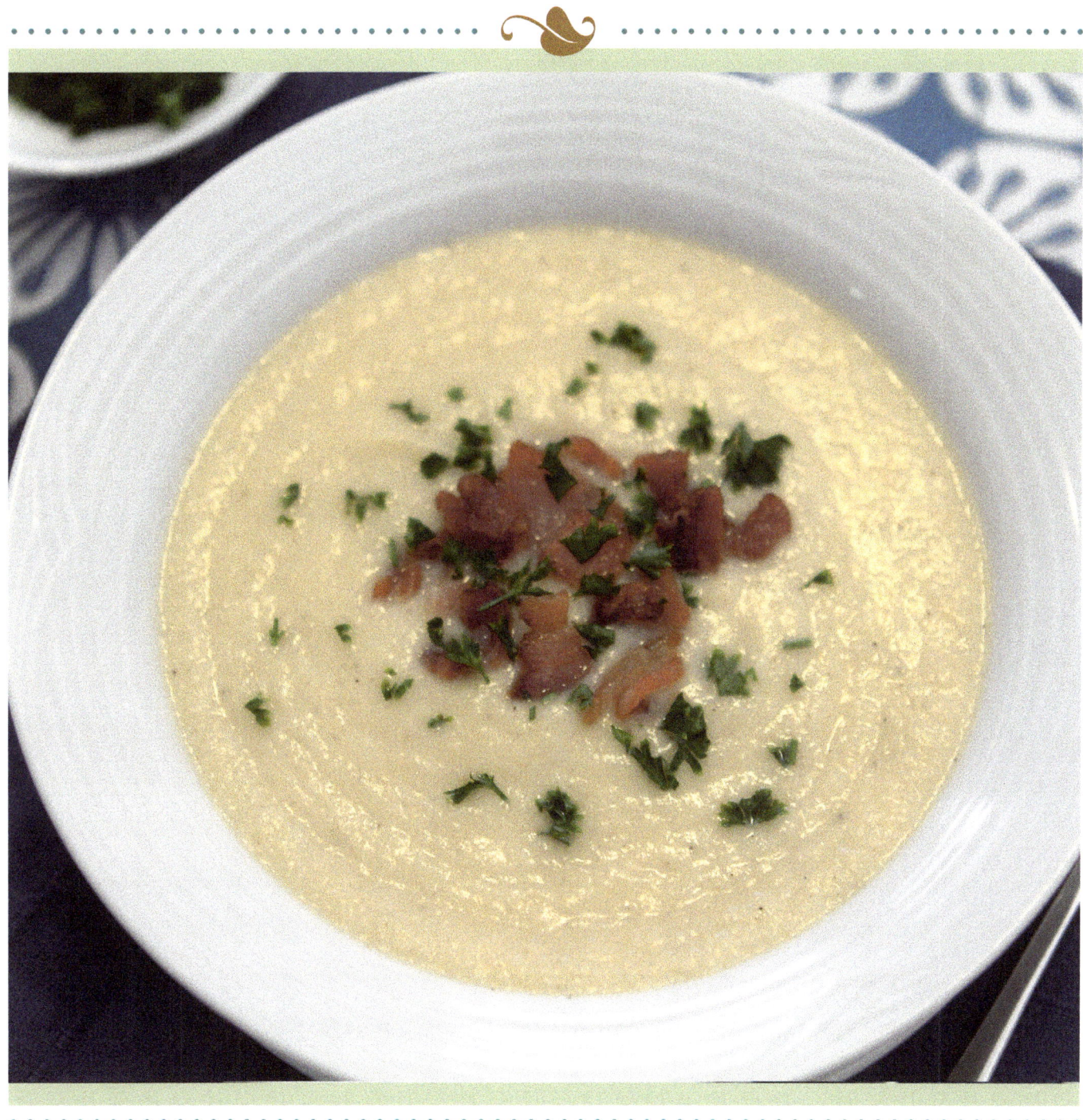

54 | SOUPS

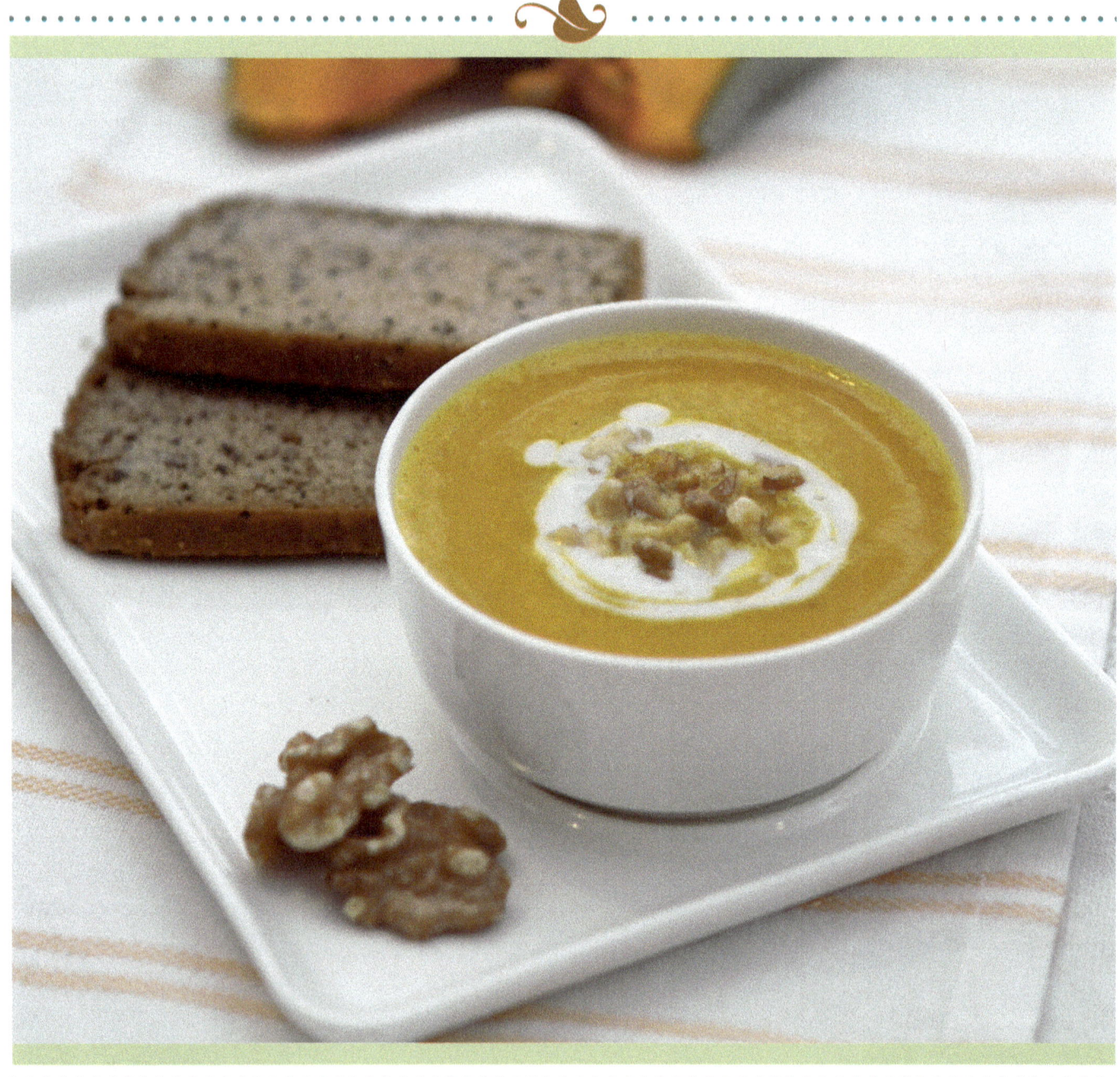

Pumpkin Soup

You will find a hint of cinnamon in my pumpkin soup. I have also drizzled it with coconut cream and topped with roasted walnuts to dress the soup up. Serve with Grain Free Sandwich bread, page 64.

Prep time: 10 minutes   Cooking time: 35 minutes   Serves: 4-6

Ingredients:

- 1½ Tbsp coconut oil
- 1 medium onion, diced
- 1 swede, diced
- 1 tsp garlic, minced
- 1½ tsp ground cinnamon
- 1.5kg/3.3lb pumpkin, chopped
- 2 carrots, chopped
- 1 L/4 cups chicken broth/stock
- 1 cup coconut milk or almond milk
- 1½ tsp coarse sea salt or to taste
- ⅛ tsp ground pepper or to taste
- ⅓ cup walnuts, toasted
- Coconut cream to garnish or cream of choice

Method:

Heat a large soup pot on medium heat, melt 1 tablespoon of oil, add onions. Cook for 3 minutes or until transparent.

Add remaining oil, swede, garlic and cinnamon. Stir and cook a further 2 minutes.

Add pumpkin and carrots. Stir them through the onion and swede mixture.

Add broth/stock and bring to a boil. Reduce to a simmer and cover.

Simmer for 25 minutes or until vegetables are tender. Add coconut milk, sea salt and pepper to taste.

While soup is cooking, preheat oven and roast walnuts until just browning. Set aside to cool, then roughly chop.

Transfer soup to a blender, blend in batches until smooth. Add extra broth if you need to adjust the consistency.

Serve with a drizzle of coconut cream or cream of choice and a sprinkling of chopped walnuts.

Taco Soup

We enjoy Taco soup as a main meal. With no corn or beans allowed, I wasn't sure I would be making it again. I've substituted with carrot and bacon and the family is happy, still lots of flavour. Don't be put off with the large list of ingredients, most are spices to create the taco seasoning minus the maize or rice flour and anti-caking concoctions. Delicious served with avocado, coriander and sliced spring onions or a dollop of dairy free sour cream, recipe page 302.

Prep time: 15 minutes   Cooking time: 55 minutes   Serves: 6

Ingredients:

- 200g bacon, chopped, (nitrate free)
- 2 medium onions, diced
- 4 tsp garlic, minced
- 2 Tbsp ground cumin
- 1½ tsp medium chili powder or to your taste
- 2 tsp dried oregano
- 2 tsp ground coriander
- ½ tsp paprika
- 800g/1.75lbs minced beef
- 400g/14oz can diced tomatoes, BPA free can
- 750ml/3 cups beef broth/stock
- 700ml/2.8 cups bottle organic passata or tomato puree
- 2 large carrots, diced
- Juice of 1 lime
- 1 Tbsp Apple Cider vinegar
- 1½ tsp coarse sea salt
- ¾ cup coconut milk or almond milk
- Avocado, coriander leaves, spring onions, chopped to serve on top

Method:

Heat a large soup pot on medium heat. Add bacon, cook until lightly browning and set aside.

Fry onions and garlic in the bacon fat for 3 minutes, add some ghee if needed. Stir in spices and herbs. Cook a further 1 minute, until spices are fragrant.

Increase heat to medium-high. Add minced beef and cook, stirring often to break up any lumps. When meat has changed colour add all remaining ingredients except for the milk and garnishes. Simmer for 40 minutes, add milk and more stock if needed.

Serve topped with chopped avocado, fresh coriander and sliced spring onions.

SOUPS | 57

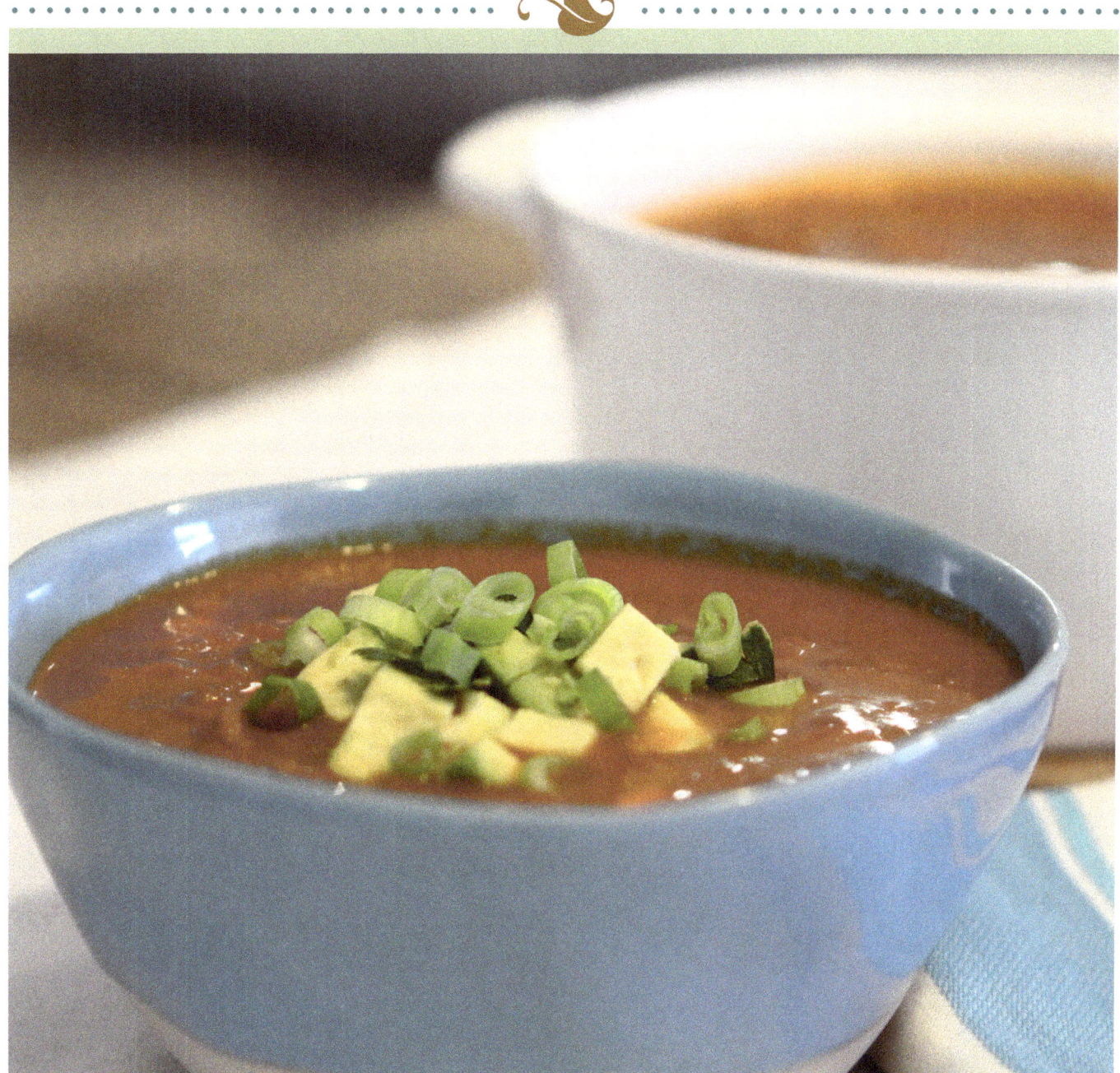

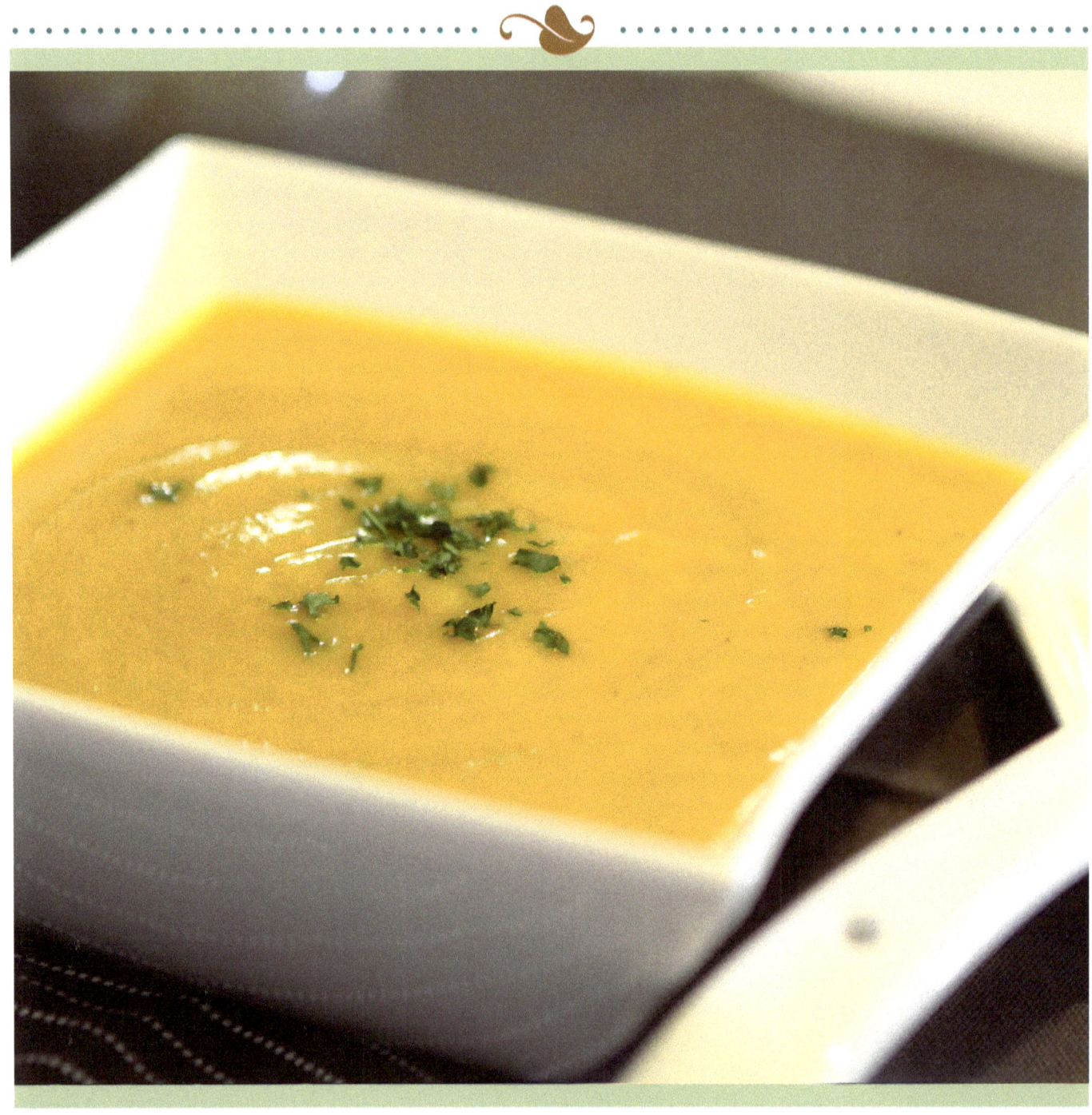

Sweet Potato and Vegetable Soup

This is a great soup to make when you want to sneak lots of vegetables into your family. Any soup that is orange, my grandchildren think of it as pumpkin soup, which they love. I blend it well so no green is showing. We love thick soup. If you find the consistency isn't to your liking, add a little extra broth when blending.

Prep time: 20 minutes Cooking time: 40 minutes Serves: 6-8

Ingredients:

- 1 Tbsp coconut oil
- 1 leek, sliced
- 1 onion, chopped
- 3 tsp garlic, minced
- 1kg/2.2lbs sweet potatoes, chopped
- 2 carrots, chopped
- 1 large zucchini, chopped with skin on
- 1 bunch broccoli
- 2L/8 cups chicken broth/stock, or amount needed to cover vegetables
- Sea salt & black pepper to taste

Method:

Heat a large soup pot on medium heat. Add coconut oil and cook leek, onion and garlic for 4-5 minutes. Add all the vegetables and broth/stock and bring to a boil, then reduce to a simmer. Cook vegetables until they are tender.

Add to a blender, and blend in batches until smooth and no green bits can be seen. Adjust consistency and seasoning to your liking.

Serve with warm Damper bread, on page 66.

Seafood Chowder

I've used vegetables to thicken the chowder and fish sauce to add that extra flavour. I added three different kinds of seafood; prawns, scallops and white fish, you choose your favourites.

Prep time: 20 minutes   Cooking time: 50 minutes   Serves: 4-6

Ingredients:

- 1 Tbsp ghee or organic butter
- 1 small onion, diced
- 2 stalks of celery, diced
- 2 garlic cloves, minced
- 350g/12ozs sweet potato, peeled cut into small pieces
- ½ head cauliflower, cut into pieces
- 1 tsp nutmeg
- ½ tsp paprika
- 1L/4 cups chicken broth/stock (or fish broth)
- Juice of 1 lime
- 1 Tbsp fish sauce
- 1 tsp sea salt
- ⅓ tsp pepper
- 2 cups coconut cream, canned
- 550g/1.2lb mixed seafood (prawns, scallops, white fish, crabmeat) divided
- 2 Tbsp fresh parsley, chopped

Method:

To a large soup pot over medium-low heat, melt the ghee. Add onion, celery and garlic.

Fry gently for approximately 4-5 minutes, stir often so onions don't brown.

Add sweet potato, cauliflower, nutmeg and paprika, cook for a few minutes until spices are fragrant.

Add the broth/stock, lime juice, fish sauce, salt and pepper.

Bring to a boil then reduce and simmer until vegetables have softened, approximately 30 minutes.

Add in the coconut cream and adjust the seasonings if required.

Add 150g/5.3ozs of mixed seafood. Increase heat to medium, for approximately 6 minutes for the seafood to cook.

Use a blender or a hand held immersion blender and puree for a few seconds. Return to pot.

Roughly chop and add the remaining 400g/14ozs of seafood to the pureed soup. Cook for a further 6 minutes.

Ladle the soup into bowls and garnish with parsley.

SOUPS | 61

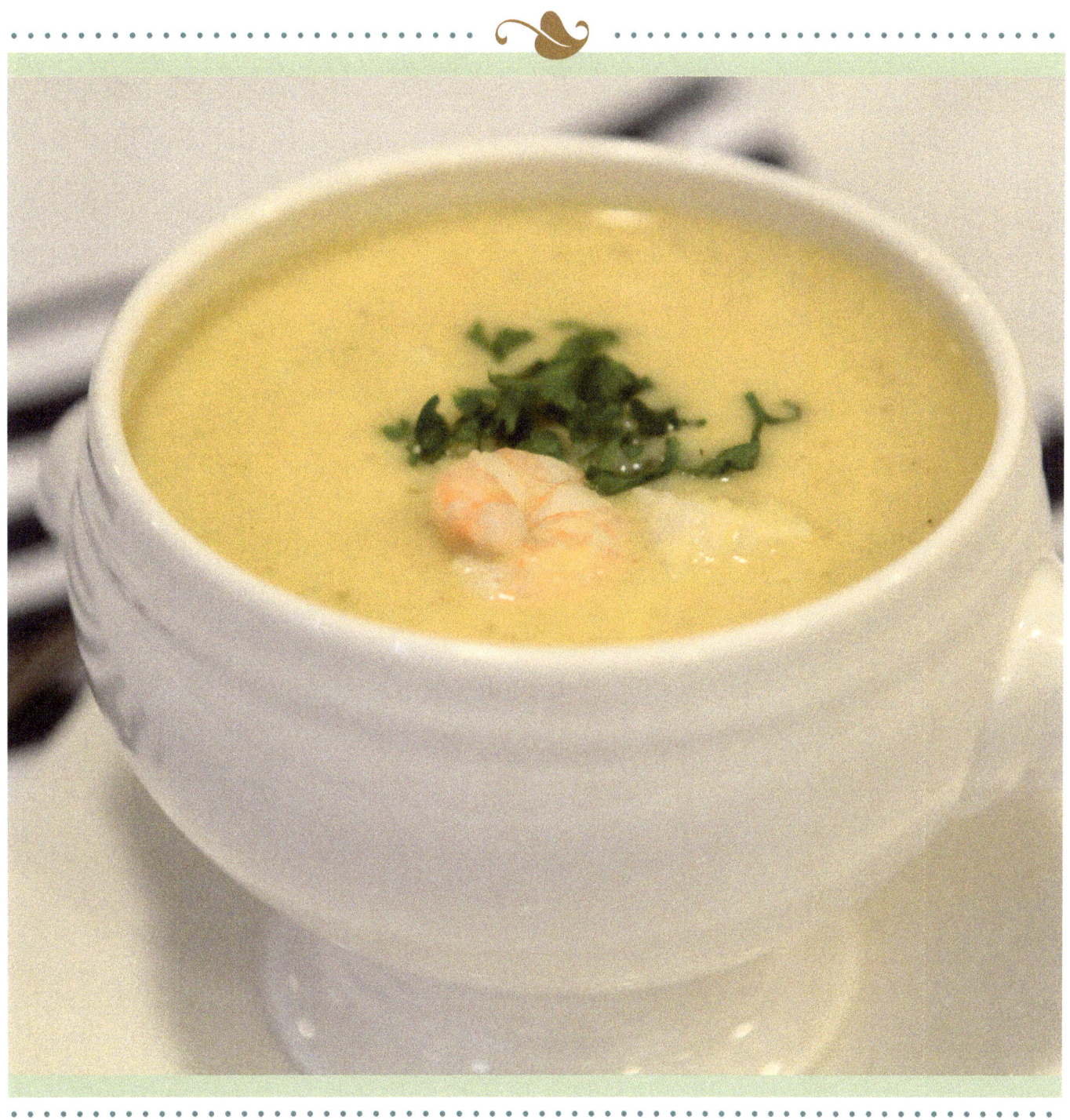

BREADS, CRACKERS & CRUSTS

Grain Free Sandwich Bread 64

Damper 66

Focaccia Style Bread 69

Hamburger Buns 70

Spinach & Feta Loaf 73

Naan Bread 74

Wraps, Tortillas or Crepes 77

Spinach Flat Bread 78

Pizza Base 80

Seed Crackers 82

Sweet Coconut Piecrust 85

Pie Crust (Use for sweet or savoury pies) 86

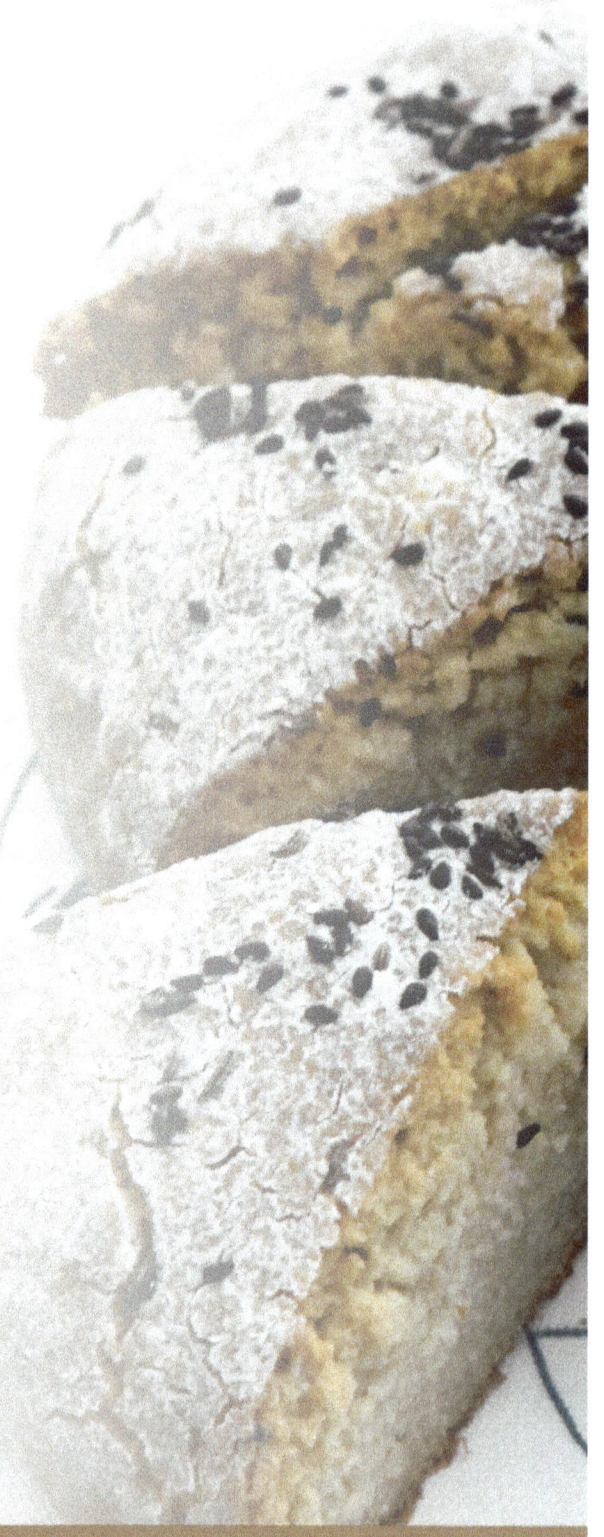

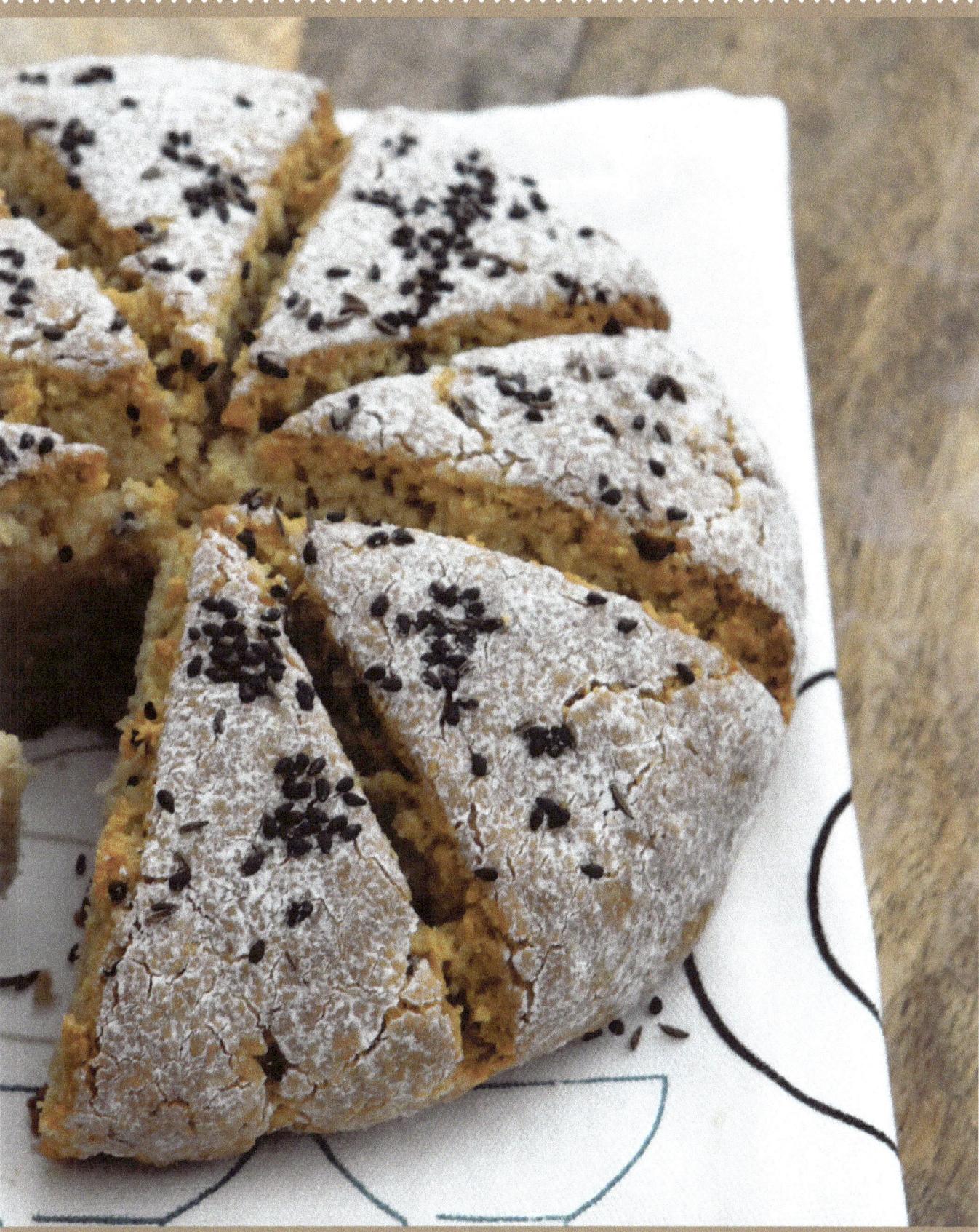

Grain Free Sandwich Bread

This bread is so delicious toasted and can be sliced thinly for sandwiches without crumbling. Double the recipe for a large loaf or use a 22 or 23cm round cake tin to make a bakers cob loaf, (bake the larger loaf for 65 minutes).

Prep time: 15 minutes   Cooking time: 45-50 minutes   Makes: 1 loaf

Ingredients:

- 2 Tbsp chia seeds
- 3 Tbsp filtered water to soak chia
- 4 large eggs
- 1 cup/250g cashew butter, recipe page 306 or a jar of store bought containing 100% cashews
- ⅓ cup cashew or almond milk, or milk of choice
- 1 Tbsp Apple Cider vinegar
- ¼ cup coconut flour
- 2 Tbsp arrowroot flour
- 1¼ tsp baking soda
- ½ tsp fine sea salt
- 2 Tbsp sesame seeds

Method:

Preheat oven to 150c/300f. Grease a loaf tin with coconut oil and line the base with baking paper.

Add chia seeds and water to a small jug and mix. Set aside to soak for 5 minutes to form a gel.

To a food processor add, eggs, cashew butter, milk, vinegar and chia mix. Process until combined, scraping down sides of bowl when needed.

Add coconut flour, arrowroot flour, baking soda and salt. Process until all ingredients are well incorporated and you have a smooth aerated batter. Add sesame seeds, pulse a couple of times to mix through.

Pour batter into the prepared loaf tin. Bake for 45-50 minutes or until golden and firm on top, insert a skewer to see if it comes out clean.

Cool in tin for 20 minutes then remove to a wire rack to completely cool. Slice before storing in an airtight container in the fridge or freezer. Keeps for up to 10 days in the fridge.

BREADS, CRACKERS & CRUSTS | 65

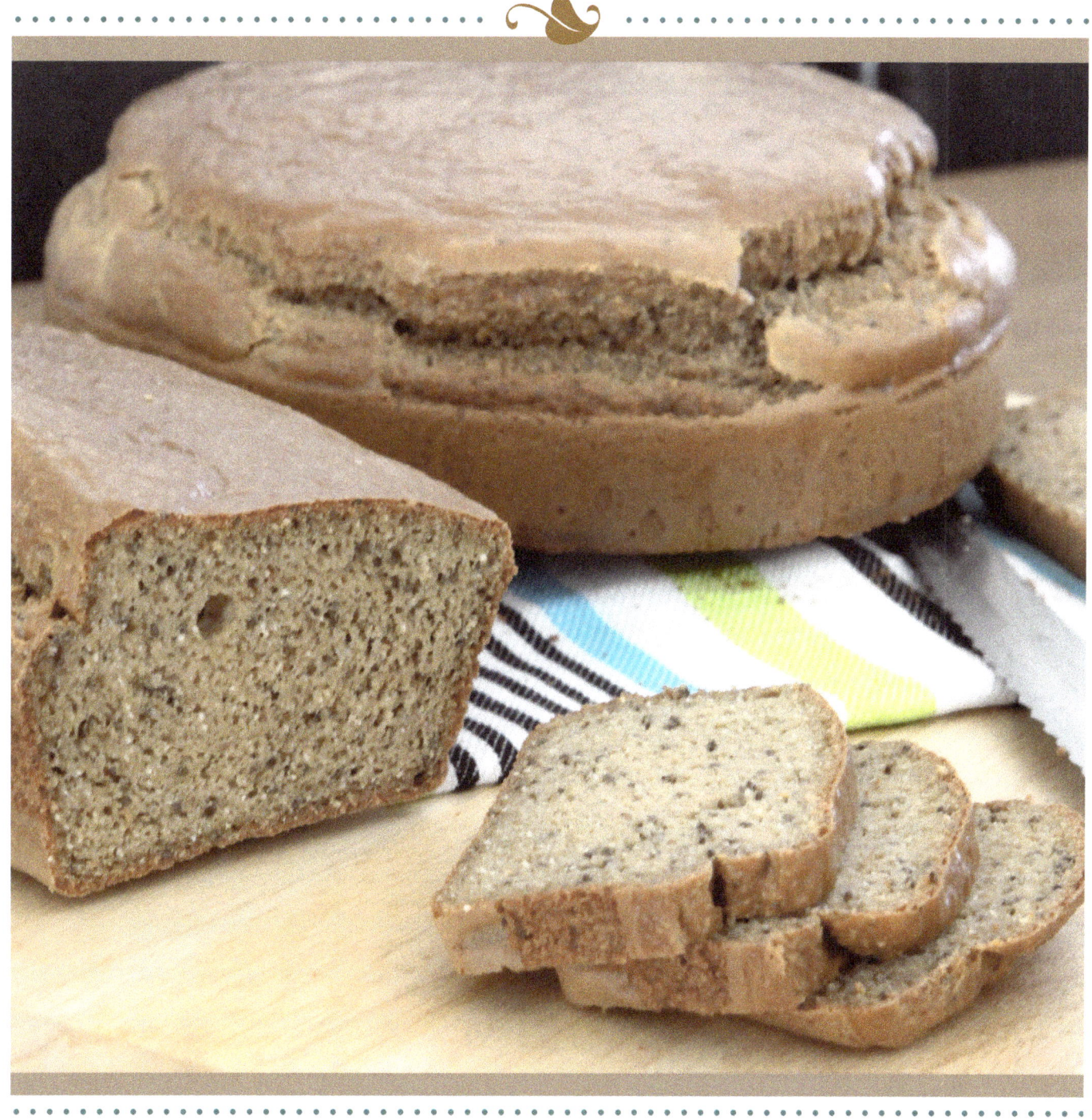

Damper

Damper is an iconic Australian food. This traditional Australian soda bread was prepared by swagmen, drovers, stockmen and travellers. It was baked in the coals of a campfire. Serve it with stews to dip into the gravy and with main meal soups. Slather with organic butter or ghee.

Prep time: 15 minutes   Cooking time: 30 minutes   Makes: 8 portions

Ingredients:

- 3 cups almond meal/flour
- ¾ cup arrowroot flour, plus extra for dusting
- 1½ tsp baking soda
- 1 tsp gluten free baking powder
- 2 tsp coconut sugar
- ½ tsp fine sea salt
- ¼ tsp caraway seeds
- 3 large eggs
- 1 Tbsp Apple Cider vinegar
- Black sesame seeds to sprinkle on top

Method:

Preheat oven to 170c/340f. Line a baking tray with baking paper.

Add to a large bowl, almond meal, arrowroot flour, baking soda, baking powder, sugar, salt and caraway seeds. Mix to combine and remove any lumps.

Add to a small bowl, eggs and vinegar. Whisk together. Pour into the dry ingredients and mix well to combine.

Using hands that are lightly dusted in arrowroot flour, place dough onto the prepared tray and shape into a circle. Approximate diameter of 15cm(6ins) and height of 3cm(1.5ins). Lightly dust top and sides of damper loaf with a very small amount of arrowroot flour. Sprinkle top with black sesame seeds. Press lightly so they stick. It's best to use less arrowroot flour so seeds stick and then dust again lightly if needed.

Using a knife, score the top. First into quarters then into eighths, make the cuts 1.5cm(0.5in) deep.

Bake for 30-35 minutes or until a hard crust has formed and brown. Let sit for 10 minutes before serving.

Serve with soup, stews or with eggs for breakfast.

BREADS, CRACKERS & CRUSTS

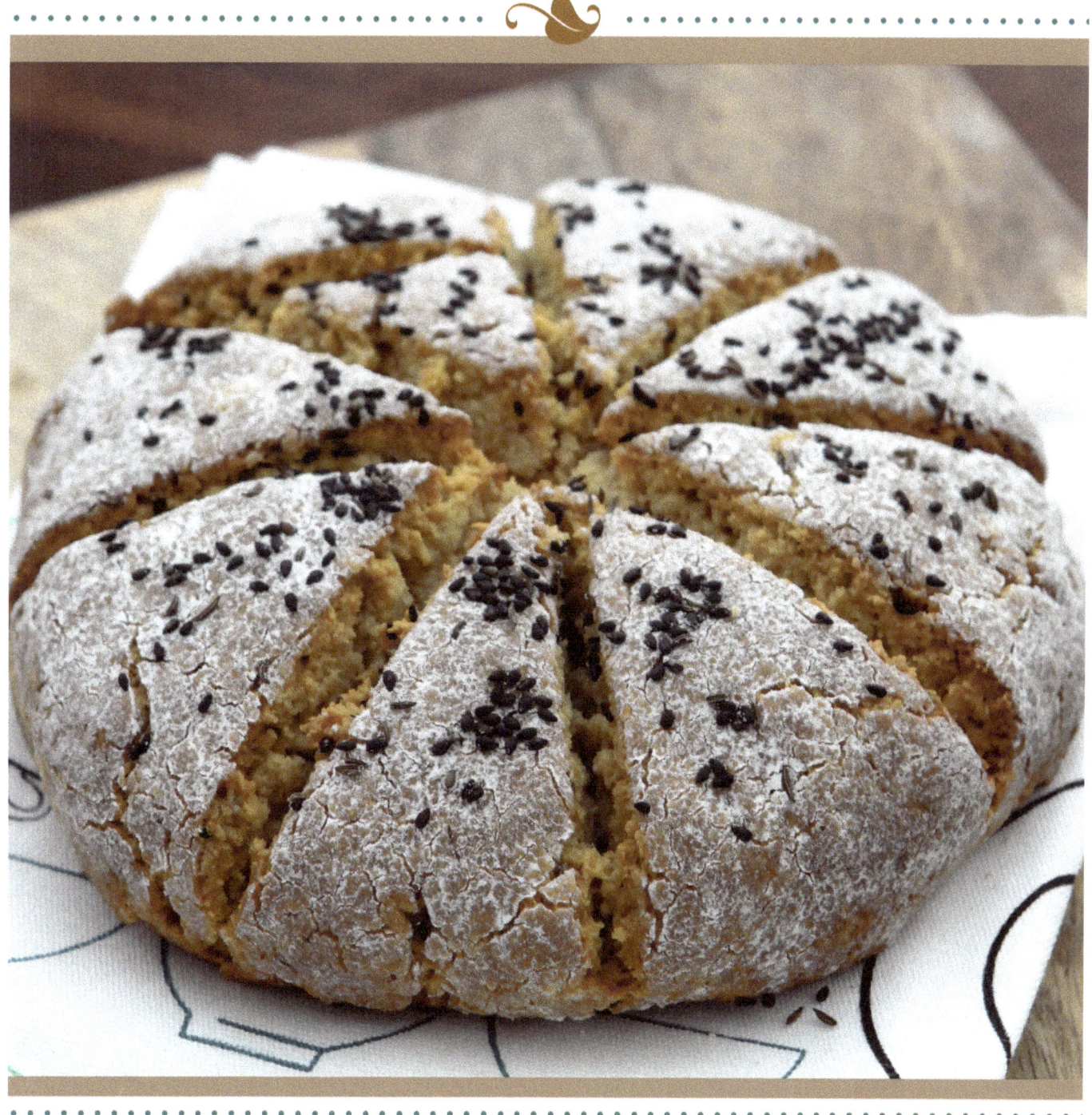

68 | BREADS, CRACKERS & CRUSTS

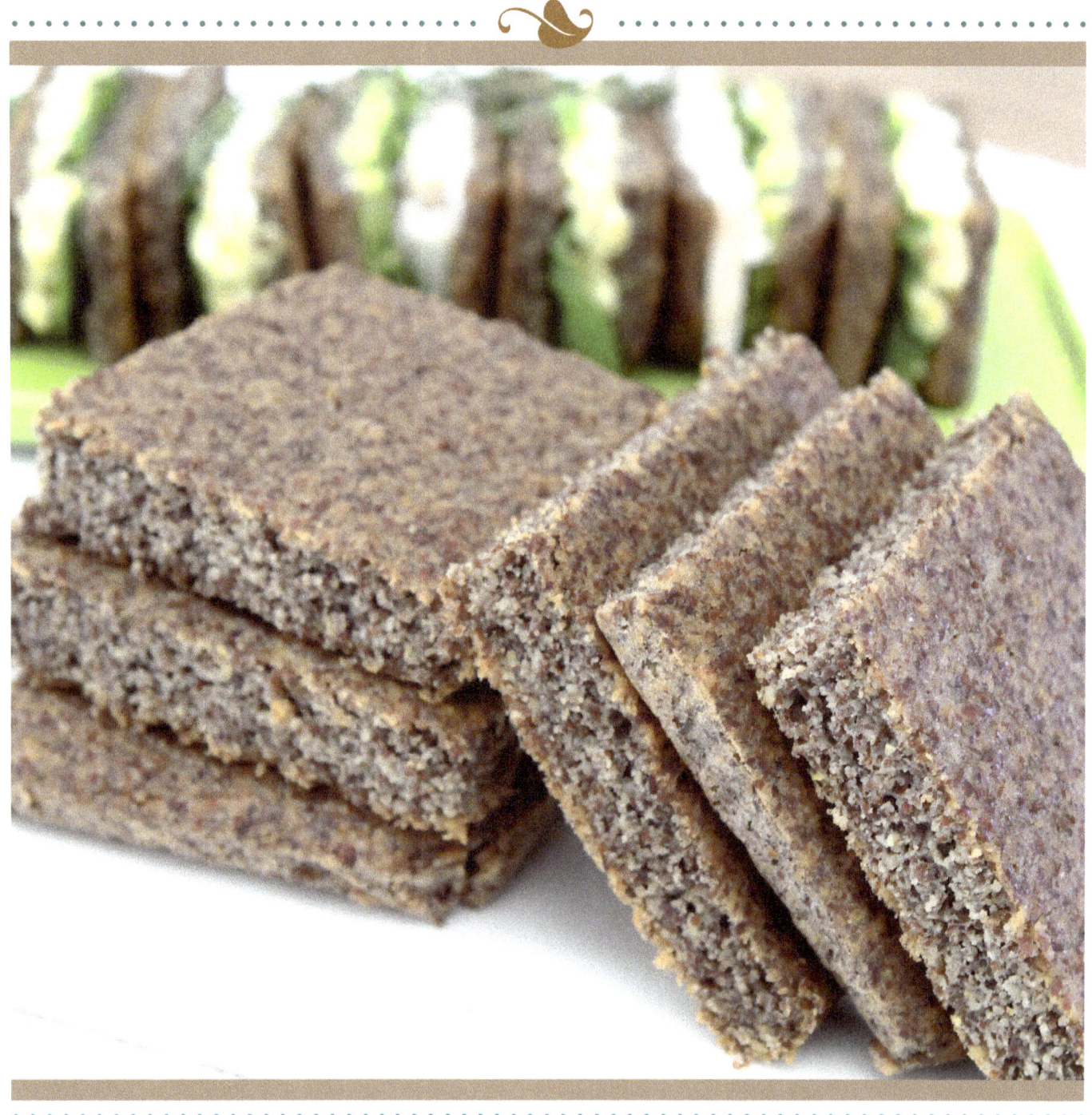

Focaccia Style Bread

This is the first bread I tackled when going grain free. It is still a great bread to use for fresh or toasted sandwiches. People often comment that it tastes like rye bread.

Prep time: 10 minutes Cooking time: 25 minutes Makes: 9

Ingredients:

- 5 large eggs
- ½ cup water
- ⅓ cup macadamia oil or coconut oil
- 2 tsp Apple Cider vinegar
- 1½ cups golden flaxseed meal
- ¾ cup almond meal/flour
- 1 Tbsp coconut sugar
- 1 tsp baking soda
- ½ tsp Herbamare seasoning salt
- ¼ tsp garlic powder

Method:

Preheat oven to 170c/340f. Line a swiss roll or lamington tin 30x25cm(12x10ins) with baking paper, leave a little extra length to cover sides of tin.

Add eggs to a medium bowl and whisk. Add water, oil and vinegar. Whisk to combine.

In a large bowl, add flaxseed, almond meal, coconut sugar, baking soda, Herbamare seasoning and garlic powder. Mix well, removing any lumps.

Make a well in the dry ingredients and stir in egg mixture. Mix well together and let stand 3 minutes to thicken.

Pour batter into prepared pan, spread out quickly as batter thickens fast. Make the thickness approximately 1cm(0.5in), smooth top with spatula. The batter won't take up the whole tin. Make a neat edge with your spatula where the batter doesn't reach the end of the tin.

Bake for approximately 25-30 minutes, or until top is lightly brown and bounces back when touched. Allow bread to cool for 30 minutes before removing. Cutting into 9 portions.

Keeps moist for days, store in an air tight container. Freezes well, best to store in a single layer when freezing and thaw before slicing in half. Great for sandwiches and for toasted filled sandwiches. (Slice with a serrated knife)

Options: Double recipe and it will fill 3 bar or slice tins 27x17cm(10.5x6.5ins), no need to shape into rectangle as batter fills tins perfectly and will be 1cm thick. 6 squares in each tin will make perfect size focaccia bread. Bun option: prepare single recipe and use 6 mini cheesecake spring pans to make bread rolls. Cut circles out of baking paper to line base of mini spring pans, and grease sides. When cooked and cooled run a spatula around the inside before opening spring.

Hamburger Buns

This nut free bread recipe has a lovely light texture. It does a perfect job of holding everything together so you can enjoy a hamburger. They are also suitable for making sandwiches.

Prep time: 5 minutes Cooking time: 20 minutes Makes: 8 or 4 sets

Ingredients:

- 3 Tbsp coconut flour
- 2 Tbsp arrowroot flour
- 1 Tbsp golden flaxseed meal
- 180g/6ozs peeled pumpkin, cubed (use a mild flavoured pumpkin like Jarrahdale)
- ⅓ tsp baking soda
- ¼ tsp fine sea salt
- Pinch of pepper
- 2 large eggs
- ⅓ cup filtered water

Method:

Preheat oven to 180c/350f. Line 2 baking trays with baking paper.

To a food processor add, flours, flaxseed and uncooked diced pumpkin. Process for 50 seconds until you have a fine mixture. Stop half way and scrap down sides.

Add baking soda, salt and pepper. Pulse to combine.

Add eggs and water and process for 60 seconds until mixture has become smoother.

Scoop 8 portions of mixture onto trays, approximately 2 tablespoons per portion. Use the back of a spoon to spread the mixture out to form a 10cm(4ins) diameter circle.

Bake for approximately 20 minutes or until firm and edges are starting to brown.

If stored in an air tight container they will keep fresh for days. Freeze in a freezer safe container, separated with baking paper.

BREADS, CRACKERS & CRUSTS | 71

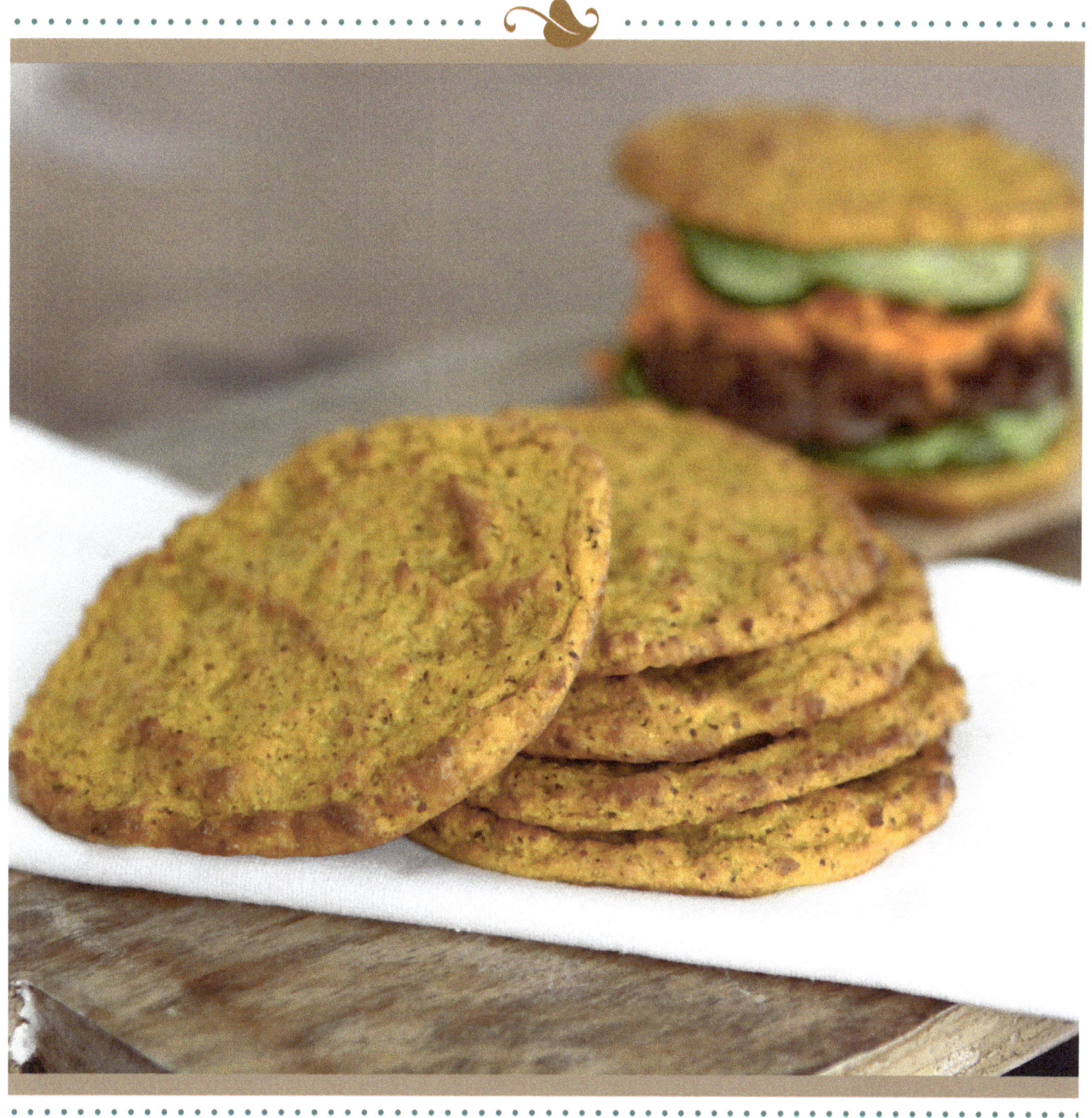

BREADS, CRACKERS & CRUSTS

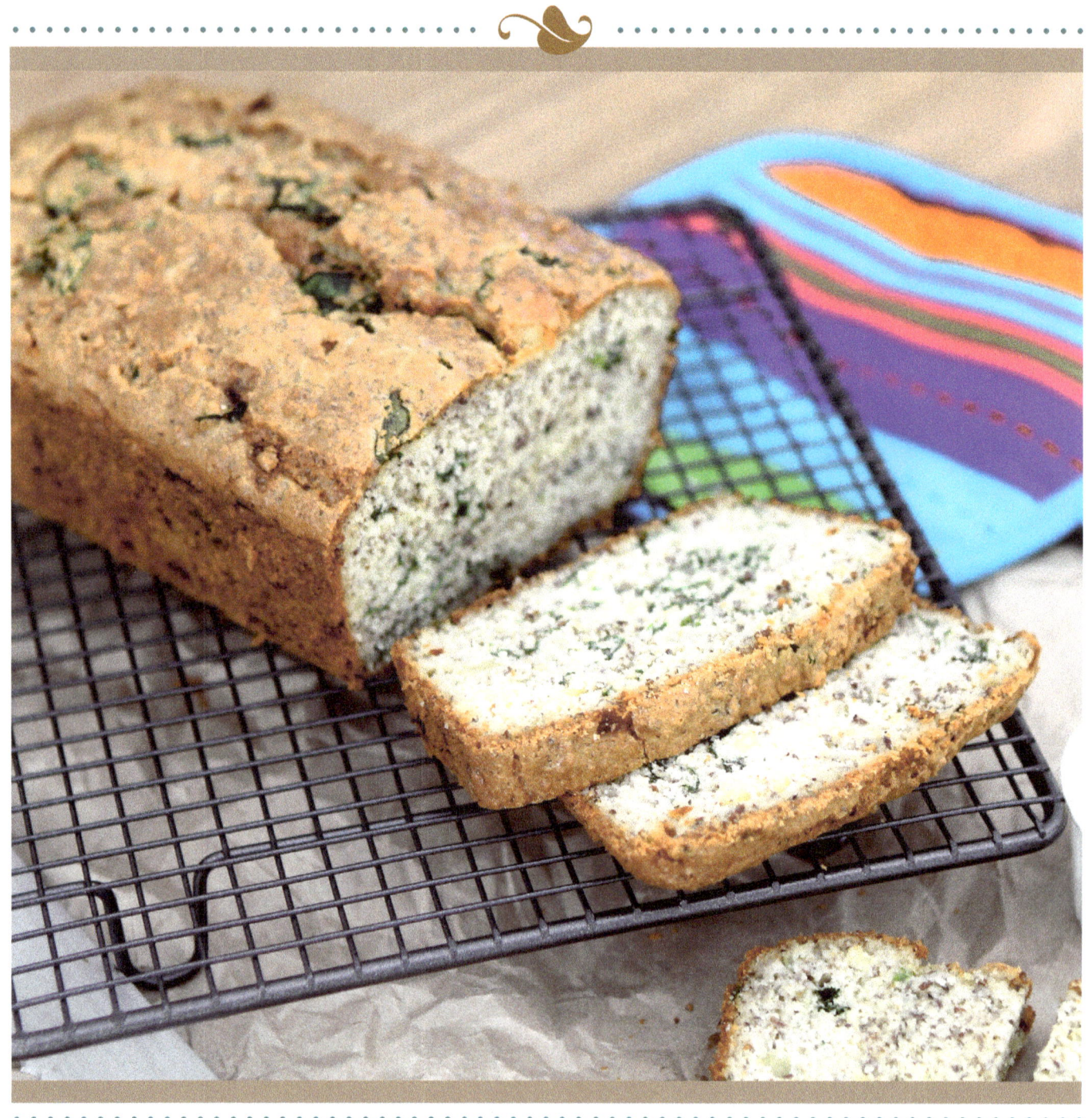

Spinach & Feta Loaf

This bread contains feta, if you cannot tolerate dairy, you have to pass this one up. For a change you can add chopped sundried tomatoes or sliced olives. Spread with organic butter or ghee for a light lunch or snack. It's delicious served with pumpkin soup.

Prep time: 20 minutes   Cooking time: 45 minutes   Makes: 1 loaf

Ingredients:

- ½ Tbsp ghee, for frying
- 1 small onion, finely diced
- 1 tsp garlic, minced
- 3 cups baby spinach, washed
- 120g/4ozs feta, crumbled or diced
- Coarse sea salt and ground pepper, to season spinach mix
- 2 cups almond meal/flour
- ½ cup golden flaxseed meal
- ¾ tsp baking soda
- ½ tsp fine sea salt
- 130g/4.5ozs sour cream (Cashew Sour cream page 302)
- 4 large eggs, beaten
- 2 Tbsp macadamia oil

Method:

Preheat oven to 170c/340f. Grease a medium loaf tin with ghee and line the base with baking paper.

Heat a large frying pan over medium heat, melt ghee. Add onion and garlic. Cook stirring, for 4 minutes or until softened.

Remove pan from heat, stir in spinach and set aside until spinach has wilted. Then add, feta, sea salt and pepper, and mix them through the onion and spinach mixture.

To a large bowl, add almond meal, flaxseed, baking soda and salt. Mix well to combine and remove any lumps. Sir in sour cream, eggs and macadamia oil, mix until smooth.

Add onion and spinach mixture to batter and mix well to combine. Make sure spinach is distributed evenly.

Spoon into prepared loaf tin and smooth surface. Check you have a little of the spinach showing on the top.

Bake for 40-45 minutes or until cooked when tested with a skewer or toothpick and golden in colour. Cool in tin for 5-10 minutes. Serve warm with organic butter/ghee or transfer to a wire rack to cool completely for later use. It's best to slice with a serrated bread knife.

Naan Bread

Serve with Indian Butter Chicken on page 188. Hope you love this as much as we do, I also use this bread to serve taco meat on top with salad and avocado. It is not like traditional wheat naan bread but so yum, as it's crunchy on the outside but soft inside.

Prep time: 10 minutes   Cooking time: 20 minutes   Makes: 6

Ingredients:

- 1 cup almond meal/flour
- ½ cup arrowroot flour
- 2 tsp psyllium husks
- ½ tsp fine sea salt
- ½ cup canned coconut milk
- ⅔ cup coconut water or filtered water
- Ghee for frying

Method:

To a medium bowl add, almond meal, arrowroot flour, psyllium and salt. Mix to combine.

Pour in coconut milk and coconut water. Beat on low using a handheld electric beater or use a whisk, until well combined.

Heat a small 20cm(8in) non-stick frying pan or crepe pan on medium heat, add ½ teaspoon ghee to coat pan.

Pour ¼ cup of batter into the heated pan. Make a circle with a diameter of approximately 14cm(5.5ins). You will need to use the back of a spoon to push out and spread the batter.

Cook first side for 4 minutes or until brown and crisp. Batter should bubble a little while cooking. Don't be tempted to turn over too soon, you want a crisp bread. Cook second side for 2 minutes. Add an extra ¼-½ teaspoon of ghee to pan each time you flip bread or as needed.

Naan bread should be crispy but soft inside.

Keep warm in a single layer while cooking the remaining batter. I use two non-stick frying pans to make the process faster.

BREADS, CRACKERS & CRUSTS

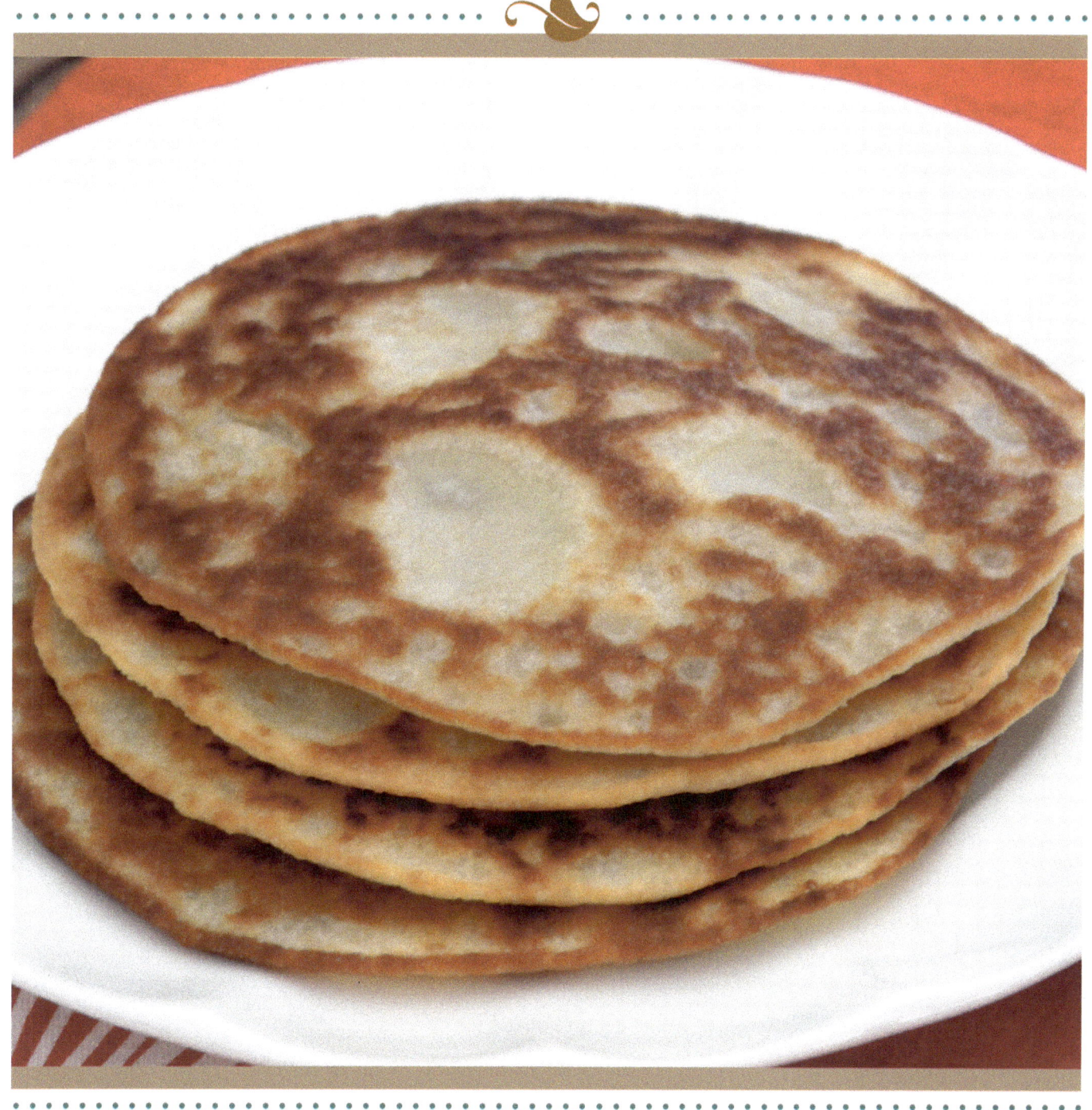

76 | BREADS, CRACKERS & CRUSTS

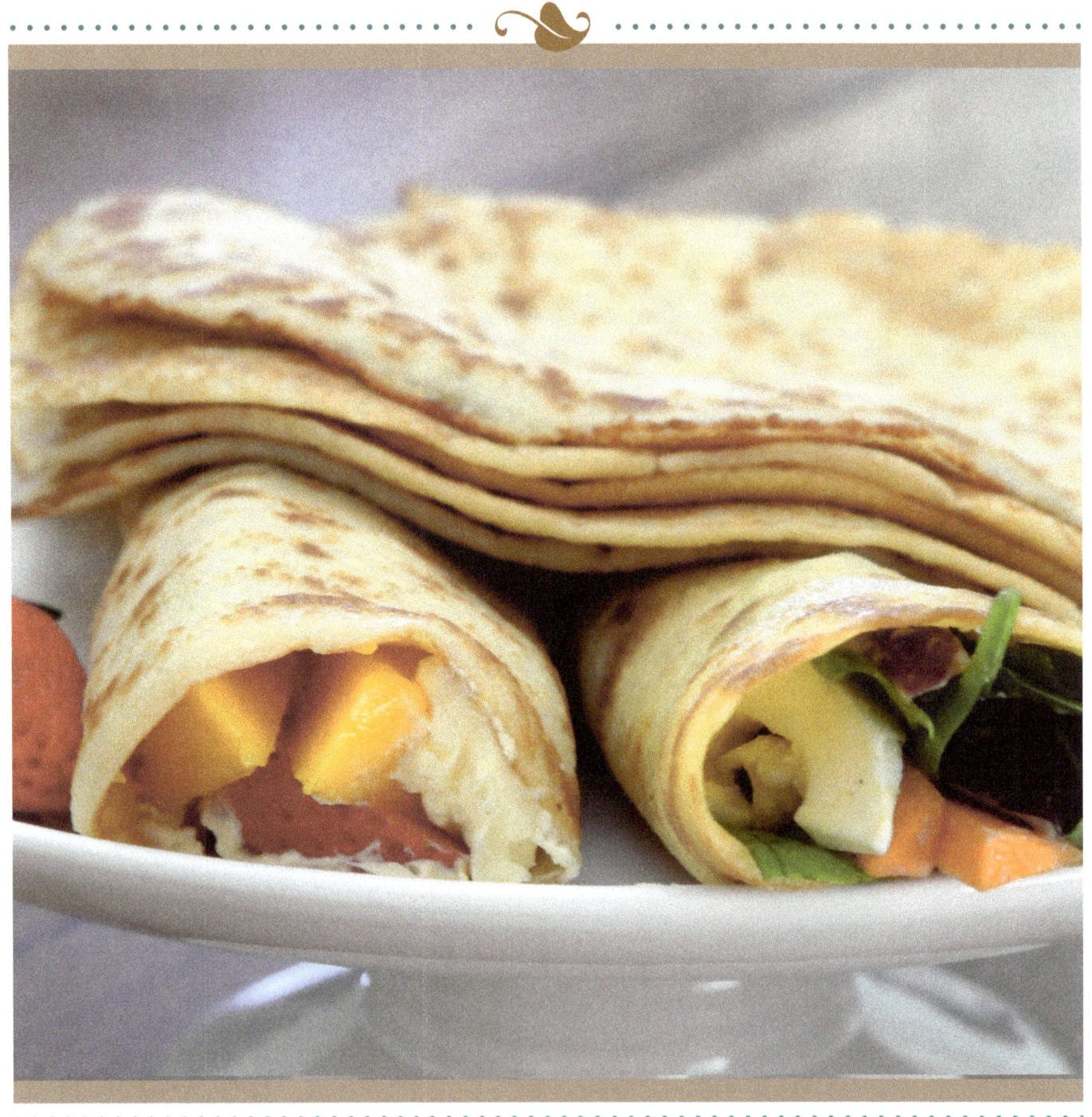

Wraps, Tortillas or Crepes

These wraps are lovely and soft and easy to roll up. Arrowroot flour is excellent for gluten free baking as it helps to make a softer and lighter texture. It has no flavour of its own to interfere with the other ingredients and it's the easiest starch to digest. Arrowroot is extracted from the root of a large perennial herb (Maranta arundinacea), which is indigenous to the West Indies. The aborigines from the West Indies, used this powder to draw out toxins from people who were wounded by poison arrows. Thus, the name arrowroot came to be.

Prep time: 10 minutes Cooking time: 20 minutes Makes: 7 medium 4 large

Ingredients:

- 1½ cup almond meal/flour
- ½ cup arrowroot flour
- ⅓ tsp fine sea salt
- ½ cup cashew or almond milk, or milk of choice
- ¾ cup coconut water or filtered water
- 1 large egg
- For Crepes;
- add 2 tsp vanilla extract and reduce salt by half

Method:

To a medium bowl add, almond meal, arrowroot flour and salt. Mix to combine.

Pour in nut milk and coconut water. Add egg. Beat mixture on low using a handheld electric beater or use a whisk, until well combined.

For crepes add 2 teaspoon of vanilla and reduce salt.

Heat a small 20cm(8in) non-stick crepe or frying pan on low-medium heat, or for larger wraps/crepes us a 23cm(9in) pan. Wipe pan over with a small amount of ghee and between each additional wrap/crepe. If you are not using a non-stick pan, add extra ghee.

Pour ⅓ cup of batter into the heated pan, making a circle with a diameter of approximately 16-17cm(6.5ins). For larger wraps use ½ cup to make a 20cm(8in) diameter. You will need to swirl pan after adding batter to help it spread. If you find it's not spreading well, reduce the heat.

Cook first side for 2½-3 minutes or until just browning and still soft. Turn over and cook second side for 1-2 minutes. Set aside to cool on a wire rack. I use two pans to make the process faster, and 2 spatulas for turning the larger wraps/crepes.

When cooled add your favourite fillings, or serve warm as a crepe with a fruit filling and cream or spread of your choice.

Spinach Flat Bread

This flat bread is so crisp you can make chips out of it for dips or nachos. The hint of sesame gives them a great savoury taste. I have also used this recipe to replace pasta in a lasagna dish.

Prep time: 20 minutes   Cooking time: 20 minutes   Makes: 8

Ingredients:

- 2 cups of firmly packed baby spinach
- Boiling water to soak spinach
- 3 Tbsp golden flaxseed meal
- ⅓ cup filtered water for soaking flaxseed
- 2 cups almond meal/flour
- ¾ cup arrowroot flour
- 1 Tbsp sesame seeds
- ¾ tsp fine sea salt
- ⅓ tsp onion powder
- ⅓ tsp garlic powder
- ⅓ tsp paprika
- Ghee for frying

Method:

Place baby spinach in a heat-proof container with lid or a saucepan. Pour over boiling water, cover with lid, set aside to soften and wilt.

In a small bowl add flaxseed and water, stir and let sit for a few minutes to thicken.

Meanwhile, add to a food processor, almond meal, arrowroot flour, sesame seeds, salt, onion and garlic powders and paprika.

Drain spinach into a metal sieve, press firmly with the back of a spoon to remove all liquid, add to food processor. Pour in flaxseed mixture. Process until dough comes together and forms a ball.

Remove dough, it shouldn't be sticky. If water was left in the spinach you will need to add extra arrowroot flour.

Using kitchen scales, weigh a 60g(2oz) ball of dough. Roll ball between 2 sheets of baking paper, to make a circle with a diameter of 16cm(6.25ins). I use a small saucepan lid as a cookie cutter to cut out circle. You could also use a plate or bowl and cut around it. Remove excess trimmings and add them back to the unrolled dough.

Heat a small non-stick frying pan or crepe pan over medium heat (I use two frying pans to save time). Melt ¼ teaspoon of ghee to coat frying pan.

Carefully peel dough off baking paper and place in pan. Cook for 2-3 minutes on each side or until lightly browning in spots and crispy. Only add ¼ teaspoon of ghee at a time, bread dries out better while cooking with less moisture. Repeat with the remaining dough.

Cool on a wire rack. Once cool you can break up into corn chip sizes pieces for using with dips.

BREADS, CRACKERS & CRUSTS

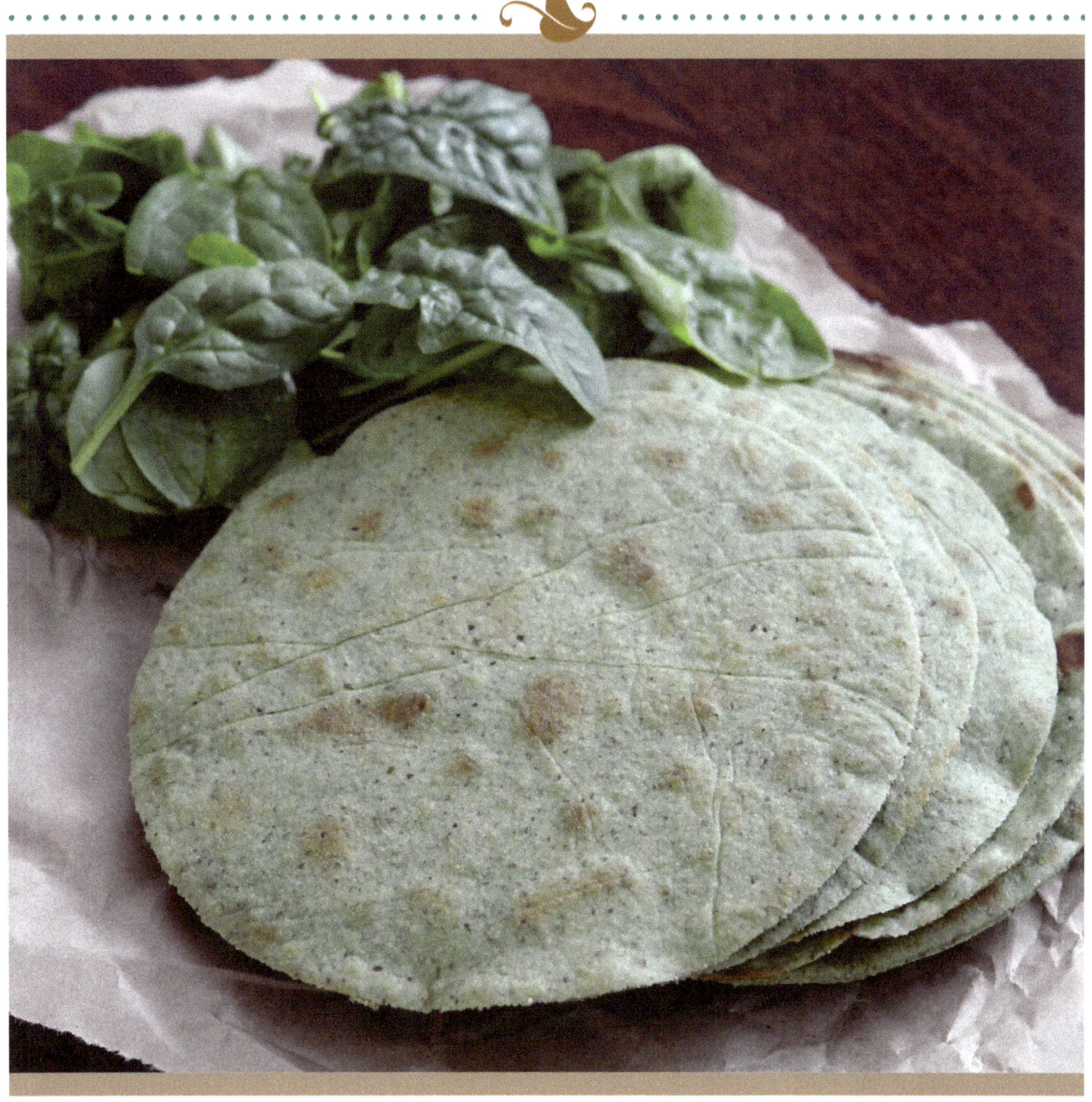

Pizza Base

This pizza dough is crisp and firm when cooked, your toppings are not going to fall off. Spread some pizza or tomato sauce over the cooked base and top with your favourite toppings and enjoy!

Prep time: 10 minutes Cooking time: 20 minutes
Makes: 1 large 30cm(12in) or 2 individual

Ingredients:

- 2 Tbsp flaxseed meal
- 3 Tbsp filtered water
- 1½ cups almond meal/flour
- ½ cup arrowroot flour
- ½ tsp Italian herbs
- ½ tsp fine sea salt
- ½ tsp baking soda
- 1 large egg
- 2 Tbsp olive oil or macadamia oil

Method:

Preheat oven to 170c/340f. Lightly grease a 30cm(12in) pizza tray with oil.

To a small bowl add, flaxseed and water. Mix and set aside for 6-8 minutes.

To a large bowl add, almond meal, arrowroot flour, herbs, salt and baking soda. Mix to combine.

Use a fork to whisk together egg, oil, and flaxseed mixture.

Pour wet ingredients into the large bowl containing the dry ingredients and mix well to combine. Dough needs to come together well. Knead dough while still in the bowl until it forms a ball.

Place dough in the centre of the pizza tray. Flatten with your palm and use your hands to press the dough out thinly to cover the 30cm tray.

Bake for 20 minutes or until golden. Remove from oven. Increase temperature to 190c/375f. Add your sauce and favourite pizza toppings, return to oven for a further 15 minutes or until toppings are piping hot and cooked.

BREADS, CRACKERS & CRUSTS | 81

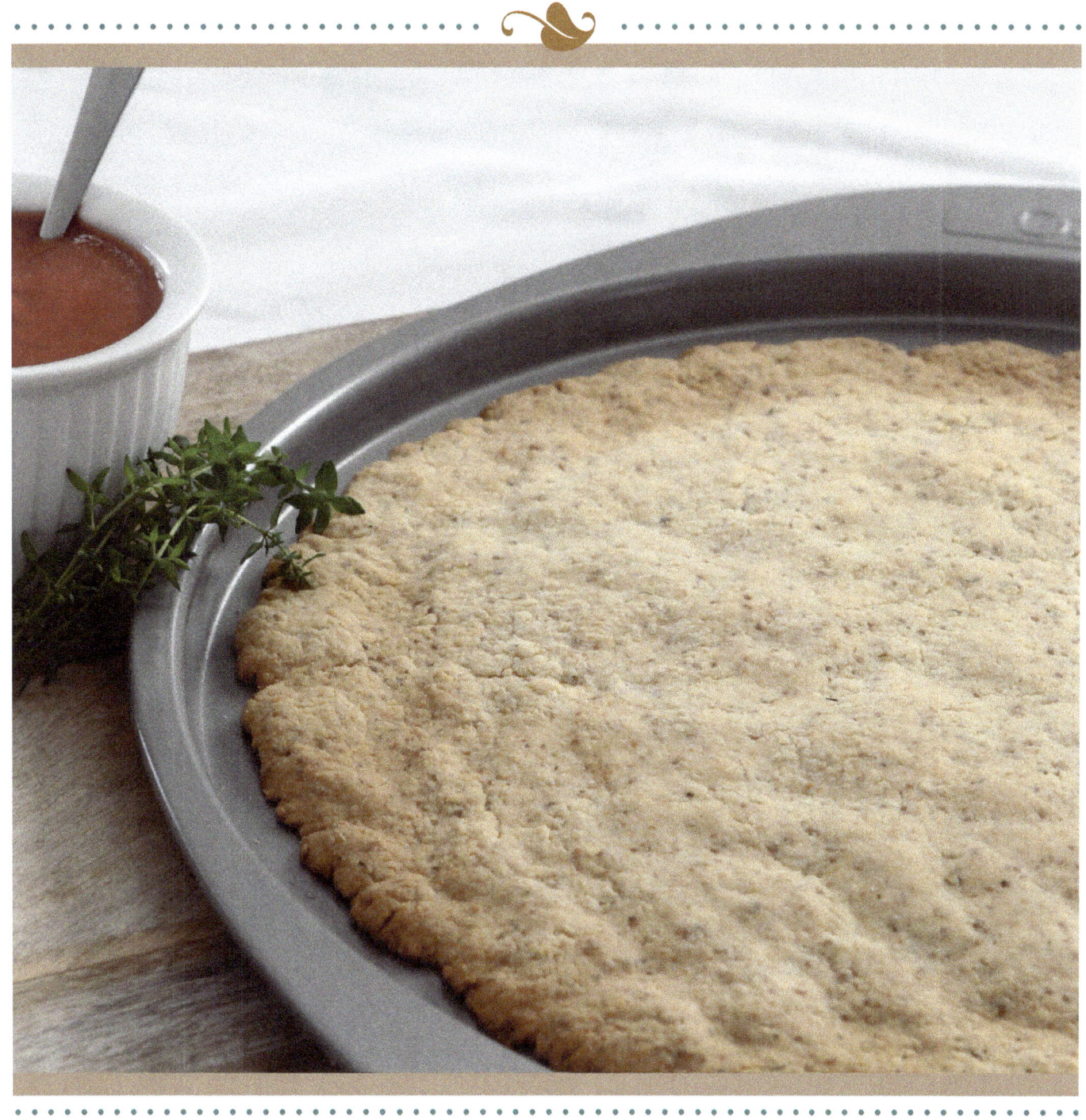

Seed Crackers

The quantity may seem large for this recipe but these crackers keep very well in an airtight glass container for weeks. You may decide to halve the recipe but they are so yummy and healthy you may change your mind next time.

Prep time: 20 minutes Cooking time: 25 minutes Makes: 50

Ingredients:

- 1 cup almond meal/flour
- 1 cup macadamia nuts or brazil nuts
- 3 Tbsp coconut flour
- ½ cup pumpkin seeds
- ½ cup sesame seeds
- ⅓ cup sunflower seeds
- 3 Tbsp whole flaxseeds
- 1 ¼ tsp sea salt
- 2 Tbsp black sesame seeds
- 2 Tbsp macadamia oil
- ⅓-½ cup water

Method:

Preheat oven to 150c/300f. You will need 3 large baking trays and 4 pieces of baking paper the size of the baking trays.

Add to a food processor, almond meal, macadamia nuts and coconut flour, pulse to mix and grind down the macadamias nuts.

Add pumpkin, sesame, sunflower and flaxseed seeds and salt. Process until they are broken up but not completely ground.

Add black sesame seeds, macadamia oil and pulse. Add water gradually until the dough forms a ball in the food processor.

Place a third of the dough between 2 sheets of baking paper. Use a rolling pin to roll out dough into a rectangle with a 2-3mm(⅛in) thickness. Remove the top piece of paper and transfer the bottom piece of baking paper with the rolled-out dough onto a baking tray. Cut the dough into 4 cm squares with a pizza cutter or sharp knife. Repeat process with the remaining portions of dough.

Bake for 20-25 minutes or until light brown and crisp. Break up the crackers once they have cooled.

These crackers keep for 3 weeks in an airtight glass container.

BREADS, CRACKERS & CRUSTS | 83

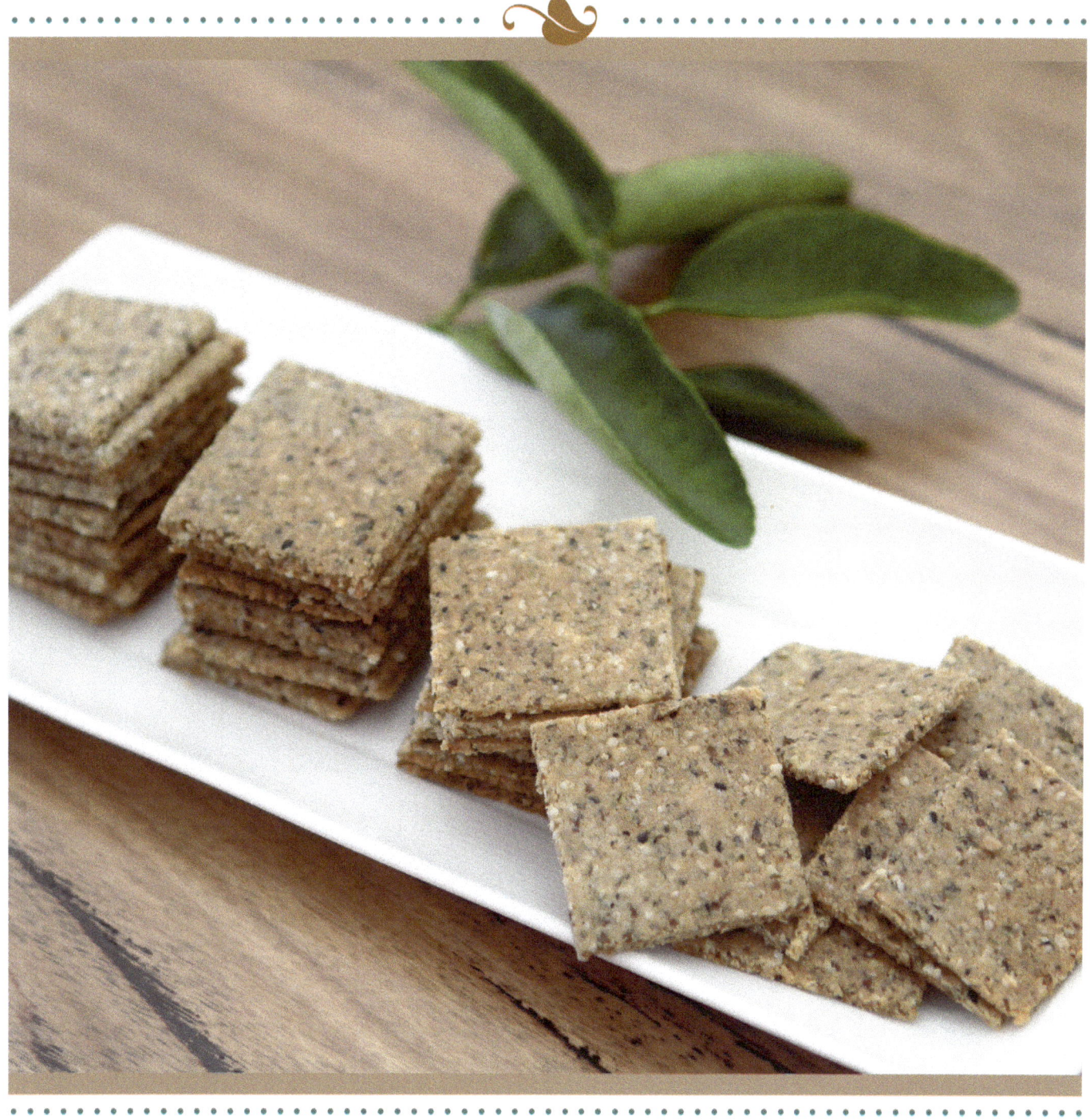

84 | BREADS, CRACKERS & CRUSTS

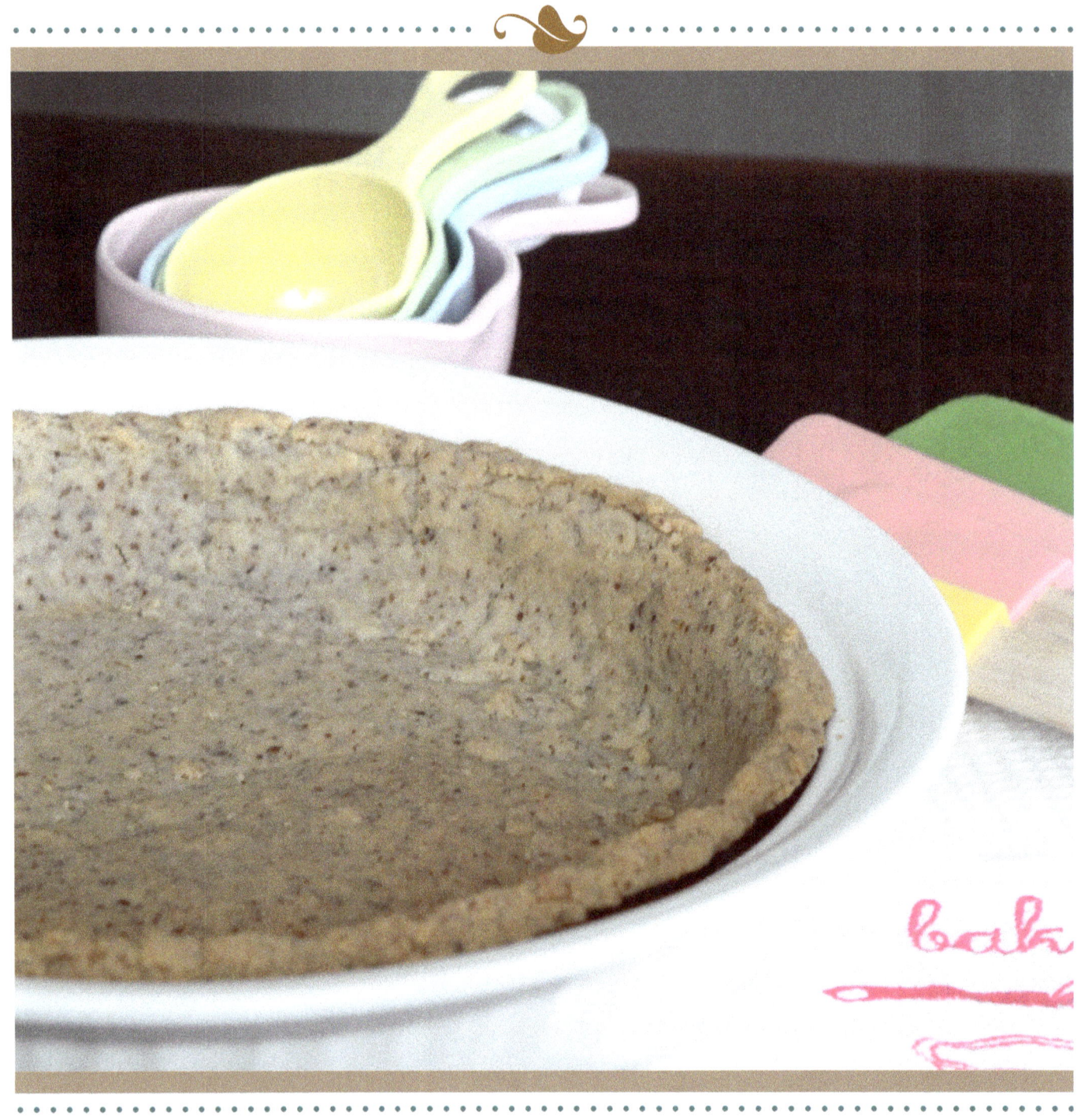

Sweet Coconut Piecrust

This is a perfect piecrust for an apple pie. It is crisp and flakier than other crusts I have made and it's nut free. The texture is very easy to roll. Pre-bake the piecrust and fill it with your favourite pie filling. Double the recipe if you are covering the top or using strips to make a crisscross pattern.

Prep time: 15 minutes Cooking time: 20 minutes Makes: 1 piecrust

Ingredients:

- 2 Tbsp flaxseed meal
- 3 Tbsp filtered water
- 2¼ cups desiccated coconut
- ⅓ cup arrowroot flour
- 1 Tbsp honey
- ⅓ tsp fine sea salt
- 1 large egg
- 1 tsp vanilla extract

Method:

Preheat oven to 150c/300f and grease a deep 23cm(9in) pie dish with coconut oil.

To a small bowl add, flaxseed and water. Mix and set aside for 8 minutes.

To a food processor add, coconut, arrowroot flour, honey and salt. Process until mixture has a fine texture, approximately 3-3½ minutes. Stop from time to time to scrape down sides of bowl.

Add flaxseed mixture, egg and vanilla. Process all ingredients together well until it becomes a soft dough and comes together, approximately 30-40 seconds.

Place the dough between two pieces of baking paper. If dough is a little sticky dust with arrowroot flour. Use a rolling pin to roll dough out, making it larger than the pie dish, approximately 33cm(13ins) in diameter.

Remove the top layer of paper and slip your hand under bottom sheet, gently turn dough over to place over pie dish. If any rips occur just press together to repair, use a knife to trim the edges.

Use a fork to prick the base of the pie in several places (this will help the dough not to rise off the bottom). Pre-bake piecrust for 20 minutes or until lightly golden, don't over cook.

Cool the piecrust before adding your filling, then bake your pie as normal.

Pie Crust
(Use for sweet or savoury pies)

This pastry has a mild flavour, it lends itself for use with a sweet or savoury pie. It has a firm texture after being baked.

Pre time: 10 minutes   Cooking time: 13-15 minutes   Makes: 1 piecrust

Ingredients:

SWEET CRUST
- 1¾ cups almond meal/flour
- 1 Tbsp coconut flour
- ¼ tsp fine sea salt
- 2 Tbsp coconut oil
- 1 large egg
- 1 Tbsp honey
- ½ tsp vanilla extract

SAVOURY CRUST
- 1¾ cups almond meal/flour
- 1 Tbsp coconut flour
- ¾ tsp Herbamare or ½ tsp fine sea salt
- 2 Tbsp coconut oil
- 1 large egg

Method:

Preheat oven to 160c/320f. Grease a 23cm(9in) pie dish lightly with coconut oil.

To a food processor add, almond meal, coconut flour and salt (Herbamare for savoury pie), pulse briefly to combined.

Add coconut oil and egg (honey and vanilla for a sweet pie), pulse until mixture comes together. If the savoury dough needs a little extra moisture, add 1-2 teaspoons of water while processing.

Using your hands, press dough evenly into pie dish. Prick base of pie dough in a few places with a fork, or cover with a circle of baking paper and some baking weights (remove weights for last few minutes of baking).

Bake for 13-15 minutes, you may like to cook a few minutes longer if you are filling with fruit or an uncooked filling which won't be returning to the oven. If the cooked base rises, press down gently with the back of spoon before it becomes firm. Make sure to let the pie crust cool completely before adding your pie filling.

BREADS, CRACKERS & CRUSTS 87

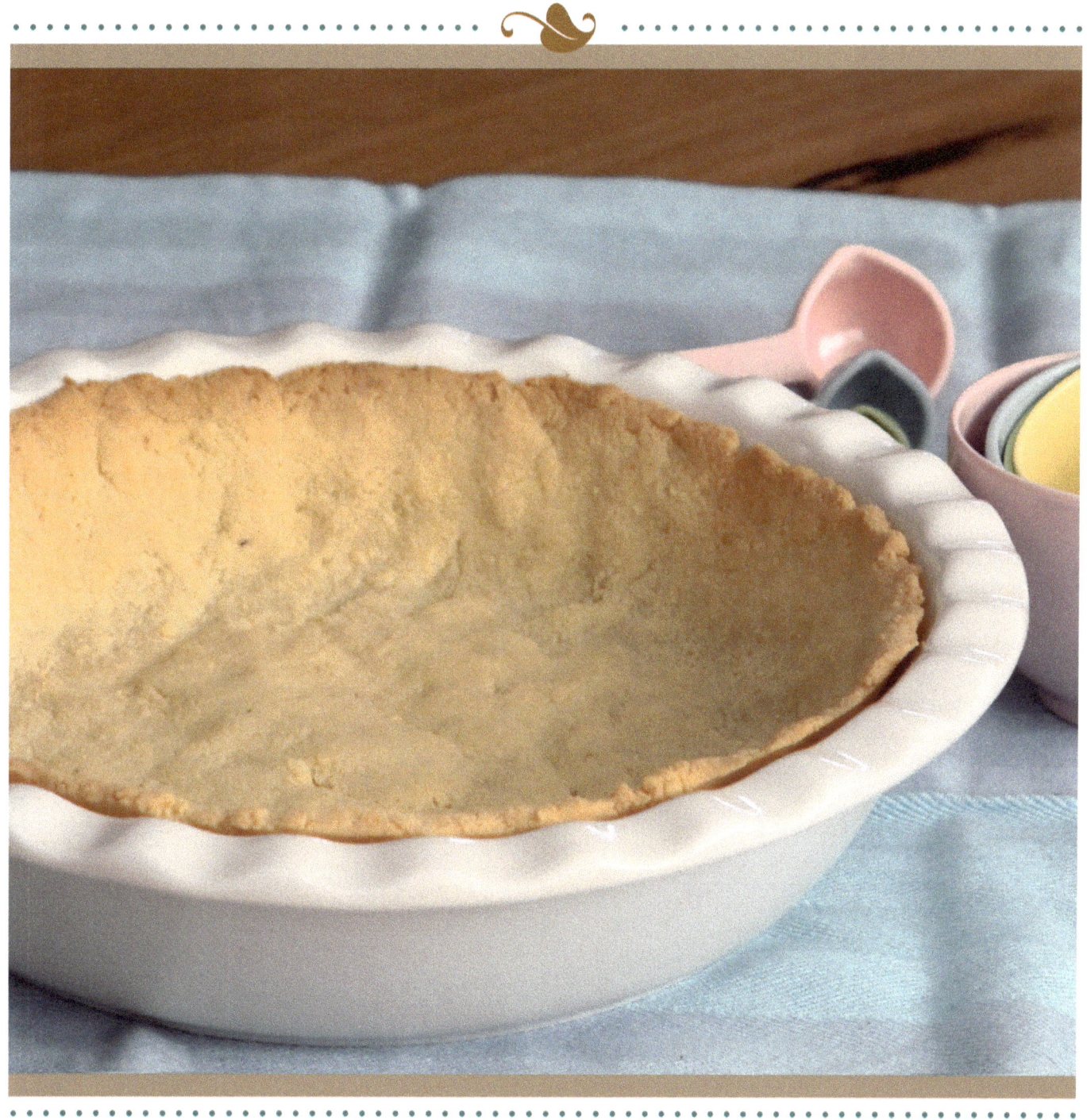

SALADS & VEGETABLES

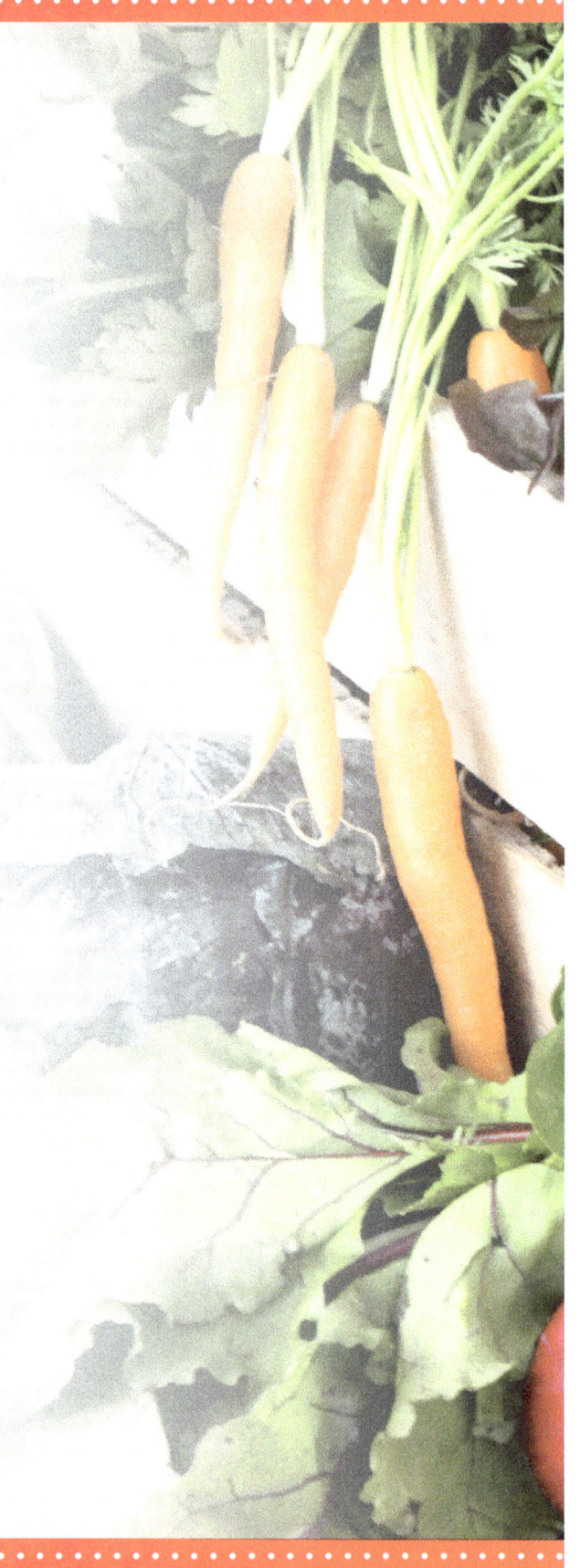

Rainbow Salad 91

Coleslaw 93

Grated Beetroot Salad 94

Broccoli Salad 97

Layered Salad 98

Sweet Potato and Spinach Salad 101

Cucumber and Tomato Salad 102

Sauerkraut 104

Winter Vegetable Bake 107

Sweet Swede 108

Mixed Steamed Vegetables with
Lemon Dressing 111

Green Beans and Water Chestnuts 113

Cauliflower and Broccoli Bake 114

Cauliflower Mash 116

Cauliflower Rice 117

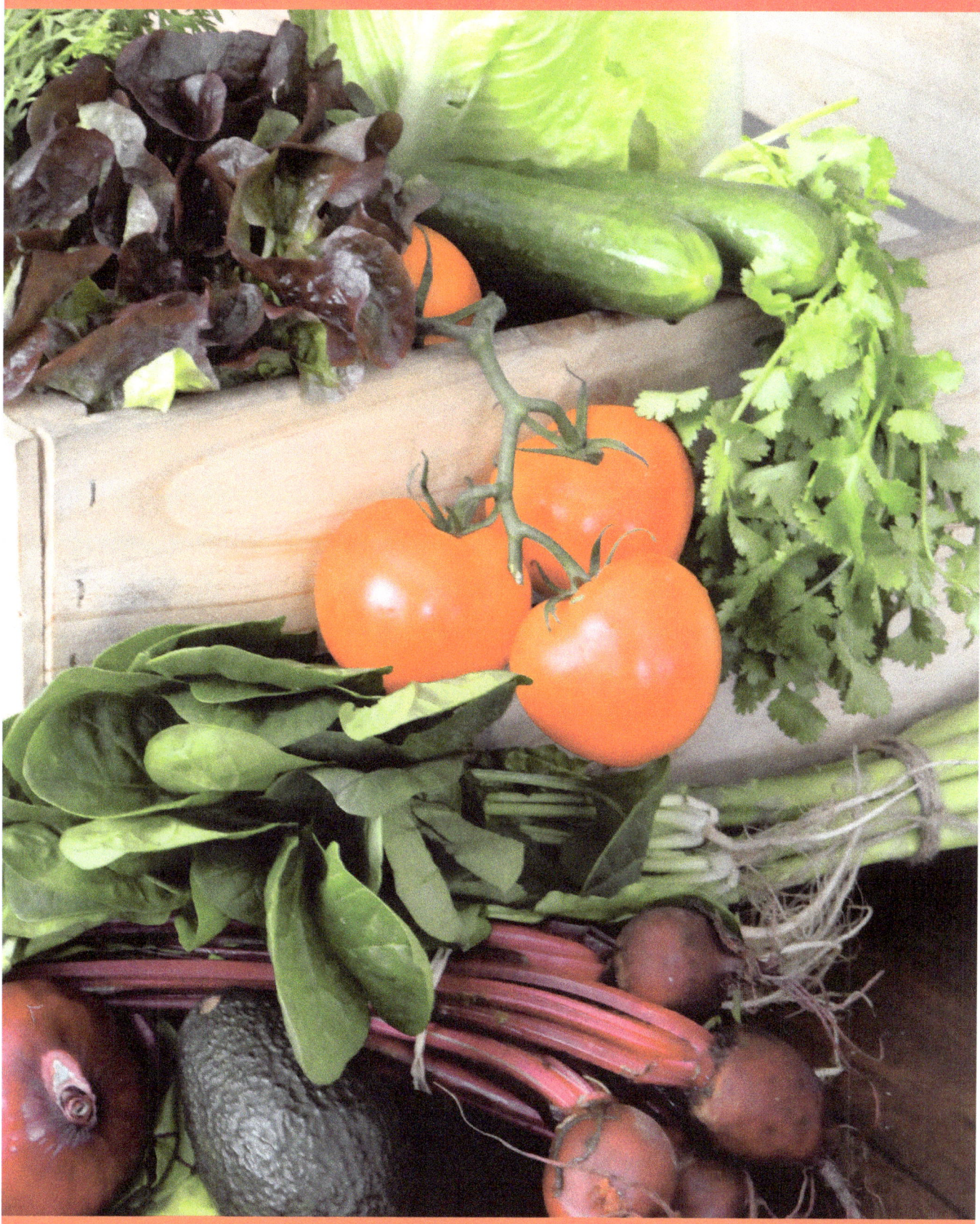

90 | SALADS & VEGETABLES

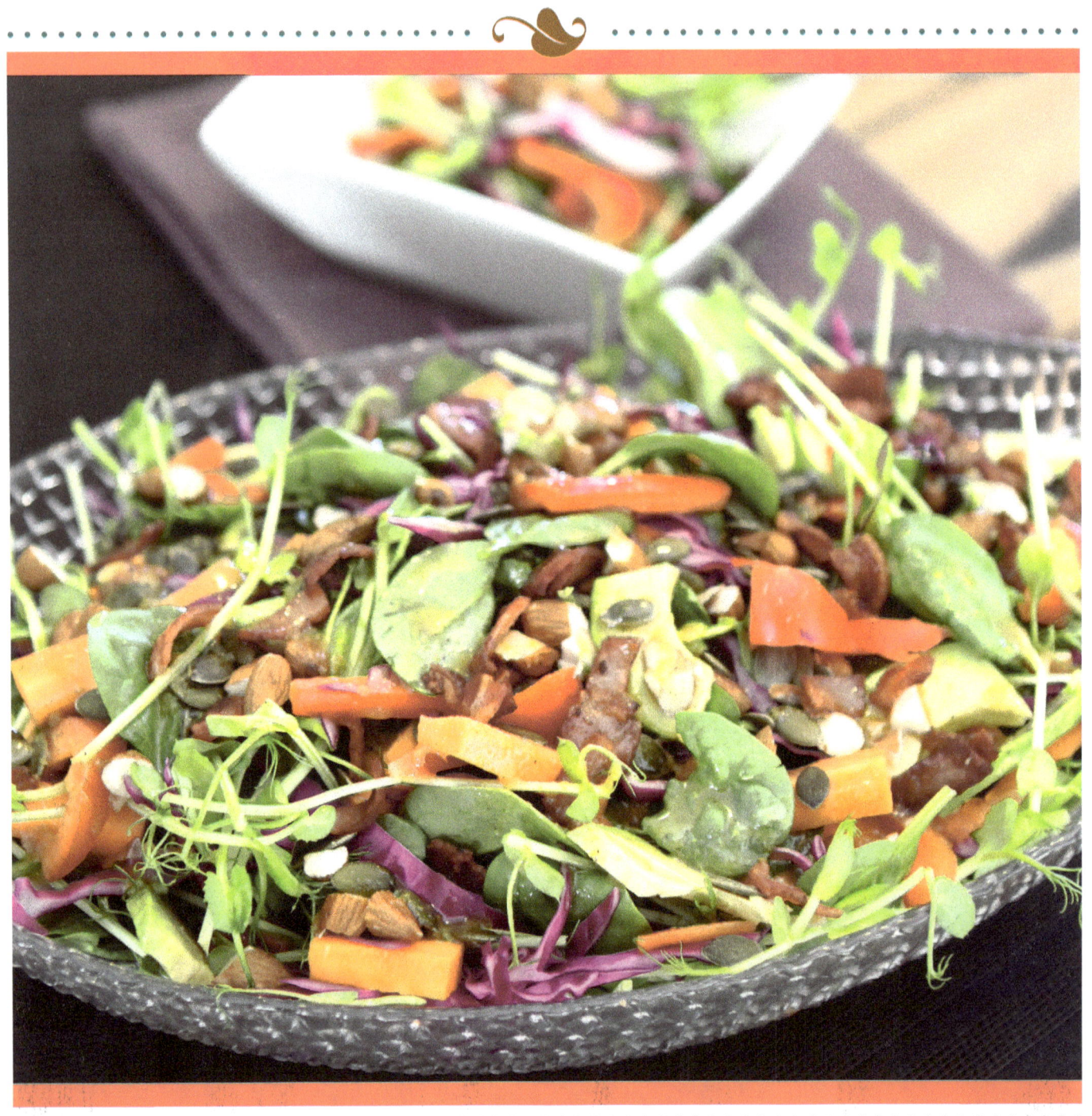

Rainbow Salad

I guess there's no question to why I named this "Rainbow salad". You get a good variety of vitamins and minerals within this bowl of different coloured vegetables. Spinach, red capsicum and carrot are all in the top 10 list of anti-oxidant vegetables. Dress the salad with Tahini Vinaigrette on page 209.

Prep time: 20 minutes Cooking time: none Serves: 6

Ingredients:

- 100g/3.5ozs baby spinach
- ¼ red cabbage, shredded
- 1 carrot, julienne
- 1 red capsicum, julienne
- 1 avocado, chopped
- A handful of snow pea sprouts
- 3 Tbsp raw almonds, roughly chopped, divided
- 3 Tbsp pumpkin seeds, divided
- Optional, cooked diced bacon to garnish
- Tahini Vinaigrette on page 209

Method:

Add all the above ingredients to a large salad bowl, except for the Tahini dressing, 1 tablespoon raw almonds and 1 tablespoon pumpkin seeds. Toss to combine.

Make the Tahini Vinaigrette.

Sprinkle the remaining roughly chopped almonds and pumpkin seeds over the salad and pour the vinaigrette over just before serving. Optional: scatter cooked diced bacon over the completed salad.

SALADS & VEGETABLES

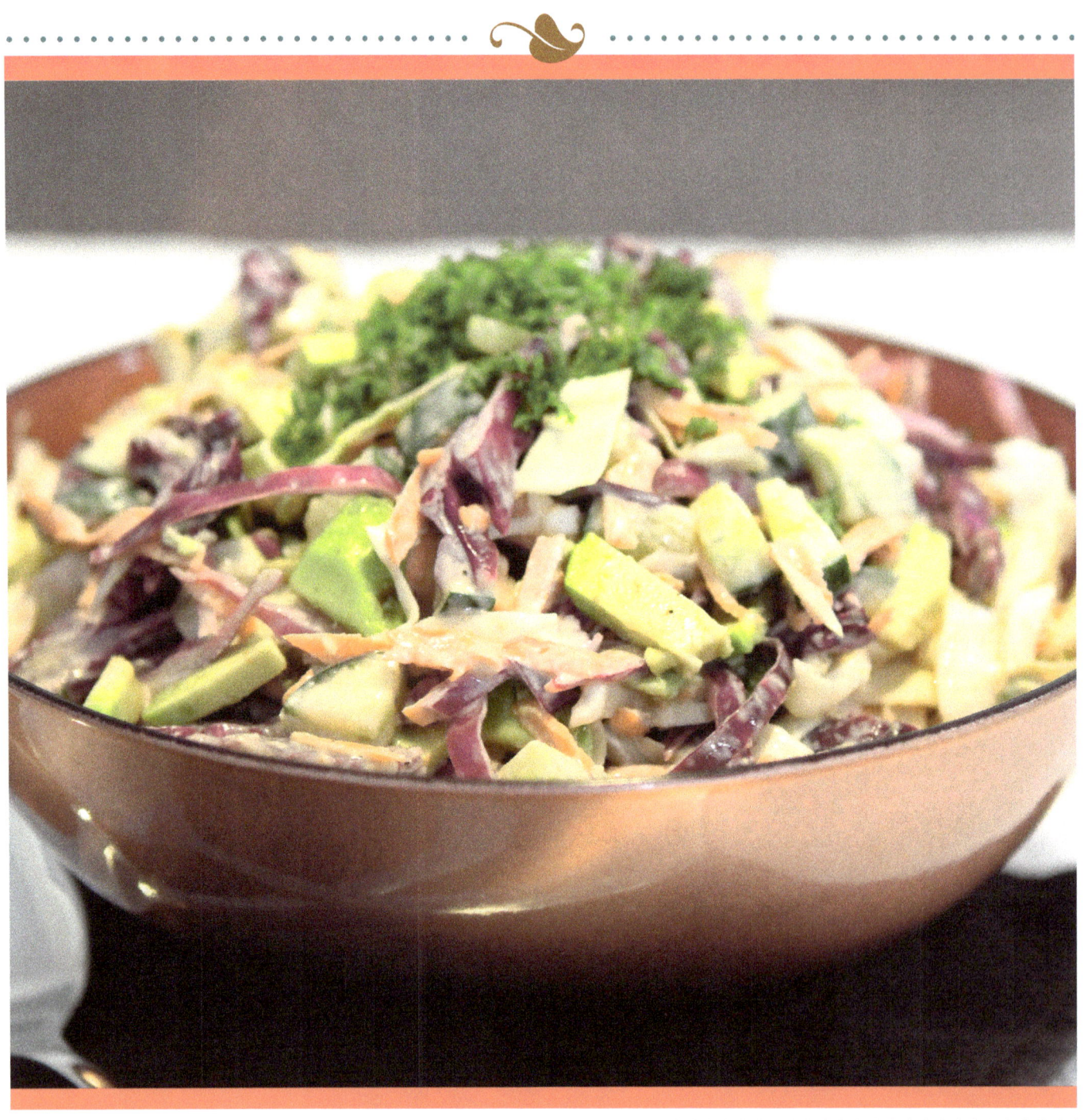

Coleslaw

A little twist on regular coleslaw. By adding cucumber my grandchildren like it and by adding avocado one of my daughters in law will eat it. Now everyone's happy! Add spring onions or any additions that will make this salad enjoyable for your family. Savoy cabbage has less water content than green cabbage, using it will prevent the watering down of your dressing.

Prep time: 15 minutes Cooking time: none Serves: 6

Ingredients:

- ¼ large red cabbage, finely shredded
- ¼ large savoy or green cabbage, finely shredded
- 1 large carrot, coarsely grated
- 2 Lebanese or 1 continental cucumber, leave skin on, finely diced
- 2 Tbsp fresh parsley, finely chopped
- 1 large or 2 small avocado, diced
- Juice of 1 small lemon
- ¼ cup mayonnaise, Egg Mayonnaise page 207
- Sea salt & black pepper to taste, be generous

Method:

To a large mixing bowl add, cabbages, carrot, cucumber and parsley, mix well.

Stir through the avocado. Add lemon juice, mayonnaise, salt and pepper. Thoroughly mix to combine, don't worry if the avocado smashes a little while mixing, it adds a lovely creamy consistency. Add more mayonnaise if required but mix well first before deciding.

To serve, transfer to a salad bowl.

Grated Beetroot Salad

The colour of this Beetroot salad makes a lovely contrast against other salads on a table. Excellent as a side dish for a summer BBQ or used as a relish on beef or lamb hamburger patties. This is made in minutes, double or triple for a larger party.

Prep time: 10 minutes Cooking time: none Serves: 4

Ingredients:

- 2 large beetroot, total weigh 500g/1.1 lbs
- 1 small or ½ large red onion, finely diced
- 2 Tbsp red wine vinegar
- 2 Tbsp extra virgin olive oil
- 2 tsp honey
- ½-¾ tsp fine sea salt
- ⅓ tsp ground pepper

Method:

Trim the beetroot and peel or scrub with a brush. Grate the beetroot. I use disposable rubber gloves to do this job and cover my chopping board with plastic wrap before I start grating on it (helps with the clean up).

Place beetroot in a sieve and squeeze out as much liquid as possible.

To a bowl add onion, vinegar, oil, honey, salt and pepper, and mix. Add the beetroot, stir to combine.

To serve, transfer to a small salad bowl.

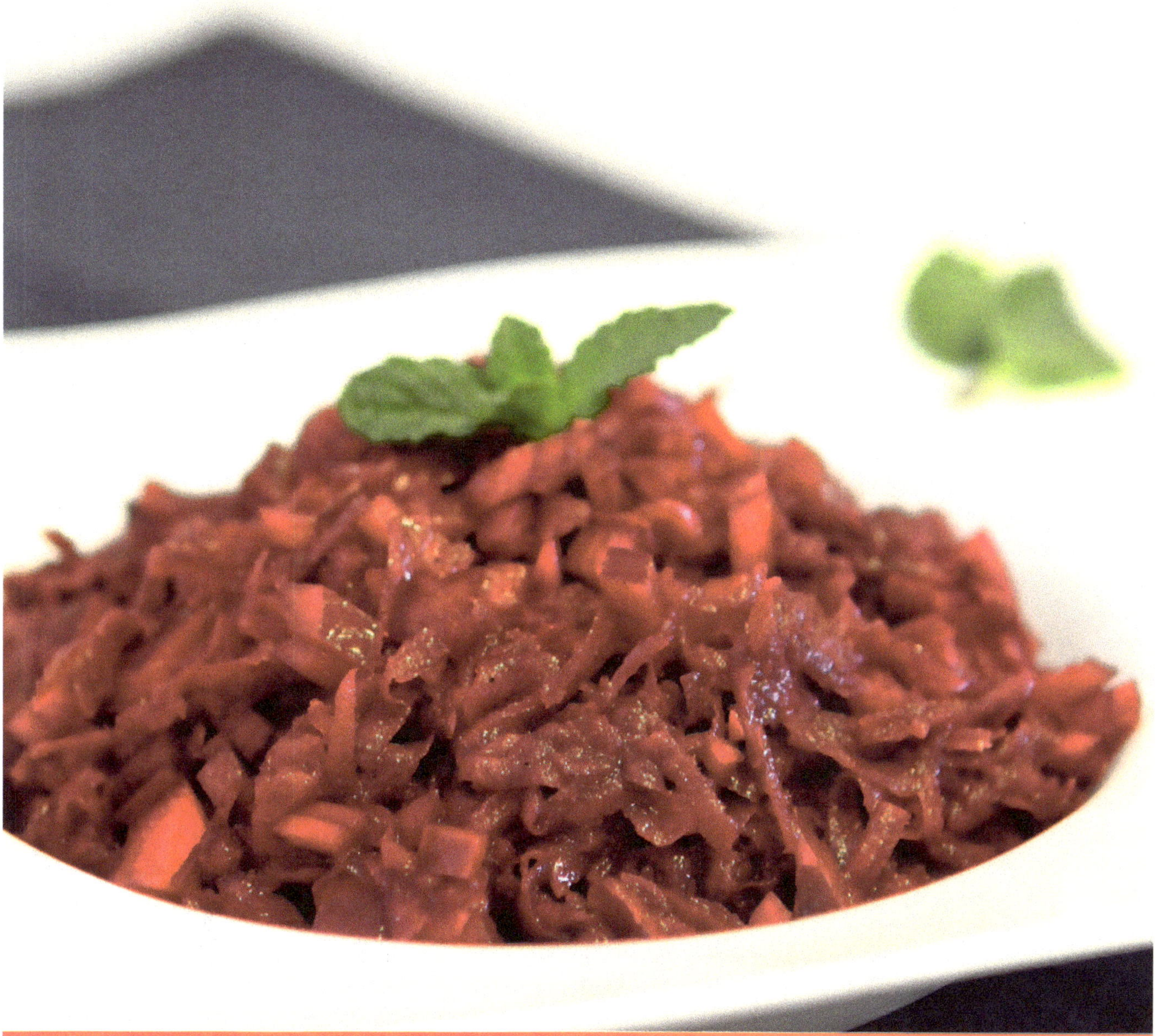

SALADS & VEGETABLES | 95

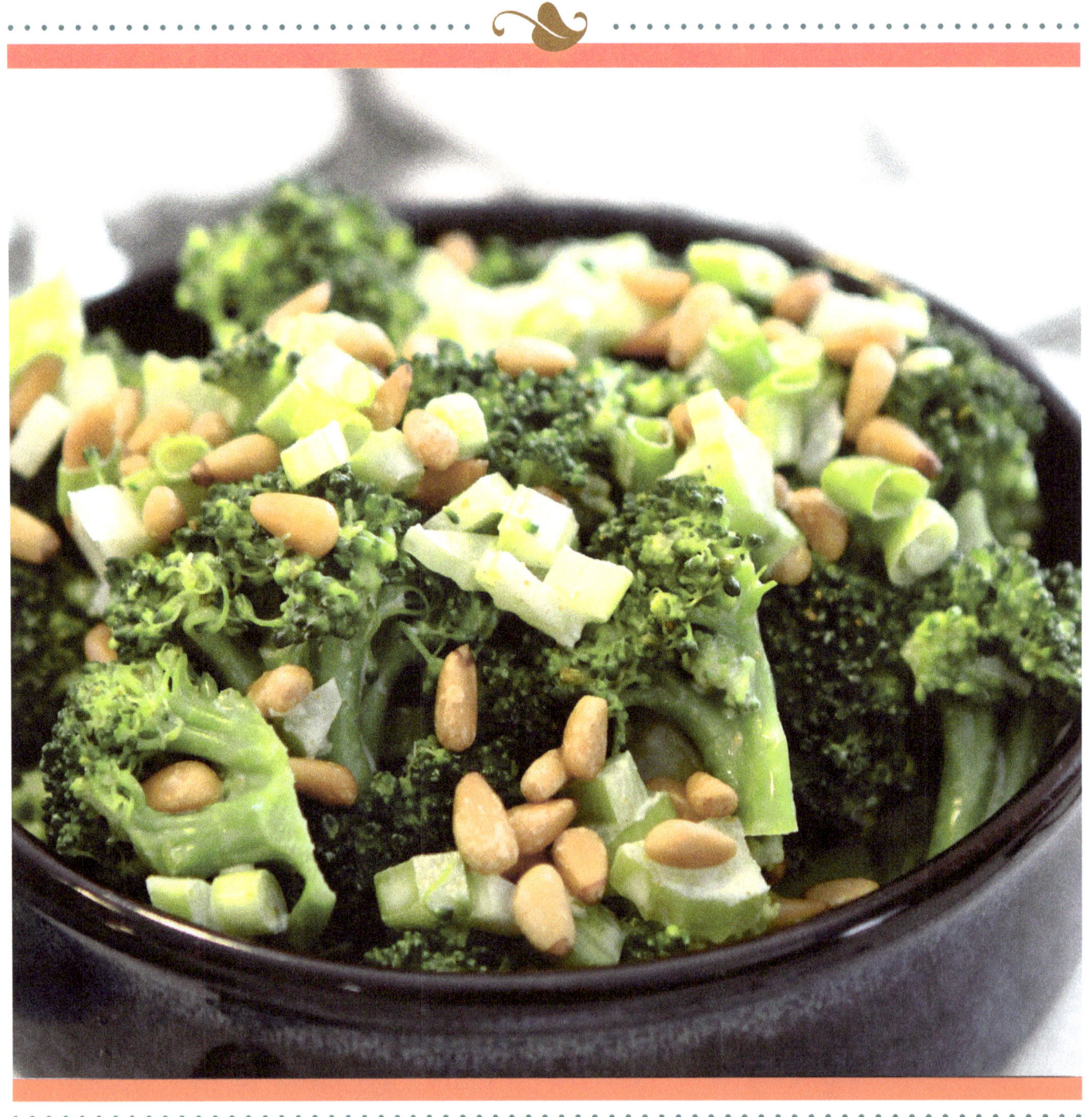

Broccoli Salad

Everyone knows broccoli is good for you, but did you know steamed is better than raw? According to "The World's Healthiest Foods" website, broccoli can provide extra health benefits when cooked by steaming. Broccoli is full of phyto-nutrients, which are known to help protect from several forms of cancer.

Prep time: 20 minutes Cooking time: 5 minutes Serves: 3

Ingredients:

- 1 large broccoli, chopped into small florets
- 2 spring onions, finely chopped
- 2 sticks celery, finely chopped
- ¼ cup pine nuts or almond slivers, toasted

DRESSING

- ⅓ cup mayonnaise, (Egg mayonnaise page 207, if using bought mayo add 2 tsp Apple Cider vinegar)
- 2 tsp honey
- 1¼ tsp curry powder, or to your taste

Method:

Steam broccoli until just starting to get tender but still firm; approximately 4 minutes from when water starts boiling under steamer.

Rinse in cold water to stop any further cooking and to keep the bright green colour. Once cold, mix with onions and celery.

Combine all dressing ingredients and mix well or use a blender. Stir dressing through the salad with ⅔ of the toasted pine nuts or almonds.

Serve in a small salad bowl, sprinkle the remaining nuts over the salad.

Layered Salad

Use a nice glass salad bowl for an effect. Seeing a delicious looking salad is almost as good as eating it. Using frozen peas keeps the lettuce from going brown. Best made a day ahead, keep refrigerated.

Prep time: 35 minutes Cooking time: none Serves: 6-8

Ingredients:

- 1 rash bacon, diced and cooked
- ½ head of iceberg lettuce, finely shredded
- 2½ cups frozen peas
- 6 hard boiled eggs, mashed (plus 3 Tbsp mayonnaise dressing)
- 1¼ cups grated tasty cheese, omit if can't tolerate dairy
- 2 carrots, grated
- ½ large continental cucumber, sliced with skin on
- 1 tomato, thin wedges
- fresh parsley, chopped

MAYONNAISE DRESSING

- 1¼ cups Egg Mayonnaise page 207 or another good quality egg mayonnaise
- 1 tsp dijon mustard
- 1 tsp garlic, minced

Method:

Mix together all the mayonnaise dressing ingredients, set aside in the fridge. If you are making my mayonnaise just for this recipe, add the extra mustard and garlic when you are blending.

Add the bacon pieces to a heated frying pan and cook until crispy, set aside to cool.

In the bottom of a glass salad bowl, add shredded lettuce, top with frozen peas, making sure the salad layers come all the way to the sides of the bowl.

Mix the mashed egg with 3 tablespoons of mayonnaise dressing, spread evenly over peas and level using a fork. Sprinkle over grated cheese (if using).

Add grated carrot and lastly cucumber slices over lapping each other as you go around the bowl. Make sure all layers look nice through the bowl. Spoon the remaining 1 cup of mayonnaise dressing over the top, smooth over with the back of spoon.

Just before serving, arrange tomato slices evenly around the top of the salad and sprinkle over bacon and parsley.

SALADS & VEGETABLES | 99

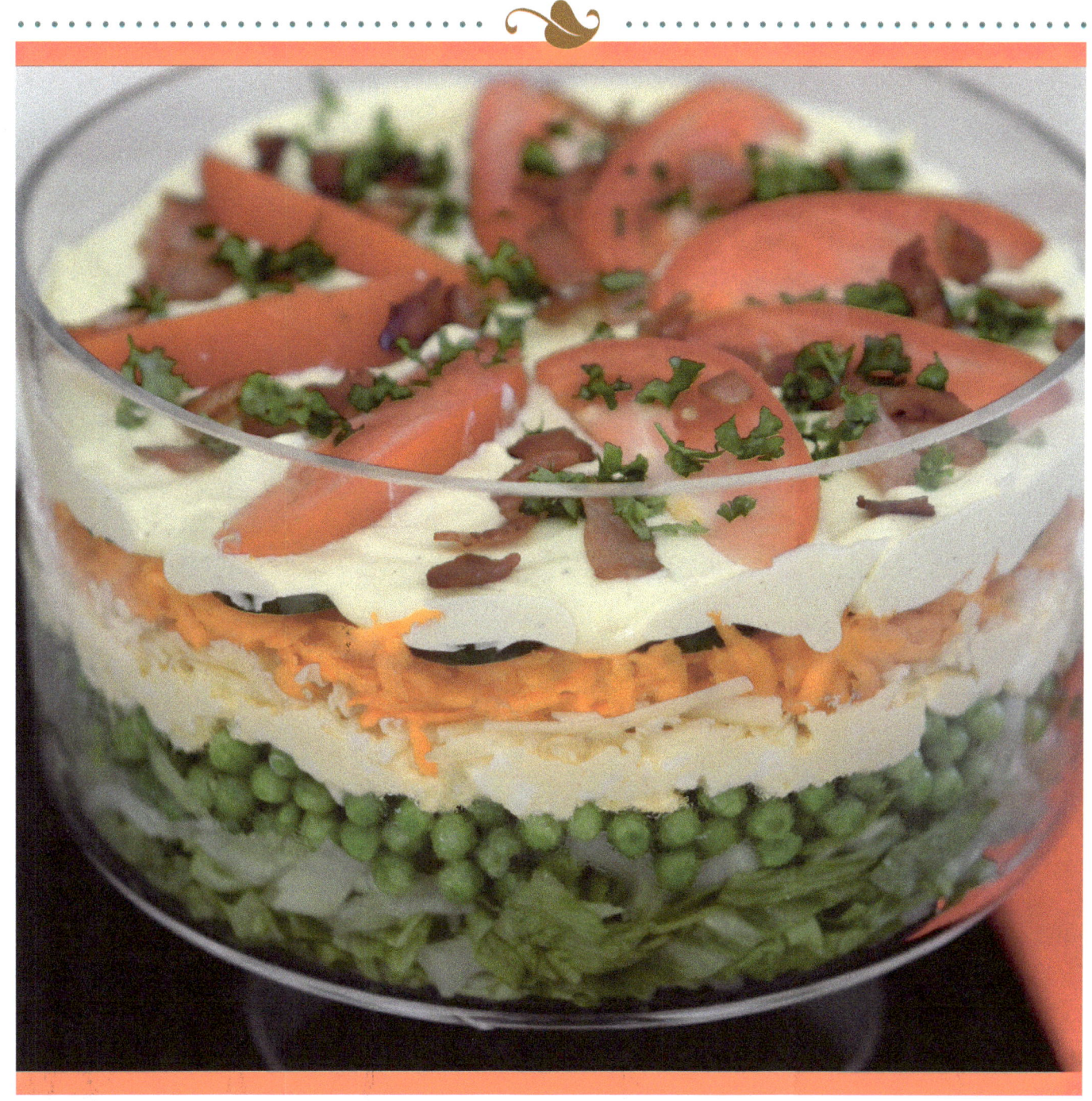

100 | SALADS & VEGETABLES

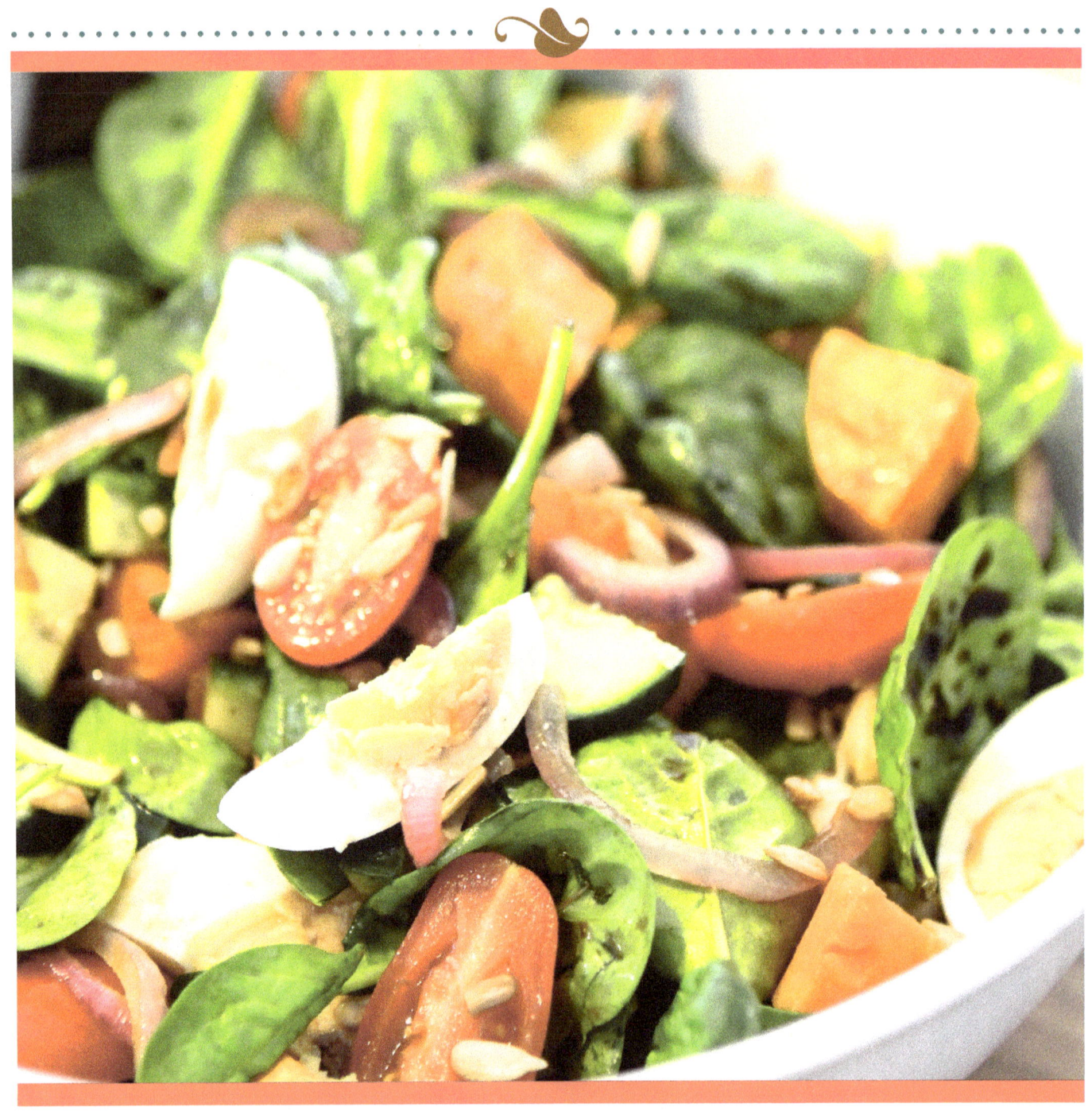

Sweet Potato and Spinach Salad

My family eats this salad often. It's great to eat in summer or winter. Sweet potato is a rich source of beta-carotene and a good source of vitamins C and E, potassium and it's full of fibre.

Prep time: 20 minutes Cooking time: 25 minutes Serves: 6

Ingredients:

- 1 medium sweet potato, 2.5cm/1in cubes
- 1 medium red onion, cut in half, sliced thinly
- 2-3 Tbsp olive oil infused with garlic, for roasting
- Sea salt and ground pepper, for roasting
- 3 Tbsp sunflower seeds, toasted
- 120g/4ozs baby spinach leaves
- 12 mini roma tomatoes or grape tomatoes, cut length ways in half
- ½ large continental cucumber, sliced in thick circles and cut into quarters
- 1 avocado, diced
- 3 hard boiled eggs, cut lengthways in half, then each half into thirds

DRESSING

- 2½ Tbsp olive oil
- 2½ Tbsp balsamic vinegar
- Sea salt and pepper, to taste

Method:

Preheat oven to 180c/350f. Place sweet potato and onion in a baking dish. Drizzle with olive oil, I use olive oil infused with garlic or you can add a little minced garlic. Season with sea salt and pepper. Use clean hands to toss the vegetables in the oil. Spread out evenly. Cook for 25-30 minutes. Keep an eye on the sweet potato, don't over cook, as it needs to hold together when tossed though the salad. Set aside to cool.

Toast sunflower seeds on a tray in the oven while the sweet potato cooks. Set aside.

To a large salad bowl, add spinach, tomatoes, cucumber, avocado, cold sweet potato with onion and sunflower seeds.

Just before serving, whisk dressing ingredients together, pour over the salad and toss to coat well. Add cut eggs, carefully mixing through with your hands, to keep yolks intact.

THE JOYFUL TABLE

Cucumber and Tomato Salad

The herbs in this salad give a very refreshing flavor, it's simple and quick to make. It can also be used as a salsa served with BBQ meat.

Prep time: 10 minutes   Cooking time: none   Serves: 4-6

Ingredients:

- 1 large continental cucumber, sliced in circles and cut into quarters (approximately 3½ cups)
- 3 large tomatoes, roughly diced (approximately 3 cups)
- 1 small red onion, finely diced
- ⅓ cup chopped fresh parsley
- ¼ cup chopped fresh basil
- 2 Tbsp olive oil
- 2 Tbsp balsamic vinegar
- 2 Tbsp fresh lemon juice
- Sea salt and pepper to taste

Method:

To a large bowl add, quartered cucumber slices, diced tomatoes, onion and fresh herbs.

Mix to combine. Add to the bowl, oil, vinegar, lemon juice, salt and pepper.

Stir to coat the salad with dressing.

To serve, transfer to a salad bowl or individual bowls.

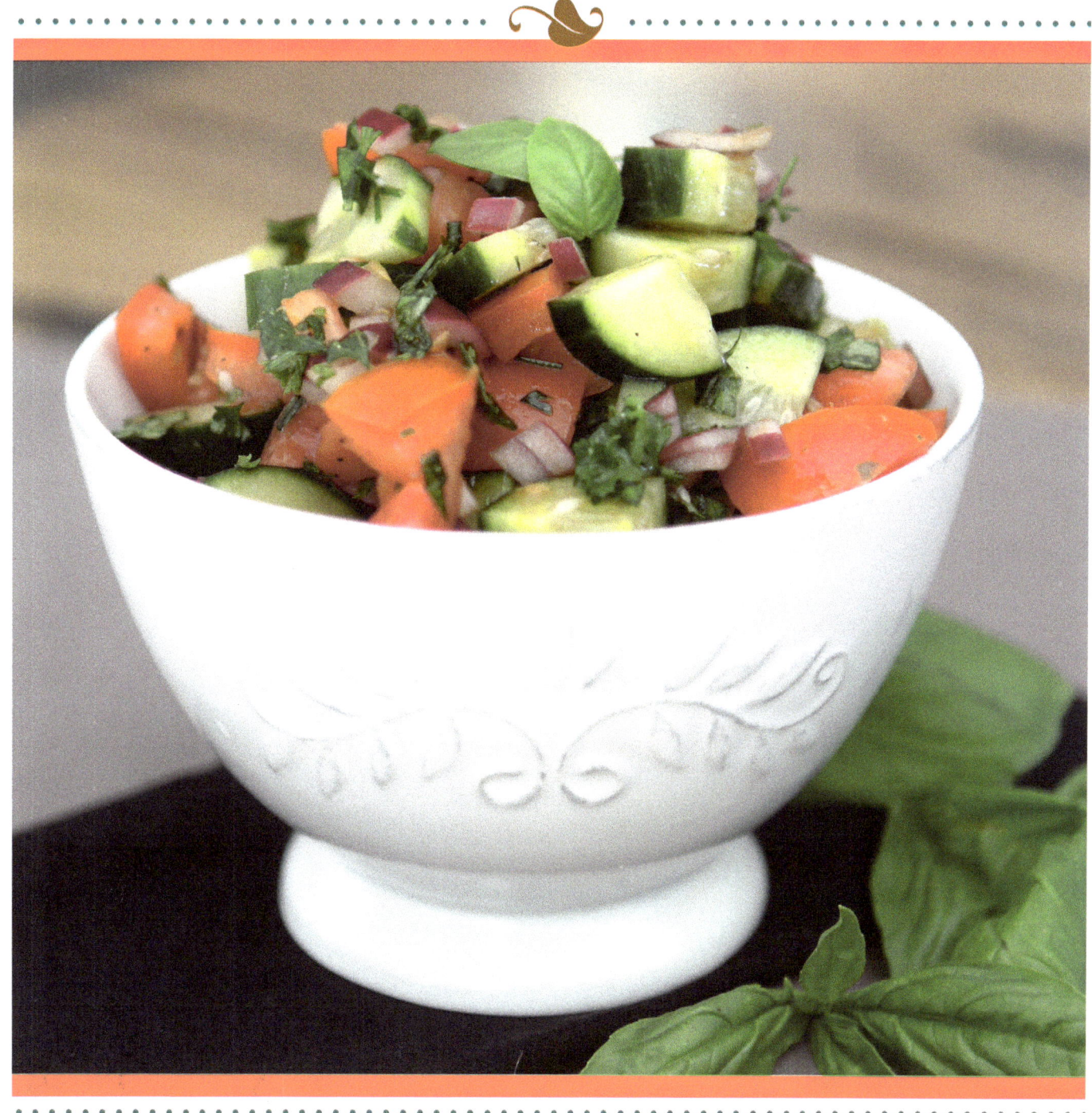

Sauerkraut

A lovely friend gave me this Russian recipe for Sauerkraut; it has been passed down through her family. I've discovered if you leave your salt sprinkled through the cabbage for two hours before starting, it makes for less work. My youngest granddaughter Ruby, has been eating sauerkraut since she was 6 months old. Fermented food is one of the most important foods we should be eating for good gut health.

Prep time: 20 minutes plus fermenting time Cooking time: none
Makes: approximately 6x2 cup pickling jars

Ingredients:

- 2 large green cabbages
- 2 heaped Tbsp fine sea salt

Method:

To shred cabbages, use a small shredding attachment on a food processor or shred finely with a knife. Place shredded cabbage into an extra large bowl. (I keep a laundry hand washing basin for this job). Sprinkle salt through the cabbage and mix well. Cover bowl or basin with a tea towel and set aside.

Come back after 2 hours and use something like a pestle (I use a large rolling pin that has a rounded end) to bash the cabbage. You will already have lots of liquid that has come out, so not too much bashing should have to happen. The juice is the important part, we want as much as possible.

Pack cabbage into a glass or ceramic container, which has a lid. You need to pack it down so tight that there are no air bubbles in it. The juice should sit a few centimeters above the cabbage. Place a small plate or bowl on top to keep the cabbage under the juice and to keep light out. If using a glass jar, cover with a tea towel. (I use a large 15 cup ceramic canister with lid and place a small tart dish on top of cabbage.)

Leave a couple of days. Then, using a long skewer, poke all the way down to the bottom of the cabbage. Bubbles of gas should start coming up (you want to get rid of the smelly gas). Poke the cabbage in several places each day. Then place the plate back and press down firmly to make liquid cover the cabbage again. Replace lid.

Continue doing this for 10-14 days in winter or 5-7 days in summer. When the smell has gone away and no gas bubbles are released when you poke the cabbage, it's ready.

Sterilize jars and place cabbage and juice in them. Seal lids and place in fridge to store. Keeps for several months in the fridge.

SALADS & VEGETABLES | 105

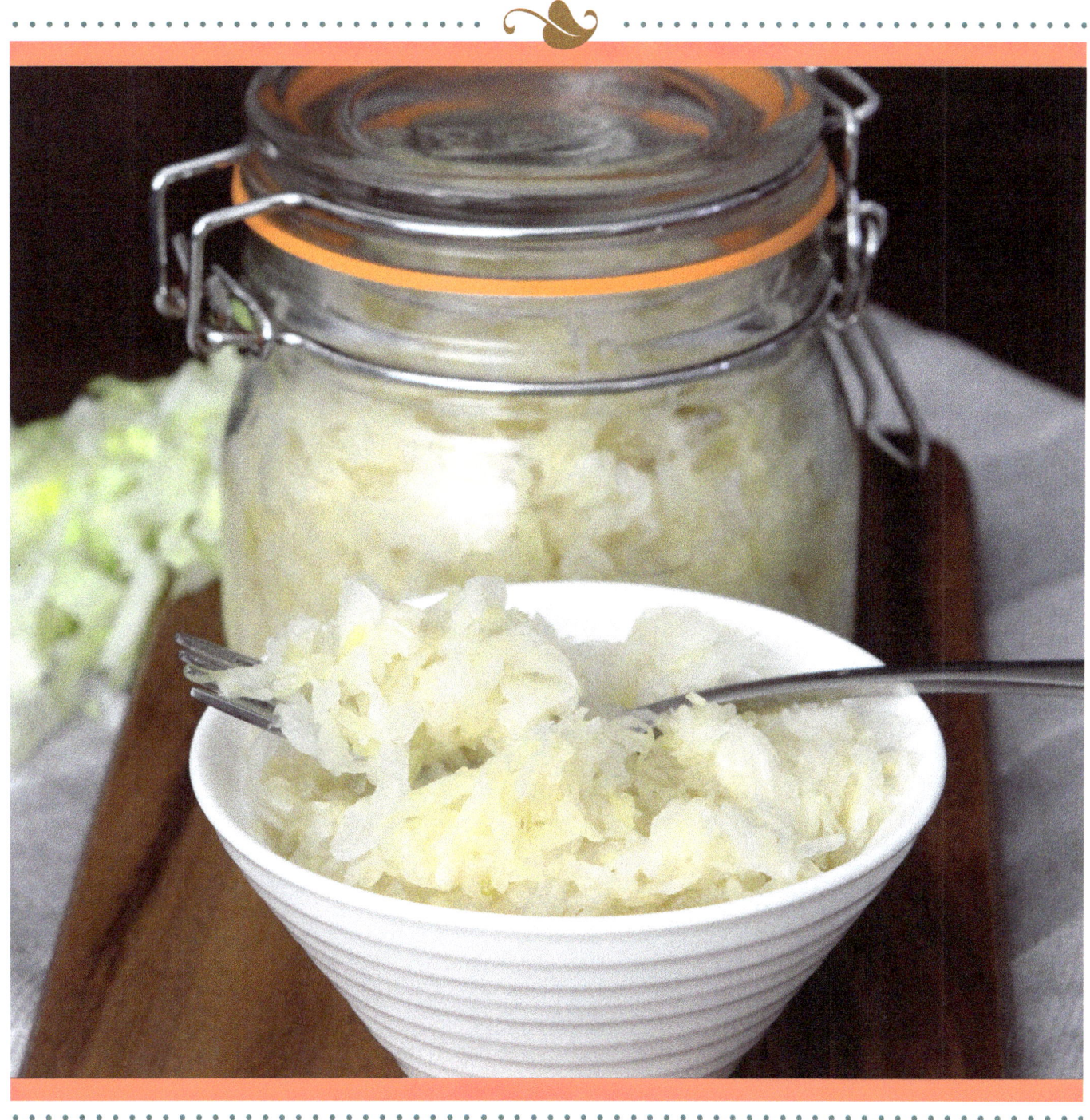

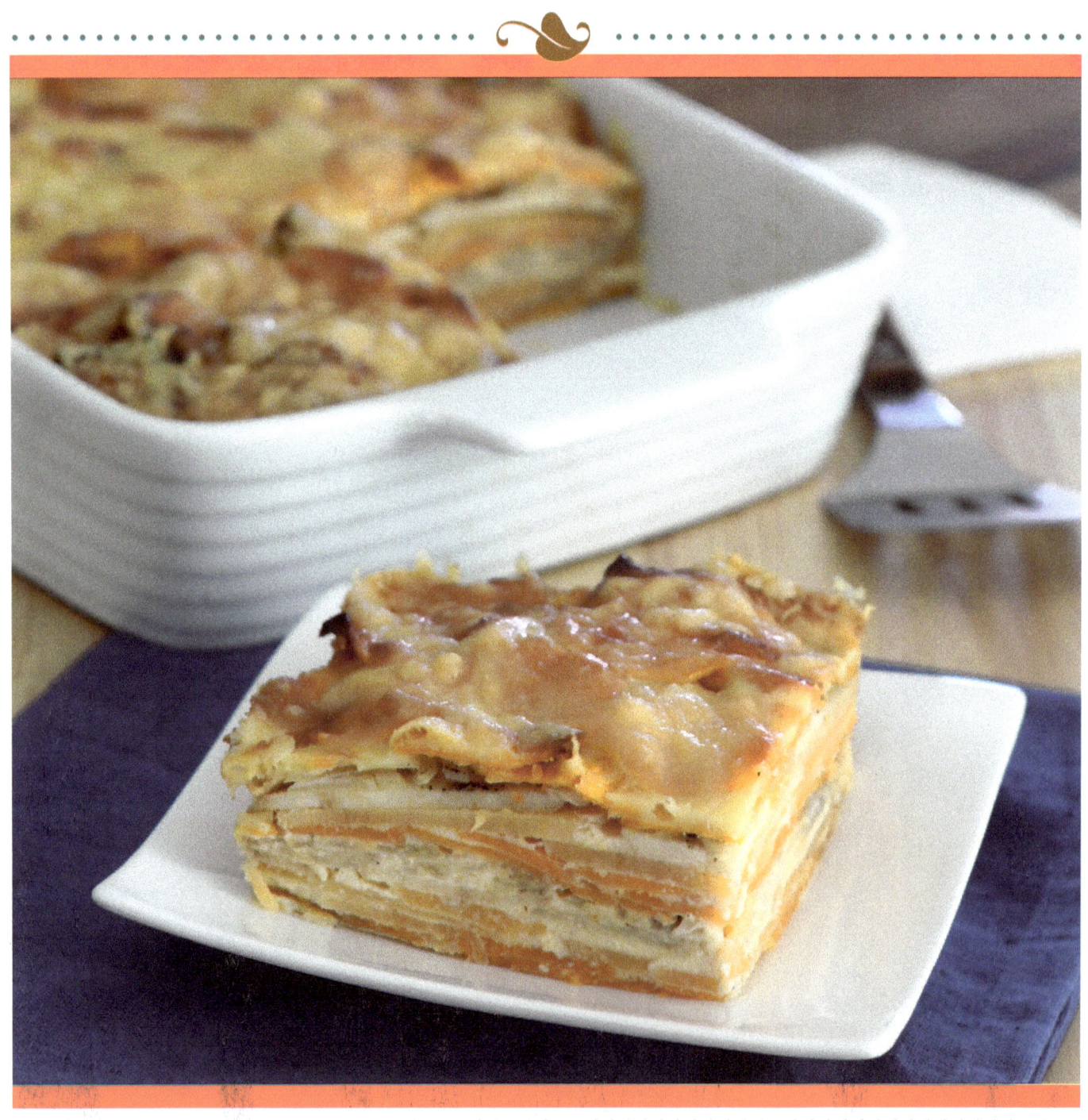

Winter Vegetable Bake

This is a delicious comfort food for the cooler months. There's a lovely creamy texture between the warm winter vegetables. Cooking time is quite long due to the several layers of vegetables, but it's certainly worth it.

Prep time: 25 minutes   Cooking time: 1 hour 10 minutes   Serves: 6-8

Ingredients:

- 2 medium sweet potatoes, thinly sliced
- 2 large swede, thinly sliced
- 2 medium celeriac, thinly sliced
- 6 large eggs
- 400ml/14oz can coconut cream
- Nutmeg, sea salt and pepper
- Optional, 2 cups grated matured cheese for topping (omit for dairy free)

Method:

Note: The vegetable quantities are approximate due to how thinly you can slice them. I use a mandolin slicer, number 2 gauge.

Preheat oven to 190c/375f. Grease a 30x20cm (12x8in) rectangle ceramic baking dish.

Peel sweet potato and swede. Cut skin off celeriac, trying to keep as much flesh as possible. Slice vegetables using a mandolin (watch your fingers), or slice vegetables very thinly. Place vegetables in separate bowls ready for assembling.

In a small bowl whisk eggs and coconut cream together, set aside.

To assemble, place a layer of sweet potato overlapping on the base, followed with a layer of swede, then celeriac. Pour half the egg and cream mixture over the vegetables. Season with a sprinkling of nutmeg, salt and pepper. Continue with the exact layers for a second time. Finish off with a layer of sweet potato. (You should have 3 layers in total of sweet potato but 2 of the other vegetables).

Pour over the remaining egg and cream mixture and sprinkle with nutmeg, salt and pepper.

Cover with foil and place in oven for 1 hour 10 minutes. Remove foil, check vegetables are tender by inserting a knife in the centre.

You may like to sprinkle with a little extra nutmeg before serving or with grated cheese (if using cheese remove from oven a few minutes earlier, add cheese and place back in oven uncover to melt).

Sweet Swede

When potatoes are off the menu, we call for swede. This simple but tasty dish can accompany any meat or fish. Tastes a lot like roast potato, but heaps better!

Prep time: 5 minutes Cooking time: 12 minutes Serves: 4

Ingredients:

- 1-1½ Tbsp ghee or organic butter
- 4 medium swede, diced
- 1½ Tbsp organic maple syrup
- Ground pepper to taste, be generous
- Chopped fresh parsley to garnish

Method:

Heat a large non-stick frying pan over medium-high heat. Melt ghee and add the diced swede.

Cook for 10 minutes. Use a spatula to turn frequently, watching not to burn the swede. I also use a fork to assist with turning each piece.

Once evenly brown, but still a little firm, drizzle over maple syrup. Reduce heat to medium and continue cooking for a further 2-3 minutes, stirring through the syrup. Add ground pepper and adjust to taste.

Serve garnished with fresh chopped parsley.

SALADS & VEGETABLES | 109

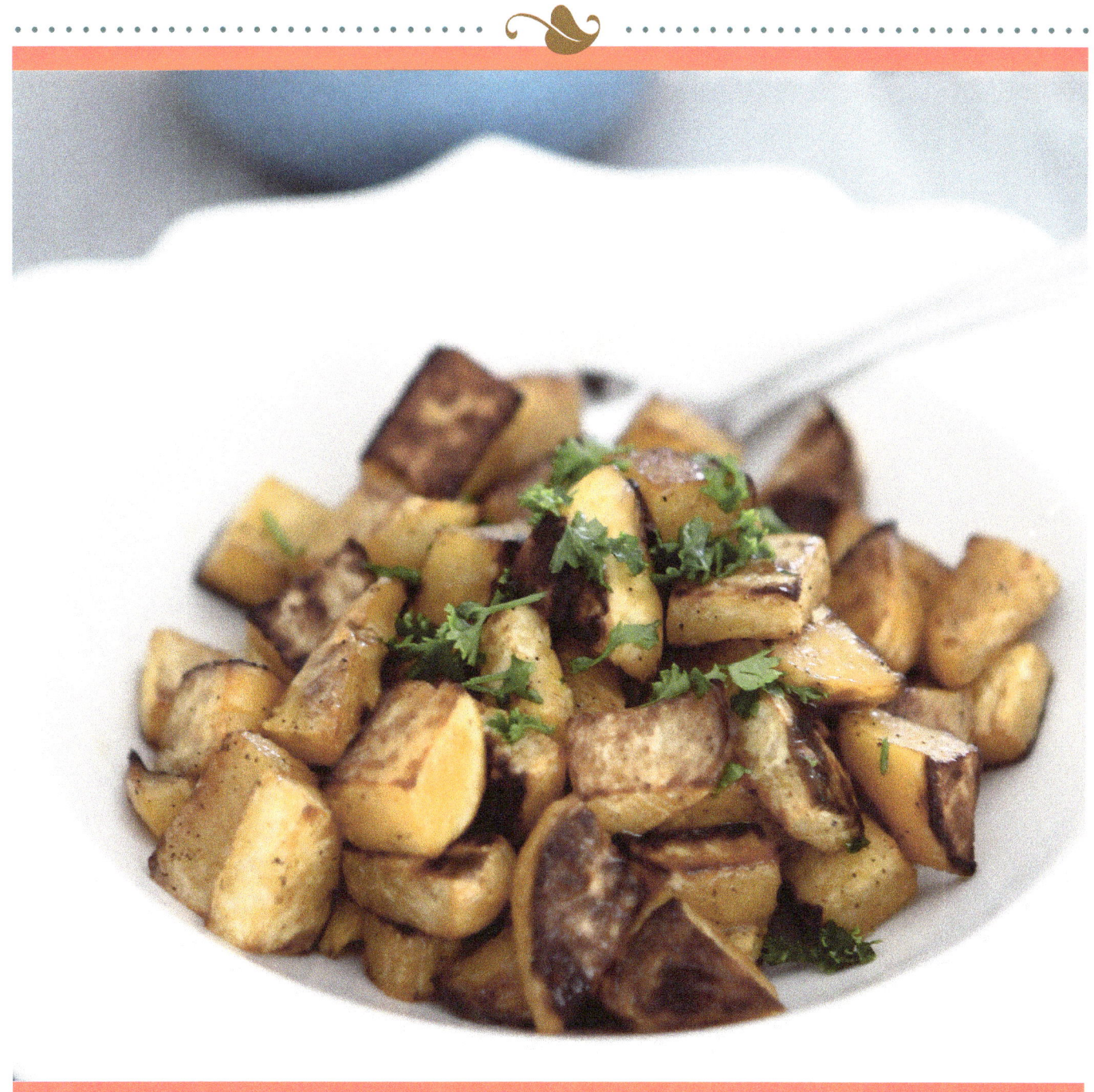

SALADS & VEGETABLES

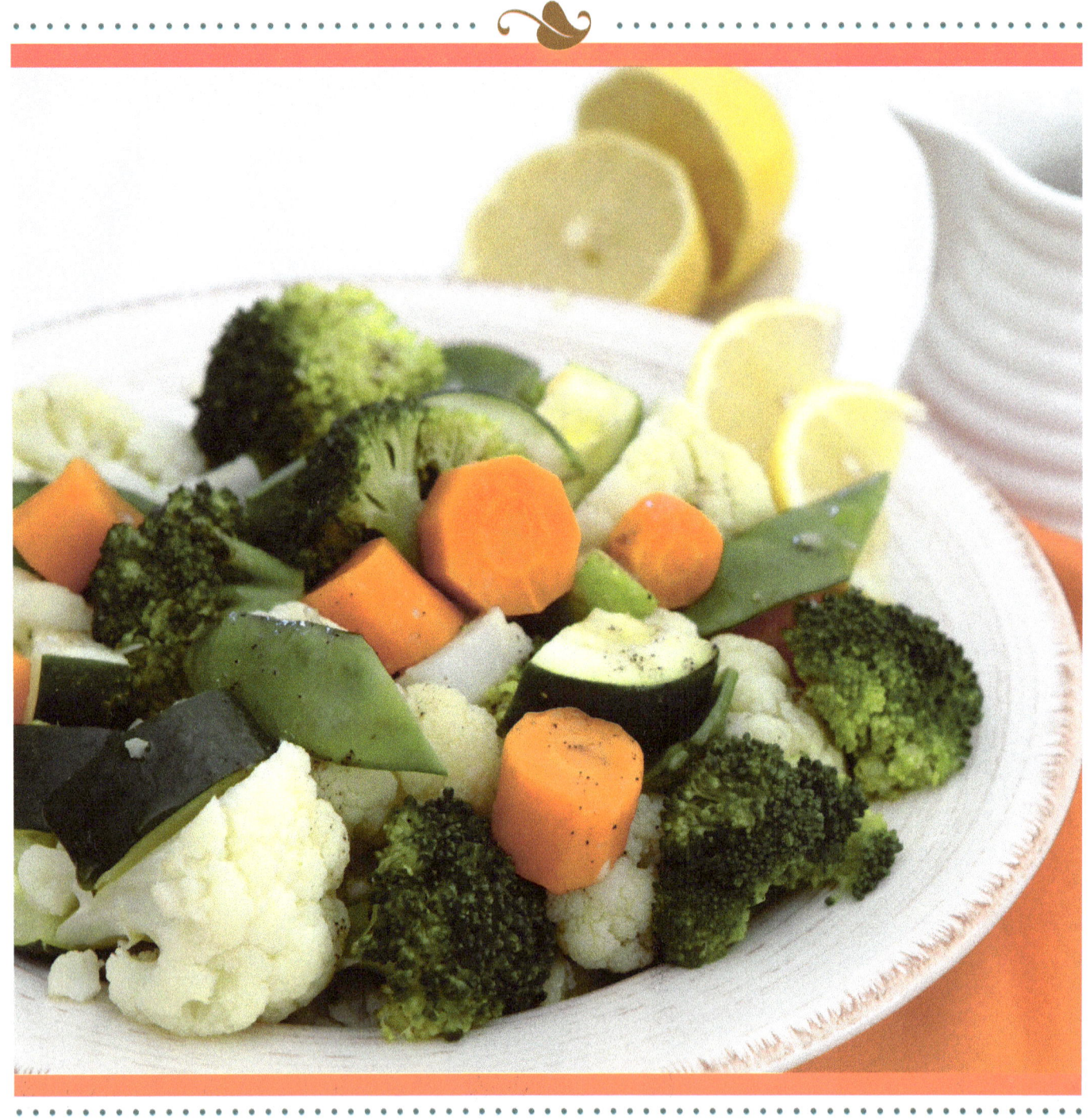

Mixed Steamed Vegetables
with Lemon Dressing

Steamed vegetables are one of those things we all know we should eat, but they can be so boring. Here's a citrus dressing to toss through plain vegetables, it adds a bit of a zing.

Prep time: 10 minutes Cooking time: 15 minutes Serves: 4

Ingredients:

2 carrots, cut in chunks
⅓ large cauliflower, small florets
1 small or ½ large zucchini, cut in chunks then cut into quarters
½ large broccoli, small florets
Small handful snow peas, trimmed and cut diagonally in half

DRESSING
Juice of 1 lemon
¼ cup olive oil
1 tsp garlic, minced
1 tsp fine sea salt
¼ tsp ground pepper

Method:

Use a large saucepan with a stainless steal steamer on top. Bring the water in the bottom to a boil, then reduce to simmering.

Add carrots first, steaming with lid on for 5 minutes. Add cauliflower to the carrots, steam for a further 5 minutes.

Add to the steamer zucchini and broccoli. After 4 minutes, check if all vegetables are just softening but still firm.

Add snow peas on top of the other vegetables, they will only take a minute or two.

While vegetables are cooking make dressing. Add all the dressing ingredients into a small jug. Whisk for 30 seconds with a fork to combine. Set aside.

Remove vegetables while still a little firm as they will continue cooking. Add to a serving dish and pour over dressing. Toss to coat vegetables, take care to not break vegetables when tossing.

SALADS & VEGETABLES

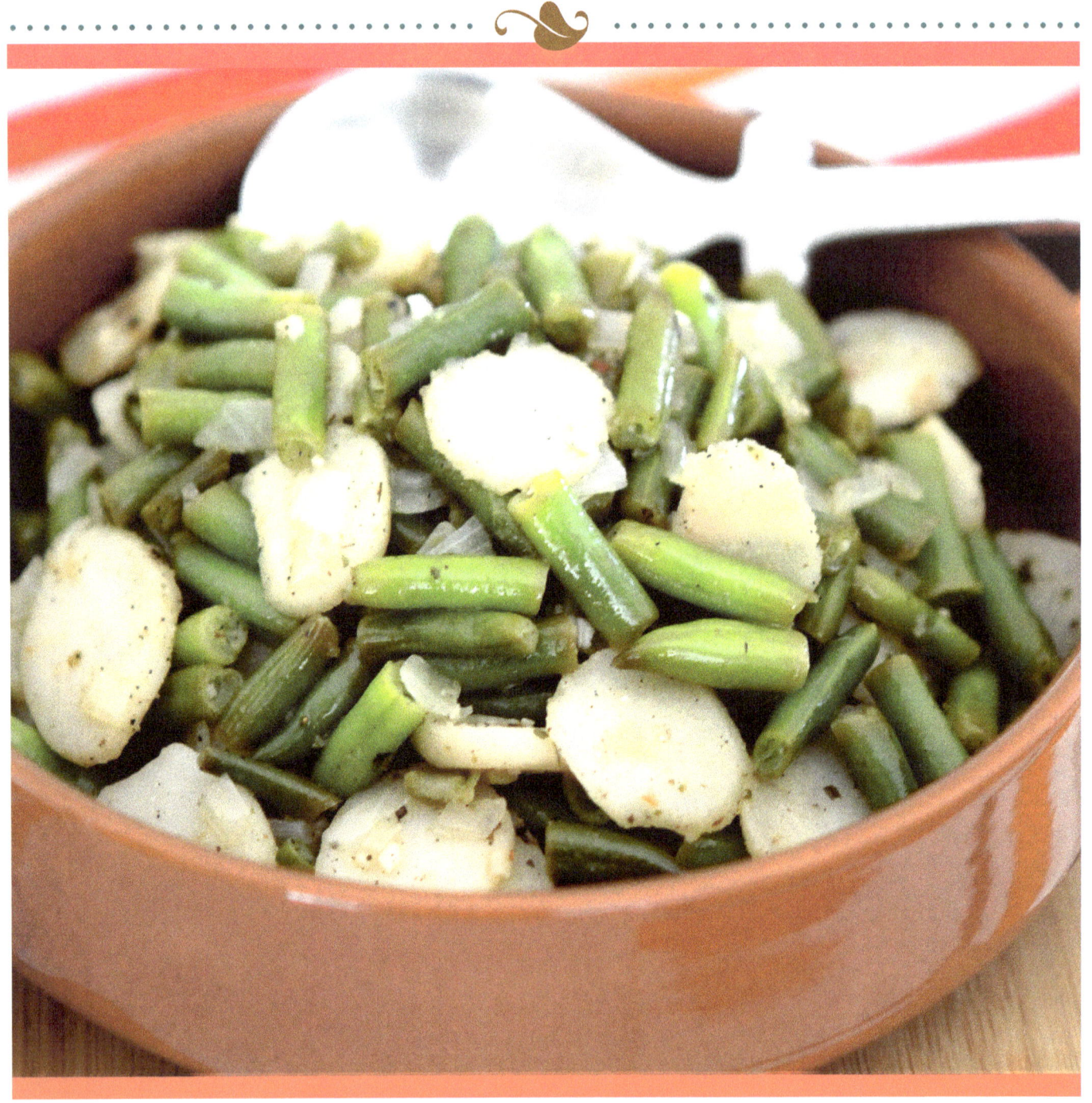

Green Beans and Water Chestnuts

Chinese water chestnuts are a vegetable (not a nut), grown in marshlands. They are unusual among vegetables because they remain crisp after being cooked or canned. This gives a great contrast when mixed with other cooked vegetables.

Prep time: 8 minutes   Cooking time: 10 minutes   Serves: 6

Ingredients:

- 500g/1.1lb green runner beans, cut into 3-4cm/1.5ins in length
- 2 Tbsp ghee, divided
- 1 onion, diced
- 1½ tsp garlic, minced
- 1 tsp ginger, minced
- 1x227g/8oz can sliced water chestnuts, (BPA free can)
- Juice of 1 lemon
- 1 tsp dried Italian herbs
- ½ tsp coarse sea salt, or to taste
- ¼ tsp ground pepper

Method:

Wash, trim and cut beans.

Add the beans to a saucepan of boiling water. Reduce heat and lightly boil for approximately 3-4 minutes, beans will still be firm. Drain, set aside.

Heat a large frying pan over medium heat, melt 1 tablespoon of ghee.

Add onion, garlic and ginger. Cook for 3-4 minutes or until onion is transparent.

Add water chestnuts, lemon juice and Italian herbs. Stir gently to prevent water chestnuts from breaking.

Add green beans, salt, pepper and remaining tablespoon of ghee. Mix all ingredients gently, heating through for approximately 3-4 minutes.

Cauliflower and Broccoli Bake

This family recipe underwent a big change, out went the can of "cream of chicken soup" and in came my new favourite white sauce recipes made from nuts or cauliflower.

Prep time: 15 minutes Cooking time: 30 minutes Serves: 6

Ingredients:

- ½ large head of cauliflower
- 1 large broccoli
- 2 cups White Nut sauce, page 211 or Cauliflower sauce, page 212
- Optional: ⅓ cup matured cheese, if you tolerate dairy

Method:

Make White Nut sauce or Cauliflower sauce and set aside.

Preheat oven to 170c/340f, grease a 30x20cm(12x8in) baking dish.

Cut cauliflower and broccoli into small florets.

Use a large steamer. Add cauliflower to the top of steamer and bring water to the boil. Steam for 4 minutes.

Add broccoli on top of the cauliflower and steam both for a further 4 minutes.

Carefully place vegetables into a greased baking dish, so they stay intact. Arrange with tops showing and colours evenly distributed.

Pour your choice of white sauce over the vegetables and top with grated cheese (if using).

Bake for 18-20 minutes or until the top is lightly browning and heated through.

SALADS & VEGETABLES

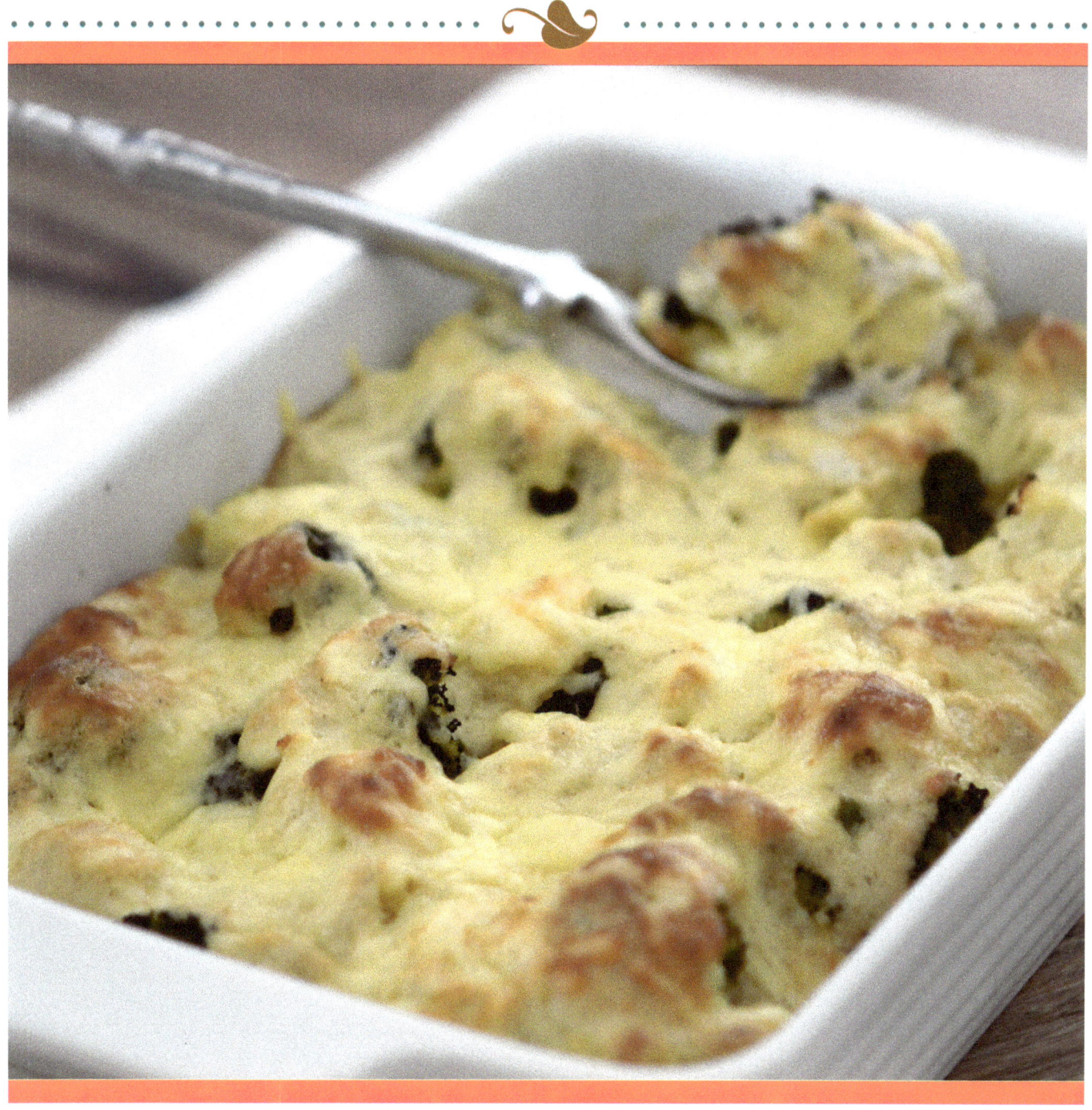

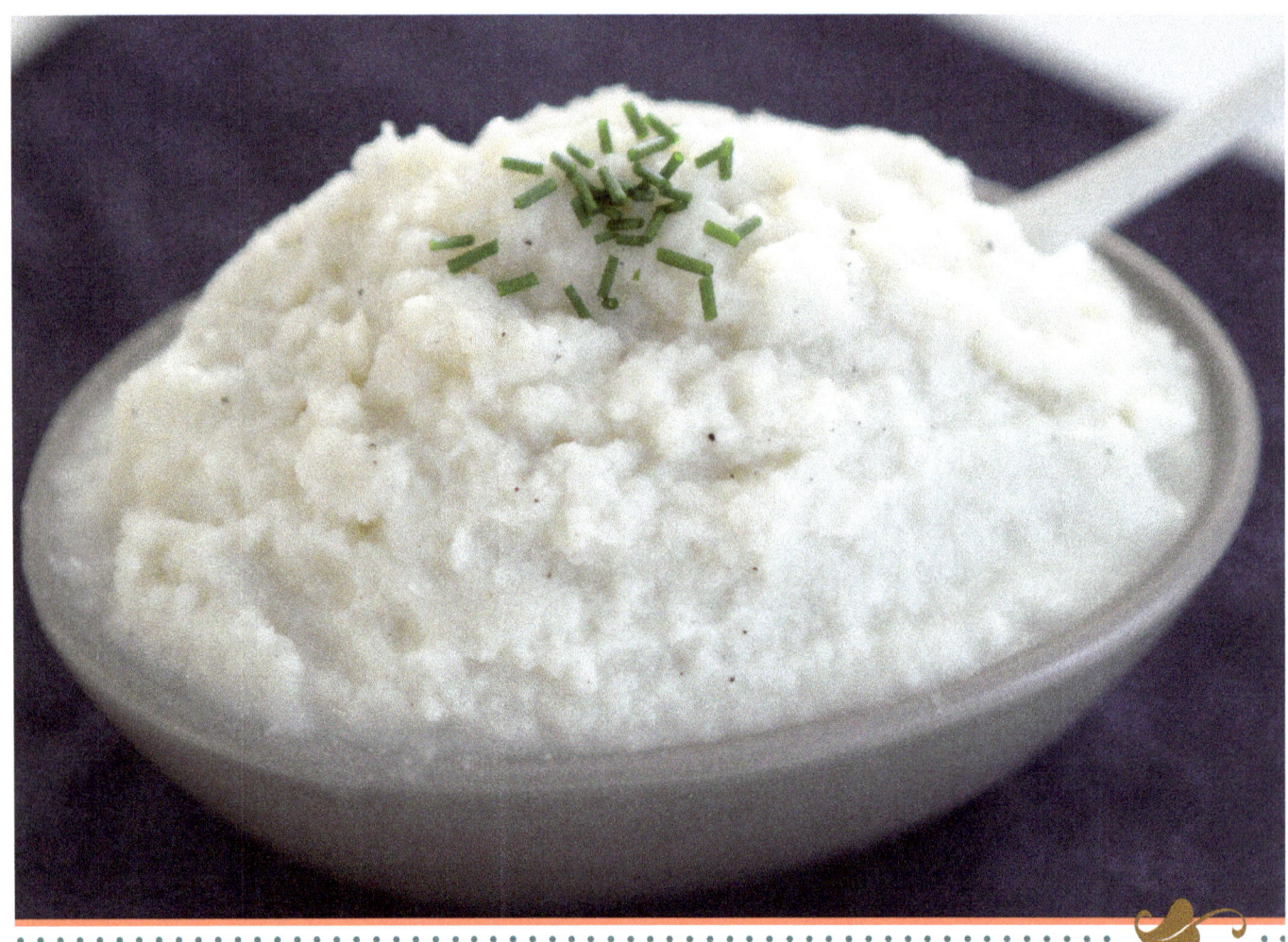

Cauliflower Mash

This is a great replacement for mashed potato. Cauliflower mash has heaps more flavour than starchy mashed potato. Pile your stew over it or have it alone with grilled meat. Extra delicious with gravy poured over it.

Prep time: 10 minutes Cooking time: 15 minutes Serves: 4

Ingredients:

- 1 large head cauliflower, cut into florets
- Sea salt and pepper, to taste
- 1½ Tbsp ghee
- 2-4 Tbsp coconut milk, depends if using blender or food processor

Method:

Use a steamer and bring water to the boil. Add cauliflower to the top of steamer. Steam for 12-15 minutes.

When cauliflower is cooked, transfer to a blender or food processor.

Add ghee, salt and pepper and blend. Add coconut milk or milk of choice, a little at a time, so you don't get a runny cauliflower mash.

If using a food processor, it won't be as soft, you will need to processor longer and add more coconut milk. Either way works fine.

SALADS & VEGETABLES | 117

Cauliflower Rice

Not quite rice, but a very good substitute and so much healthier. Serve with your Asian and Indian recipes.

Prep time: 10 minutes Cooking time: 10 minutes Serves: 4

Ingredients:

- 1 large head cauliflower, chopped into small evenly sized pieces
- 1½ Tbsp ghee
- ½ onion, diced
- 1 tsp garlic, minced
- Sea salt and pepper, to taste

Method:

Add cauliflower pieces to a food processor and pulse until the cauliflower looks like rice. Watch you don't puree it, if a few pieces on top haven't totally broken down, remove and finely hand chop.

Heat a large frying pan on medium heat. Add ½ tablespoon of ghee and cook onion and garlic for 3 minutes or until onion is transparent.

Add remaining tablespoon of ghee. Transfer cauliflower to the frying pan. Add salt and pepper to taste.

Using a spatula, flip cauliflower over several times as it cooks and dries out approximately for 5-6 minutes. Use in place of regular rice.

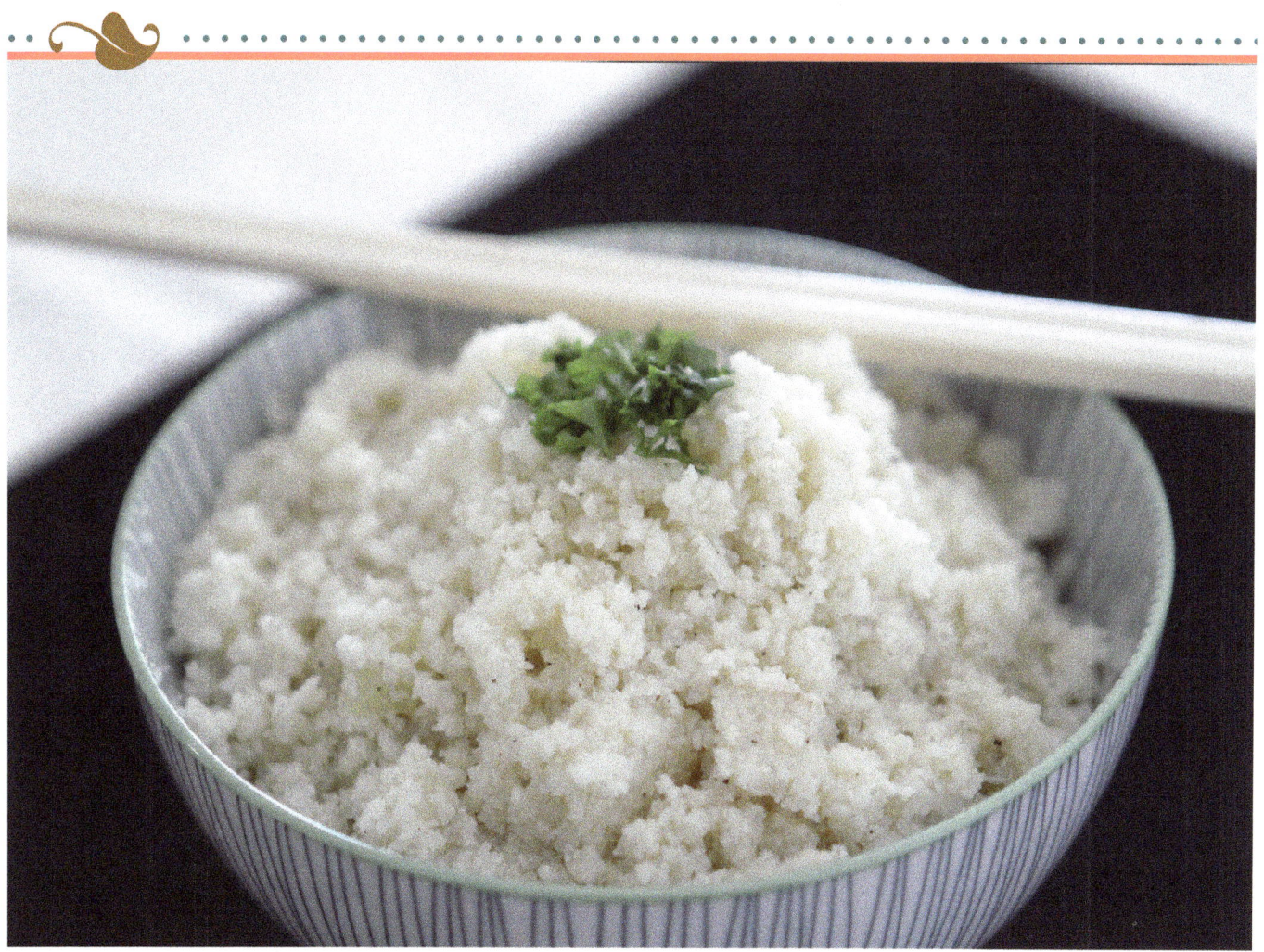

SNACKS & DIPS

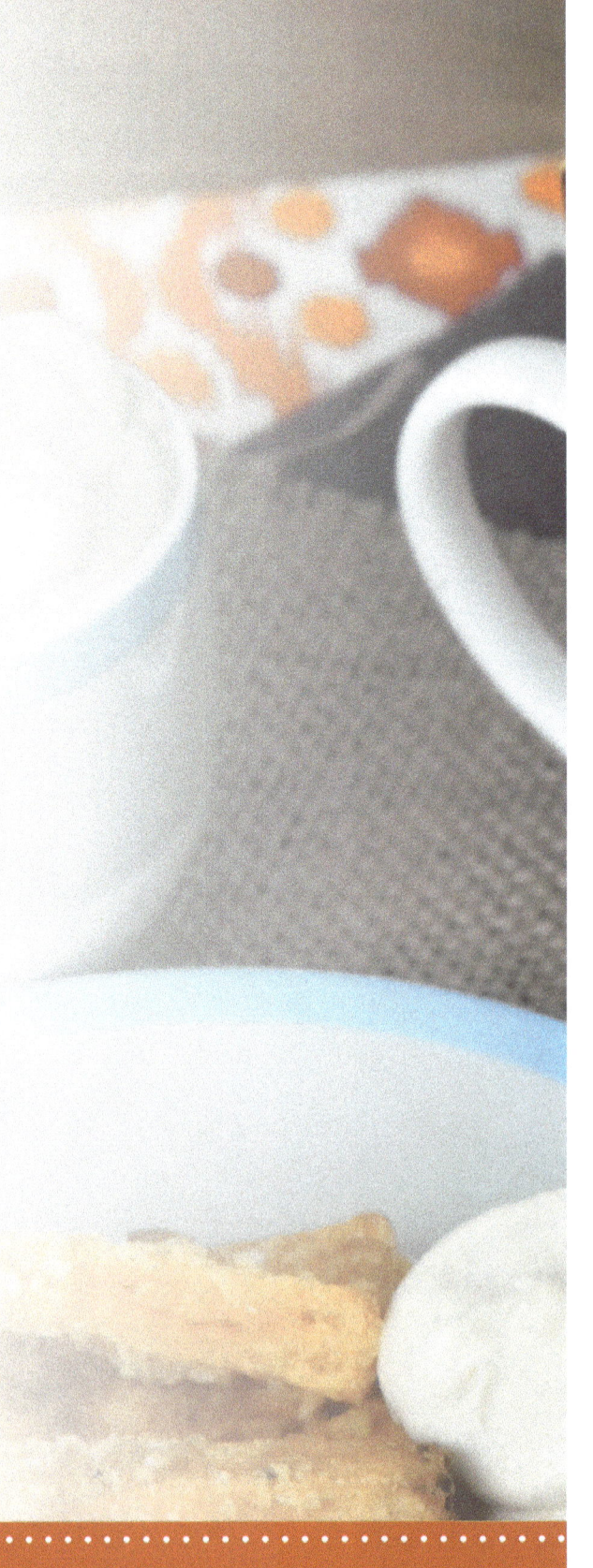

Nut and Seed Mix 121

Nut Bars 122

Seasoned Fries 122

Fruit and Nut Fingers 125

Goji Berry Energy Bites 126

Butter Balls 128

Sesame Snaps 129

Protein Balls in Coconut 130

Jaffa Bites 131

Pumpkin "Hummus" 133

Avocado Dip 133

Aioli Dipping Mayo 134

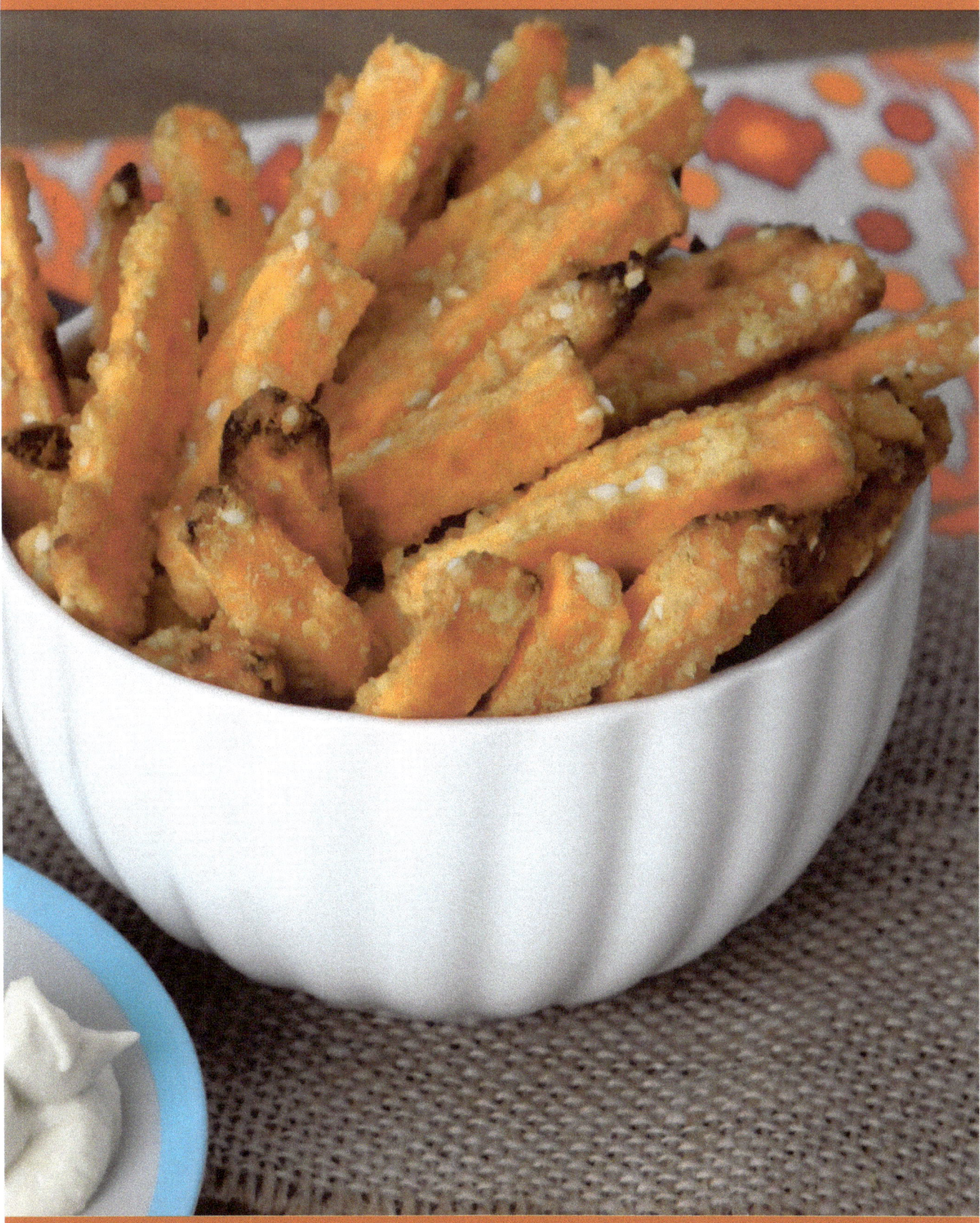

SNACKS & DIPS

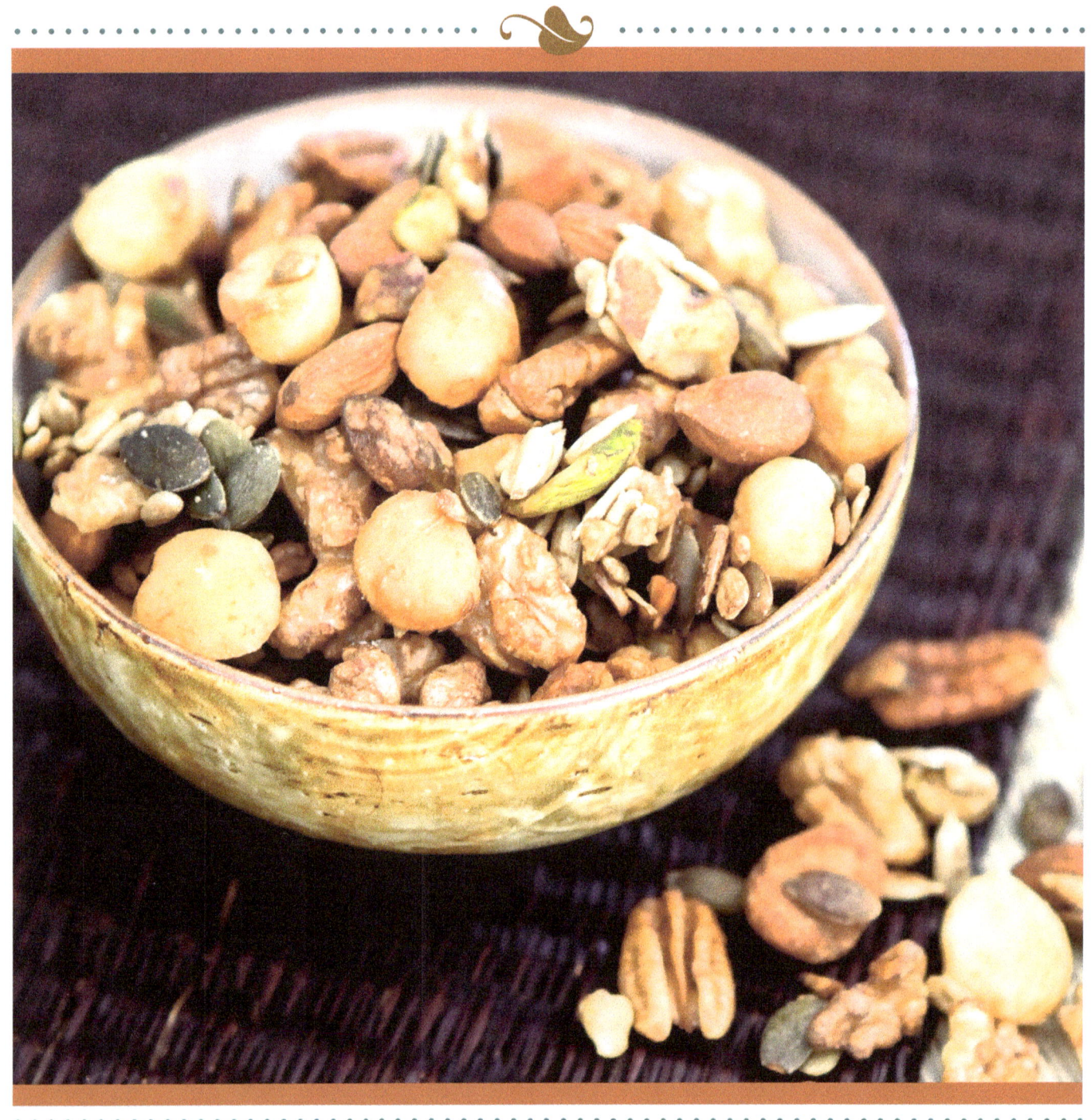

Nut and Seed Mix

I make this mix every week for my husband to snack on. There are no nasty additives like the bags of potato chips he use to eat. (I use Coconut Aminos but if you prefer to use organic tamari, omit the salt.)

Prep time: 5 minutes   Cooking time: 20 minutes   Makes: 5½ cups

Ingredients:

- 1 cup almond
- 1 cup pecans
- 1 cup walnuts
- 1 cup macadamia nuts, halved
- ½ cup pistachios
- ½ cup pumpkin seeds
- ½ cup sunflower seeds
- ¼ cup coconut aminos
- ½-¾ tsp fine sea salt or to taste (I use ¾ tsp we like them salty)

Method:

To a large bowl add all the nuts and seeds. Sprinkle with sea salt and pour over coconut aminos.

Mix well to coat. Let nuts sit for 10 minutes to soak up some of the coconut aminos, mix frequently.

While nuts are sitting, preheat oven to 150c/300f. Line 2 large oven trays with baking paper.

When oven has reached its temperature, spread mixture evenly over the trays.

Bake for approximately 20 minutes or until lightly brown and dry. If outer nuts start to brown too fast, remove the trays and mix those nuts and seeds into the centre. Try to get a nice even colour but don't let them burn.

While the nuts cool on the trays, they will continue to crisp a little more. Store in an airtight container. (You can exchange any of my nuts with your favourites).

SNACKS & DIPS

Nut Bars

A light textured raw snack full of protein that's suitable to eat anytime of the day. Storing them in the fridge will keep them nice and firm.

Prep time: 10 minutes   Cooking time: none   Makes: 15

Ingredients:

- 1 cup almonds
- 1 cup walnuts
- 10 medjol dates, pitted
- ¾ cup desiccated coconut
- 2 Tbsp coconut oil, soft
- 1 tsp cinnamon
- ⅓ tsp nutmeg
- ¼ tsp fine sea salt

Method:

Add the almonds and walnuts to a food processor and blend until you have a grainy texture.

Add dates, coconut, softened coconut oil, cinnamon, nutmeg and salt. Process until the ingredients are well combined. The mixture should be slightly sticky. The texture will look like breadcrumbs.

Place the mixture into a 22cm(8.5in) square lined baking tin. Use a spatula or the back of a spoon to pack mixture firmly into the baking tin.

Place in the fridge to set for 2 hour or freezer for a faster setting time.

Slice into squares or bars. Store in an airtight container in the fridge.

Seasoned Fries

A delicious snack for watching a good movie. Serve fries with Aioli Dipping Mayo on page 134. There are lots of reasons to love sweet potato. It's high in vitamins B6 and C, contains vitamin D, iron and magnesium. A good source of potassium and rich in carotenoids.

Prep time: 15 minutes   Cooking time: 30 minutes   Serves: 2

Ingredients:

- 550g/1.2lbs sweet potato, cut into thin sticks
- ¼ cup macadamia nuts
- 2 tsp sesame seeds, divided
- ¾ tsp fine sea salt
- ¼ tsp ground cumin
- ¼ tsp ground coriander
- ⅛ tsp dried oregano
- 1 Tbsp arrowroot flour
- 2 Tbsp coconut oil, melted

Method:

Preheat oven to 190c/375f and line 2 large oven trays with baking paper. Add macadamia nuts to a blender for a couple of seconds to crush. Add 1 teaspoon of sesame seeds and spices, blend for a few seconds to combine.

Transfer to a large bowl and add the arrowroot flour and remaining teaspoon of sesame seeds. Add melted coconut oil and mix well. Add cut potato sticks and toss to coat using your hands, mix for 1 minute, the heat from your hands will help the coating to stick.

Line up in single layers on prepared oven trays, leaving space between fries. Bake for 30-35 minutes. Turning over after 15 minutes to brown both sides.

Enjoy straight from the oven while crisp.

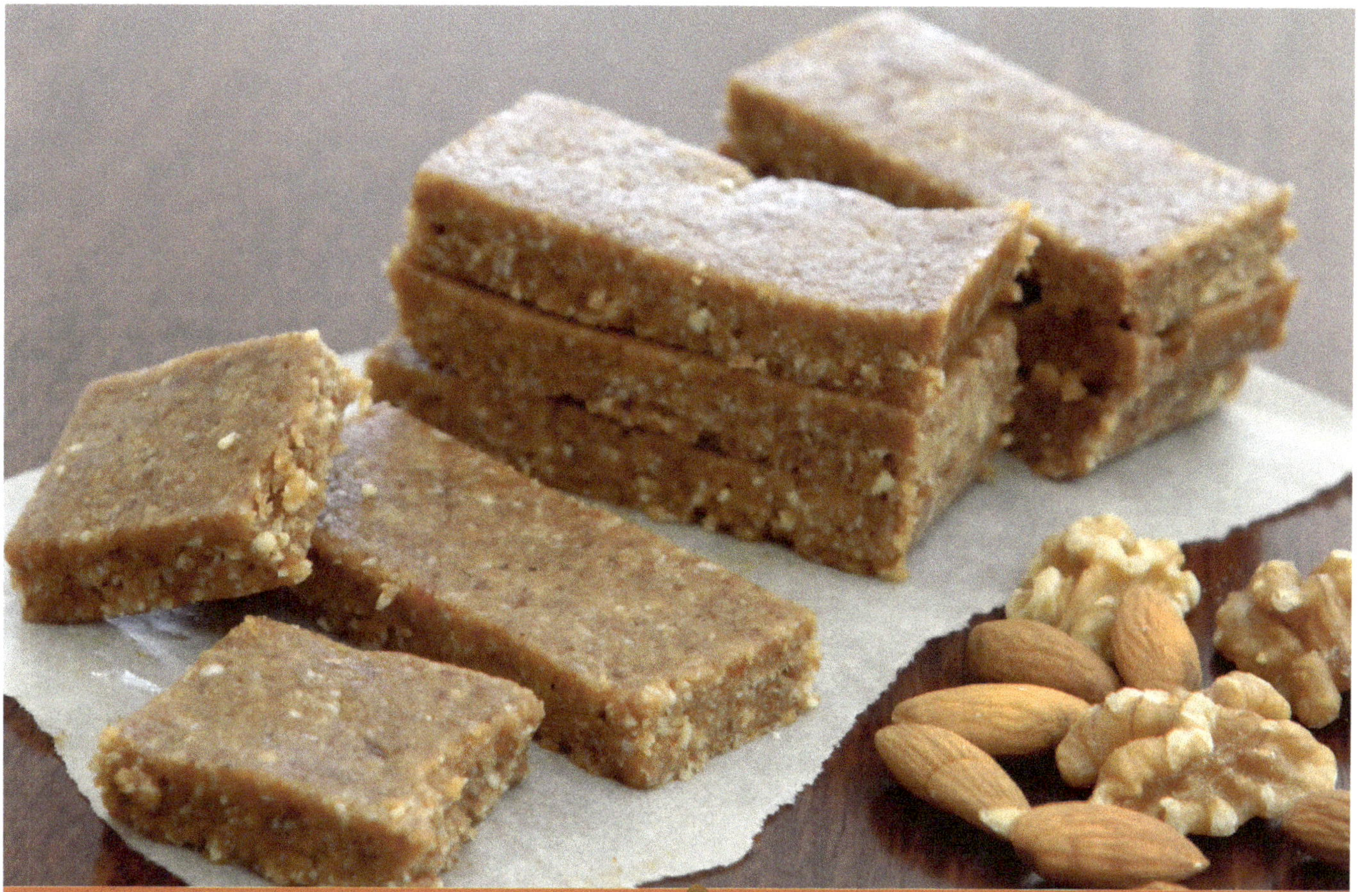

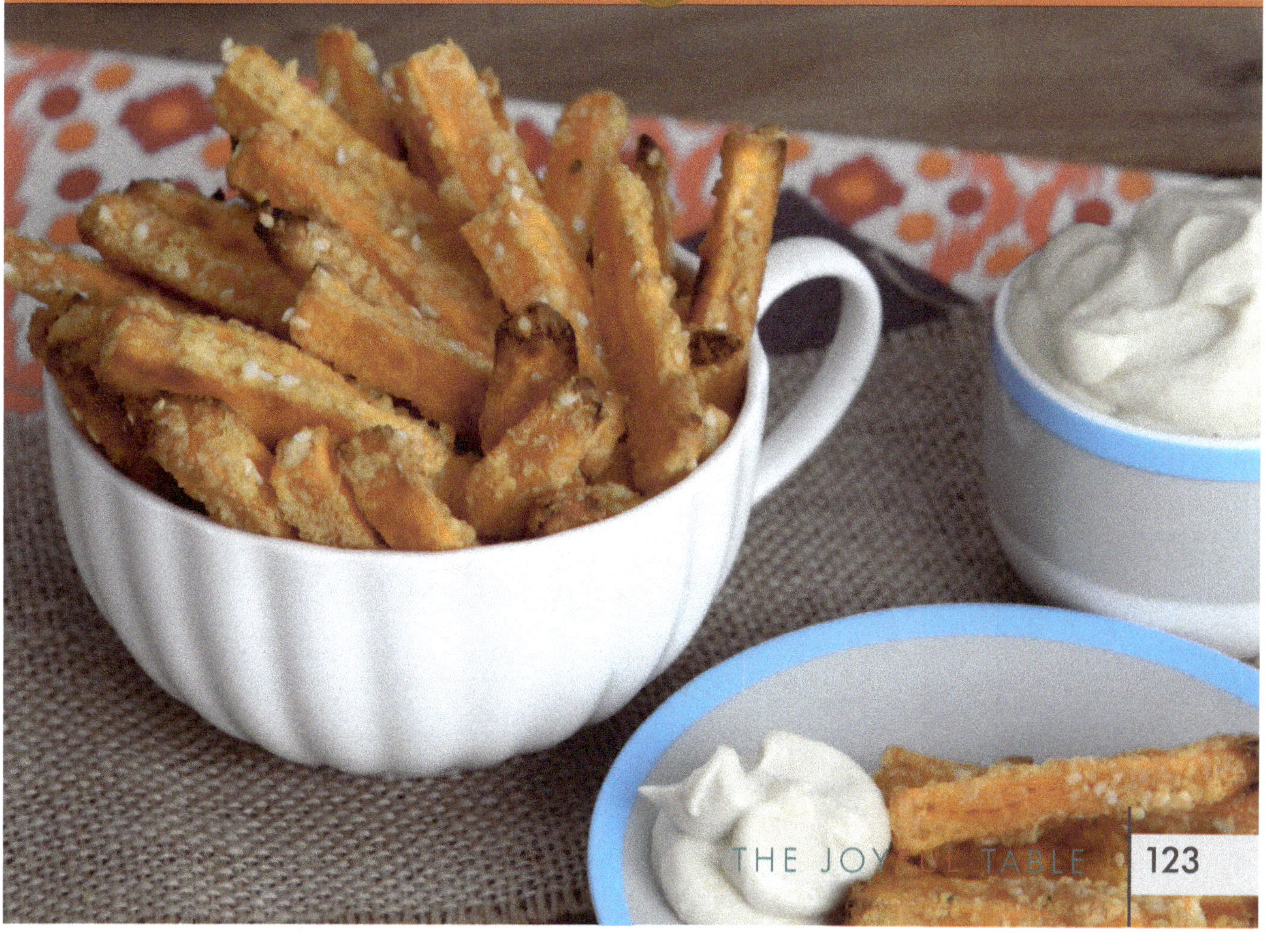

THE JOYFUL TABLE

124 | SNACKS & DIPS

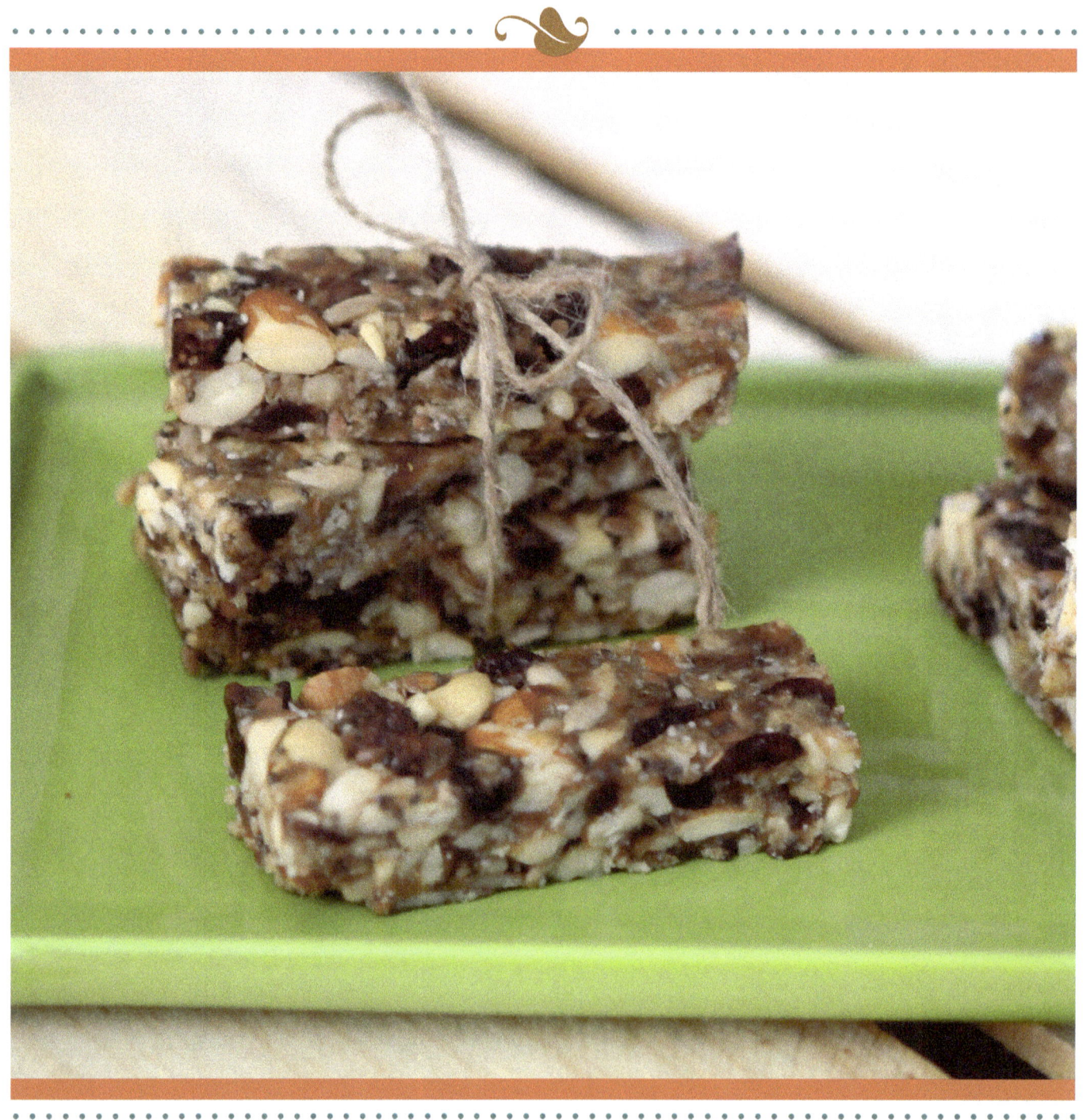

Fruit and Nut Fingers

This is a great paleo snack filled with a variety of natural healthy fruit, nuts and seeds. Eat in moderation as there are concentrated sugars in dried fruit. Use organic dried fruits to prevent packing your healthy snack with sulphur (preservatives) and additives. I have snuck some chia and linseed in for omega 3.

Prep time: 15 minutes   Cooking time: 4 minutes   Makes: 18

Ingredients:

- 8 medjool dates, pitted
- ½ cup organic cranberries
- ½ cup organic sultanas
- 2 Tbsp chia seeds
- ½ cup almonds
- ½ cup walnuts
- ½ cup cashews
- ¼ cup desiccated coconut
- ¼ cup sunflower seeds
- 3 Tbsp linseed
- ⅓ tsp fine sea salt
- ¼ cup almond butter
- 3 Tbsp coconut oil
- 2 Tbsp honey
- 1 tsp vanilla extract

Method:

Line a 27x17cm (10.5x6.5in) slice tin with baking paper, leave an overhang for easy removal. To a food processor add, dates, cranberries, sultanas and chia seeds. Process for 15 seconds, to break up fruit.

Add nuts, coconut, seeds and salt. Process for 18-20 seconds or until nuts and fruit are roughly chopped. Transfer to a large bowl and set aside.

To a small saucepan add, almond butter, coconut oil, honey and vanilla. Bring to a slow boil, reduce heat and allow to gently simmer while continuously stirring for 2 minutes. Mixture will look like it's foaming while gently simmering. Pour immediately over ingredients in bowl. Mix well to thoroughly combine.

Scoop mixture into prepared slice tin. Spread out evenly over the base. Use the back of a metal spoon to push mixture very firmly down, dampen spoon with water to prevent sticking.

The mixture needs to be well compacted, just to make sure, use a piece of baking paper to fit the size of your slice tin. Press down onto the paper with your hands and smooth over several times as you press down firmly.

Place in freezer to harden before cutting. Remove mixture from tin by lifting the overhang of baking paper. Place on a chopping board. Use a large sharp knife to cut 9 even finger strips, turn and cut once down the middle to make 18 fingers.

Store in the fridge and best served straight from the fridge.

Goji Berry Energy Bites

This is a really healthy snack but I love them even more with chocolate on their bottoms. Goji Berries are an excellent wholefood source of naturally occurring antioxidants, proteins, phyto-nutrients, amino acids and vitamins.

Prep time: 20 minutes Cooking time: none Makes: 24

Ingredients:

- 1 cup/10 medjool dates, pitted
- ½ cup macadamia nuts
- ½ cup whole almonds
- 2 Tbsp sesame seeds
- 2 Tbsp ground flaxseed
- ¾ cup organic goji berries
- ½ cup pumpkin seeds
- 2 Tbsp honey
- 1 tsp vanilla extract
- Optional: ½ cup dark chocolate chips, melted (soy free, paleo friendly) to coat base of bites

Method:

Line a 27x17cm (10.5x6.5in) slice tin with baking paper, leave an overhang for easy removal.

To a food processor add, dates, macadamia nuts, almonds, sesame seeds and flaxseed. Process for approximately 1 minute until combined.

Add the Goji berries, pumpkin seeds, honey and vanilla. Process for a further 10-20 seconds to combine but you still want to see some whole goji berries and pumpkin seeds.

Press mixture into a slice pan. Press down firmly and flatten the top with your hand or back of a spoon.

Place in fridge or freezer to firm up, then remove from pan by lifting the baking paper. Cut into squares on a chopping board pressing down firmly with a large sharp knife (try not to drag the knife through). If the mixture isn't cold enough it will break apart as you cut.

Melt chocolate chips over a double saucepan. Use a flat edged knife to spread chocolate over the base of the bites. Place upside down on a lined baking tray to set. When chocolate is set, place in a sealed container and store in the fridge. Serve straight from the fridge.

SNACKS & DIPS

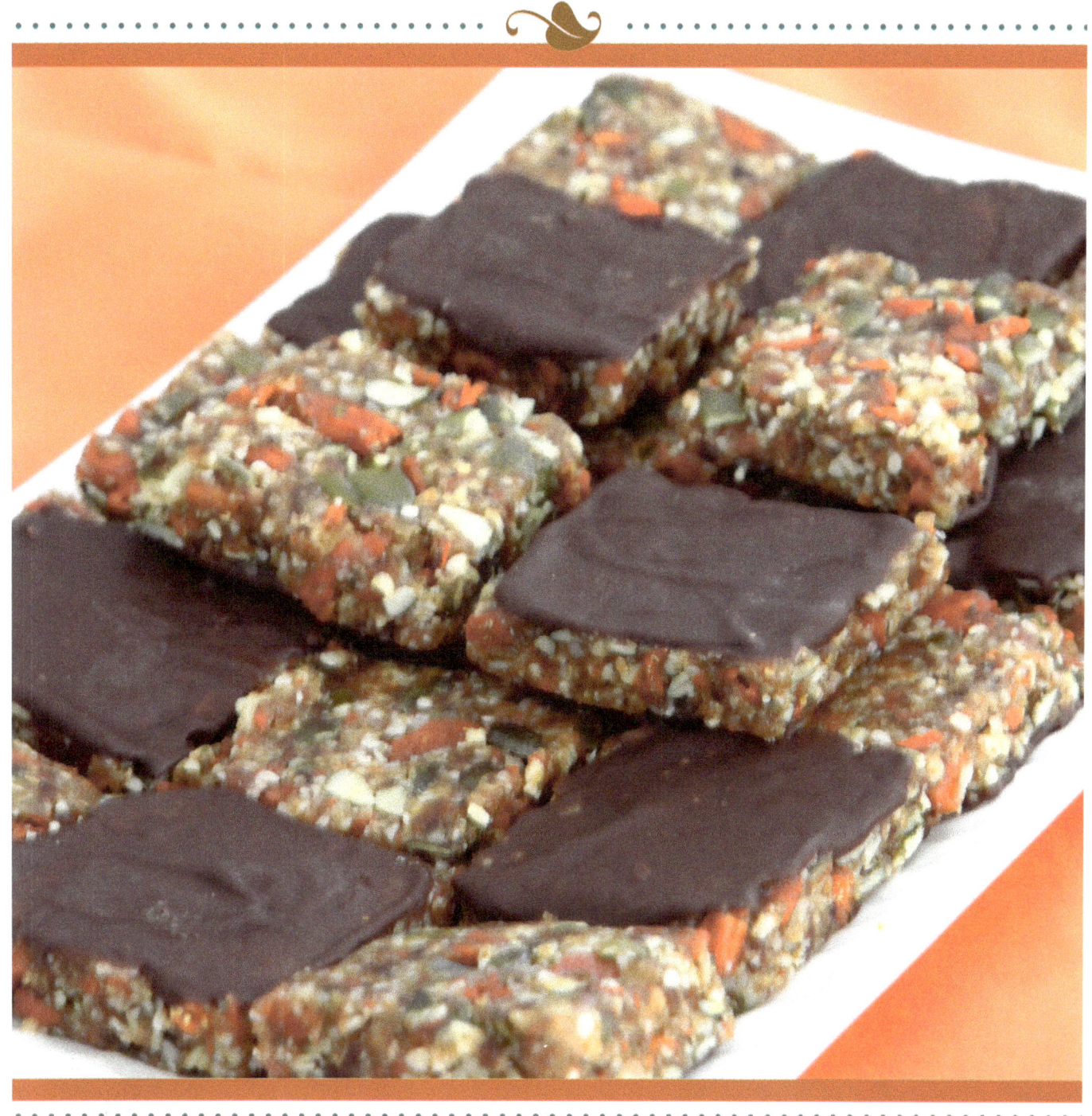

SNACKS & DIPS

Butter Balls

You may like to double this recipe, so moreish. I love these Butter Balls with a cuppa or just as a snack on the run.

Prep time: 15 minutes   Cooking time: none   Makes: 15 snack size balls

Ingredients:

- 8 Medjool dates, pitted
- ½ cup raw almonds
- ½ cup raw cashews
- ⅓ cup almond butter/spread
- 1-2 Tbsp honey
- 1 tsp ground cinnamon
- ½ tsp fine sea salt
- ¼ cup sesame seeds for coating

Method:

To a food processor add dates and blend for 10-15 seconds to break them up, scrape sides down.

Add almonds and cashews, blend for a further 20 seconds. Mixture should look like coarse breadcrumbs.

Add remaining ingredients, except for sesame seeds. Blend for approximately 15 seconds, mixture should still look like breadcrumbs. It's ready when you press mixture between your fingers and it comes together nicely. Remove blade and scoop up heaped tablespoons of mixture and roll into 15 balls.

Place sesame seeds on a plate. Scoop some into your palm and using both hands to roll each ball around to coat evenly. Continue for each Butter ball. Place in the fridge to firm up.

The balls will keep for up to 2 weeks in the fridge, if they last that long.

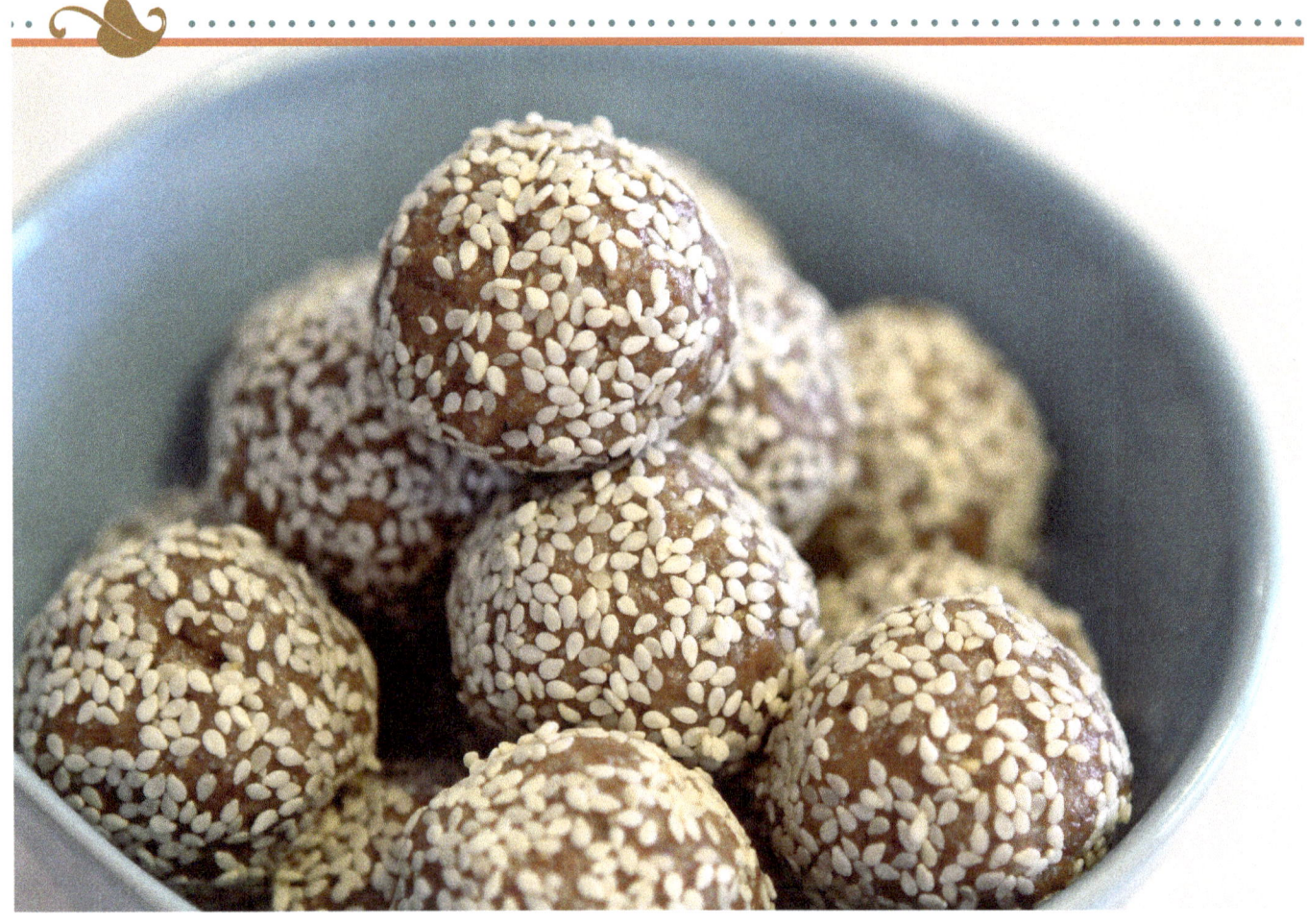

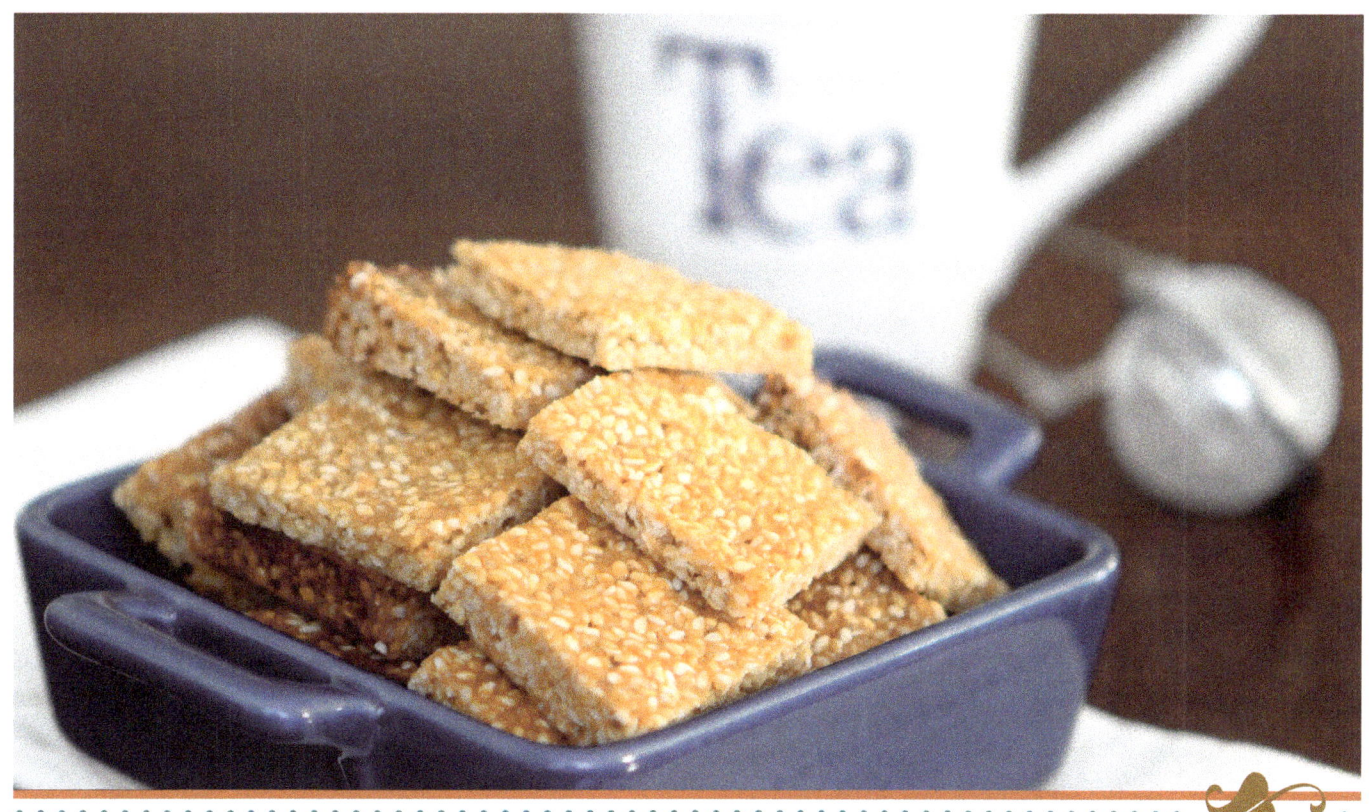

Sesame Snaps

A great lunchbox treat for kids and grown ups. Sesame seeds are a good source of copper, manganese, magnesium and calcium.

Prep time: 15 minutes Cooking time: 18 minutes Makes: 25 bites

Ingredients:

- 1 cup sesame seeds
- ¼ cup almond meal/flour
- ⅓ tsp fine sea salt
- ¼ cup honey
- 2 Tbsp coconut oil
- 1 Tbsp cashew or sunflower butter

Method:

Preheat oven to 160c/320f. Line a square 22cm(8.5in) baking tin with baking paper. Leave an overhang to make removing from the tin easier.

Add to a bowl, sesame seeds, almond meal and salt. Mix to combine. Heat honey and coconut oil slightly, just until oil melts. Mix cashew butter into the warm oil mixture. Stir until combined into a creamy mixture. Pour into the sesame mixture and stir until well combined.

Pour into prepared tin, spread out mixture with the back of a spoon. Once it's spread as well as you can with a spoon, place a piece of baking paper over the mixture. Use your hands to press and spread out without getting sticky.

Bake for 18 minutes or until golden brown. Turn during cooking for an even colour. Allow to cool and firm up completely before cutting.

Use the baking paper overhang to remove cooled sesame slab. Place on a chopping board. Use a large sharp knife to cut into square bite size pieces, approximately 3.5cm(1.5ins). Store in an airtight container at room temperature.

Protein Balls in Coconut

These Protein Balls are great before or after exercise. I would make them non-stop for number 3 son, who attends the gym regularly. Now he's married, I have happily handed over this job to his beautiful wife. They can be frozen or stored for up to 3 weeks in the fridge.

Prep time: 20 minutes   Cooking time: none   Makes: 20

Ingredients:

- 1½ cups raw cashews
- 1 Tbsp coconut sugar
- 1½ cups desiccated coconut
- 3 Tbsp cacao powder
- ¼ cup vanilla organic pea protein powder
- ½ tsp fine sea salt
- ¾ cup organic sultanas
- 1 Tbsp vanilla extract
- 2 Tbsp coconut oil, softened
- 1 Tbsp filtered water
- Extra coconut for coating

Method:

Add cashews to a food processor and blend until broken up. Add coconut sugar, coconut, cacao powder, pea protein powder and salt. Blend to mix. Add sultanas and blend well. Add vanilla, coconut oil and 1 tablespoon water. Blend well.

Press mixture between your fingers to check it comes together but not sticky. If more moisture is needed, add extra water 1 teaspoon at a time.

Take a rounded tablespoon of mixture and mold together in your palm, then roll into a ball.

Pour extra coconut for coating onto a plate. Coat each ball evenly with coconut (I place coconut in the palm of one hand and add protein ball, then use both hands to coat and press into the ball). Repeat for each ball. I make them approximately the size of a small golf ball. Or you can coat with chopped nuts of your choice.

Store in an airtight container in the fridge for up to 3 weeks or freeze.

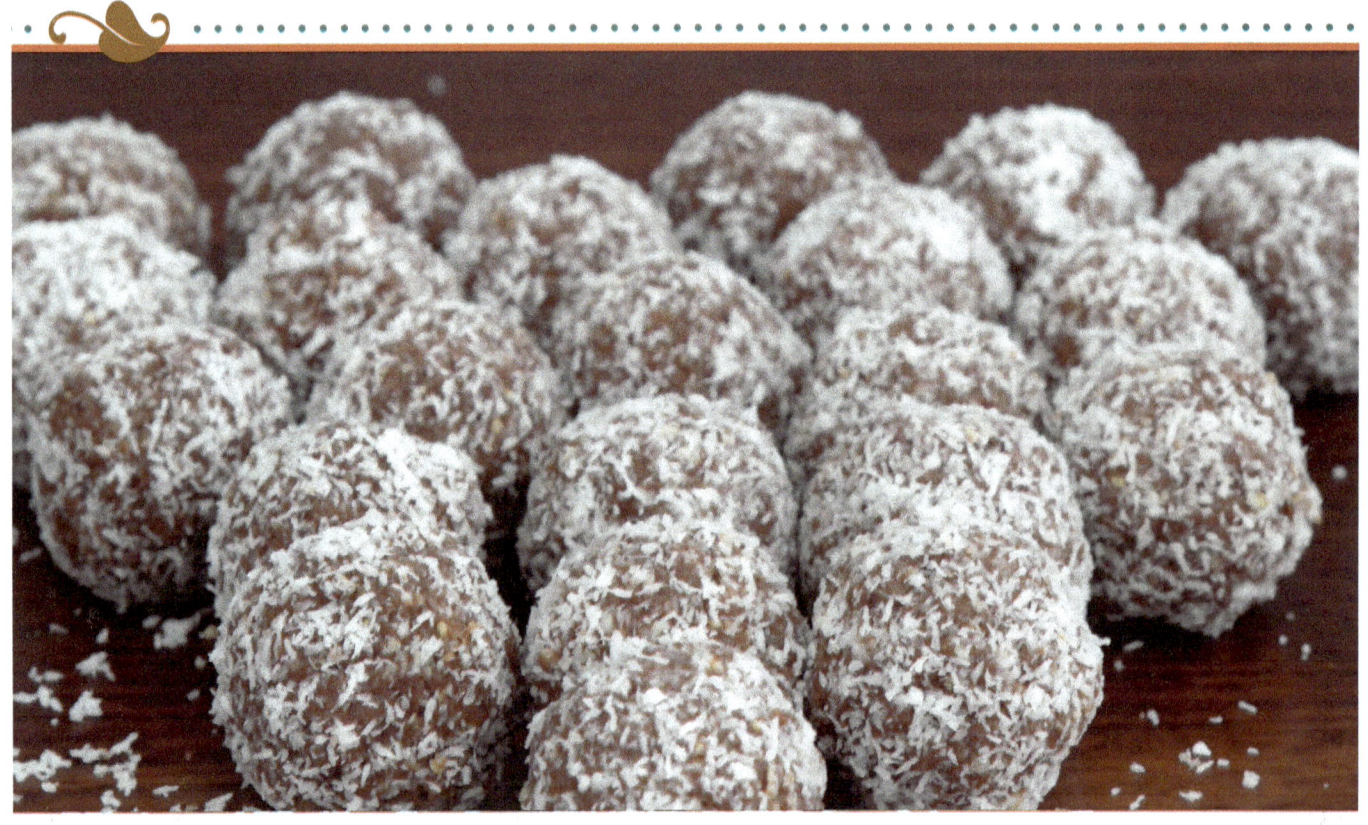

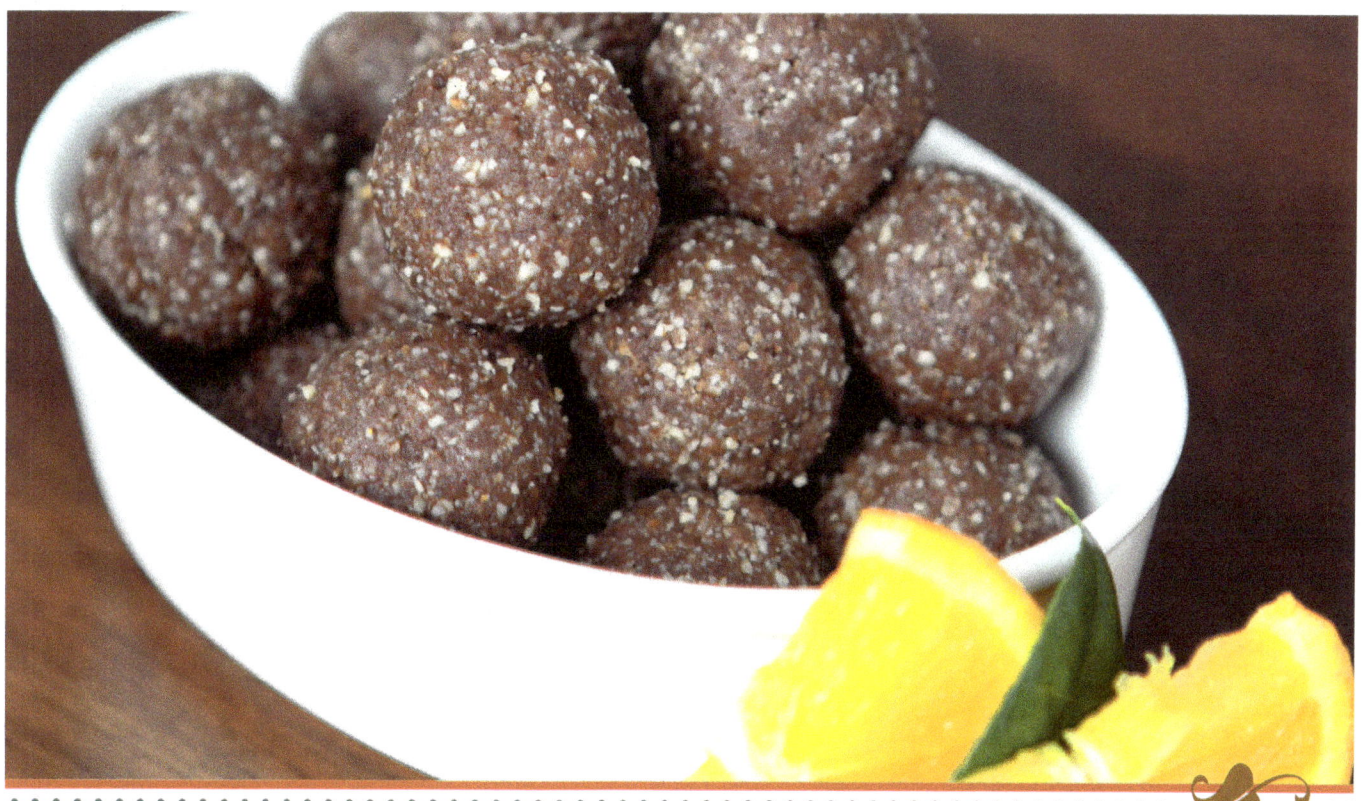

Jaffa Bites

This is a fun recipe, these bites can be made into any flavoured snack you would like. This recipe is flavoured with orange and chocolate. At Christmas time I add plum pudding spices and top with organic white chocolate and place a goji berry on top to make Christmas Pudding Bites. Add mint extract and have a chocolate mint flavour. Below is a Choc Brownie Bite version.

Prep time: 20 minutes Cooking time: none Makes: 18

Ingredients:

- 1½ cups raw almonds
- 10/1 cup medjool dates, pitted
- ½ cup desiccated coconut
- 3-4 Tbsp cacao powder
- 1½ tsp organic orange extract
- 1-3 tsp filtered water

Method:

To a food processor add, all the ingredients except for the water. Process until mixture resembles breadcrumbs. Add water 1 teaspoonful at a time while the food processor is running. Stop between additions to check mixture, it will depend on the moisture in the dates.

Press mixture between your fingers, if it sticks together you have the right consistency.

Roll mixture into small balls, a little smaller than a golf ball. Store in an airtight container in the fridge.

CHOC BROWNIE BITES

Use all the above ingredients for Jaffa Bites except for the orange extract, substitute with 2 teaspoons of vanilla extract. You may only need 1 teaspoon of water due to the extra liquid from the vanilla.

Use the same method and storage instructions for Jaffa Bites.

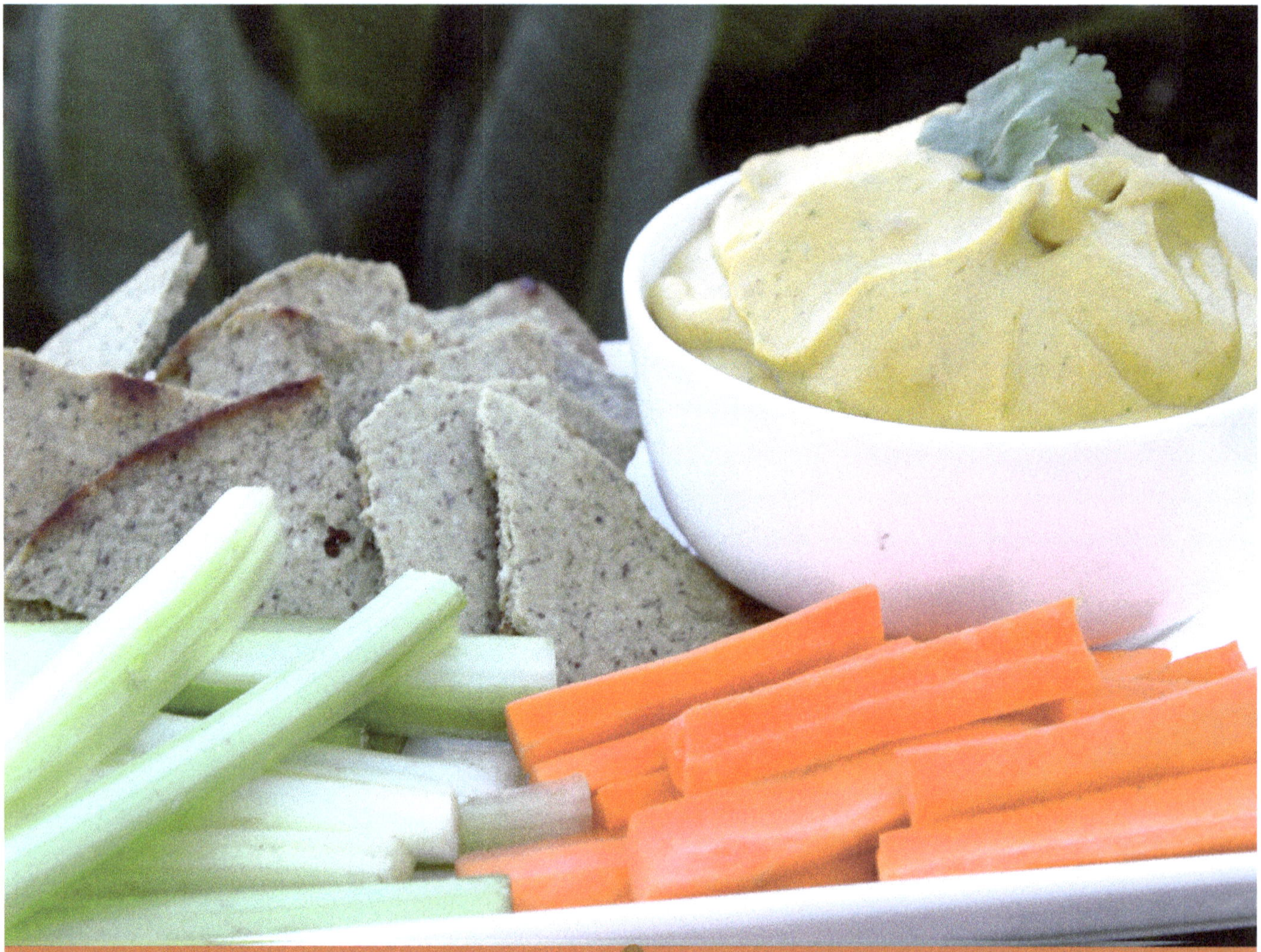

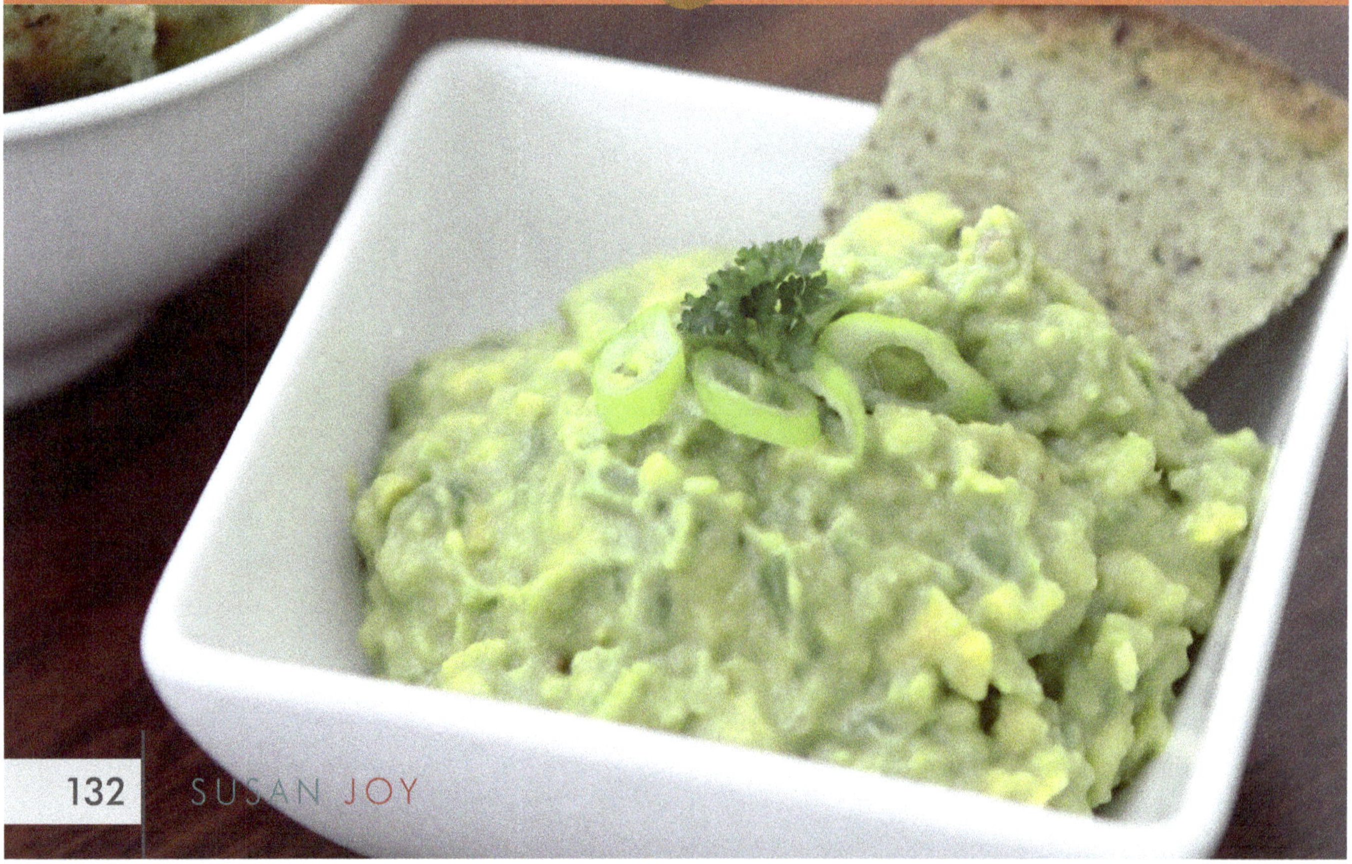

132 SUSAN JOY

Pumpkin "Hummus"

I enjoy the taste better than real chickpea hummus. Serve with vegetable sticks, Spinach Flat bread chips, page 78 or Seed crackers, page 82.

Prep time: 10 minutes plus soaking time Cooking time: 20 minutes Makes: 2 cups

Ingredients:

- 1½ cups cashews
- Water for soaking nuts, include a pinch of sea salt
- 250g peeled pumpkin
- 3 Tbsp tahini
- 1½ Tbsp fresh squeezed lemon juice
- 1 tsp ground cumin
- 1 tsp garlic, minced
- 3 Tbsp fresh coriander leaves
- ¼ tsp sea salt, adjust to taste

Method:

Soak cashews in a bowl with enough water to cover them by an extra 5cm(2ins) and sea salt for up to 1 hour. Then drain off soaking water using a metal sieve and rinse well with fresh water.

While the cashews are soaking, cut the pumpkin into small pieces and steam until just soft, don't overcook.

To a blender add the drained cashews. Use the tamper stick to push nuts onto the blade to help break them up. Add your steamed pumpkin, and the remainder of your ingredients to the blender. Blend until well combined. Garnish with a coriander leaf before serving.

Avocado Dip

This is my go to dip when I am in a hurry. I also use it to dollop on Mexican meals.

Prep time: 10 minutes plus soaking time Cooking time: 20 minutes Makes: 2 cups

Ingredients:

- 2 large ripe avocados
- ¾ tsp garlic, minced
- 2 Tbsp Cashew sour cream page 302
- 1-2 Tbsp organic mild chili sauce or salsa
- Juice of ½ lemon
- Fine sea salt to taste

Method:

In a medium bowl, mash avocados with a fork. Stir in remaining ingredients and mix well. (If you tolerate dairy you can replace Cashew sour cream with regular sour cream.)

Serve with Spinach flat bread page 78, broken into corn chip size pieces or with raw vegetable sticks.

Aioli Dipping Mayo

This is a great dip to use with raw vegetables or to dip your sweet potato fries into. Use in place of Tar tare sauce with your fish. It's an excellent base to add your own flavours to create delicious dips and sauces.

Prep time: 8 minutes plus soaking time Cooking time: none Makes: 1 cup

Ingredients:

- 1 cup raw cashews, soaked in filtered water with a pinch of salt for 30-60 minutes
- Juice of 1 lemon
- 1 Tbsp Apple Cider vinegar
- 1 tsp garlic, minced
- 1 tsp Nutritional Yeast Flakes
- ½ tsp Dijon mustard
- ½ tsp fine sea salt
- ¼ cup filtered water

Method:

Drain and rinse soaked cashews in fresh filtered water. Add to a high-speed blender along with the remaining ingredients.

Blend on high until smooth and creamy, with no grainy bits. Stop and scrape down sides once while blending.

Store covered in the fridge. Remove from fridge and allow to come to room temperature before serving to bring out the flavours.

SNACKS & DIPS | 135

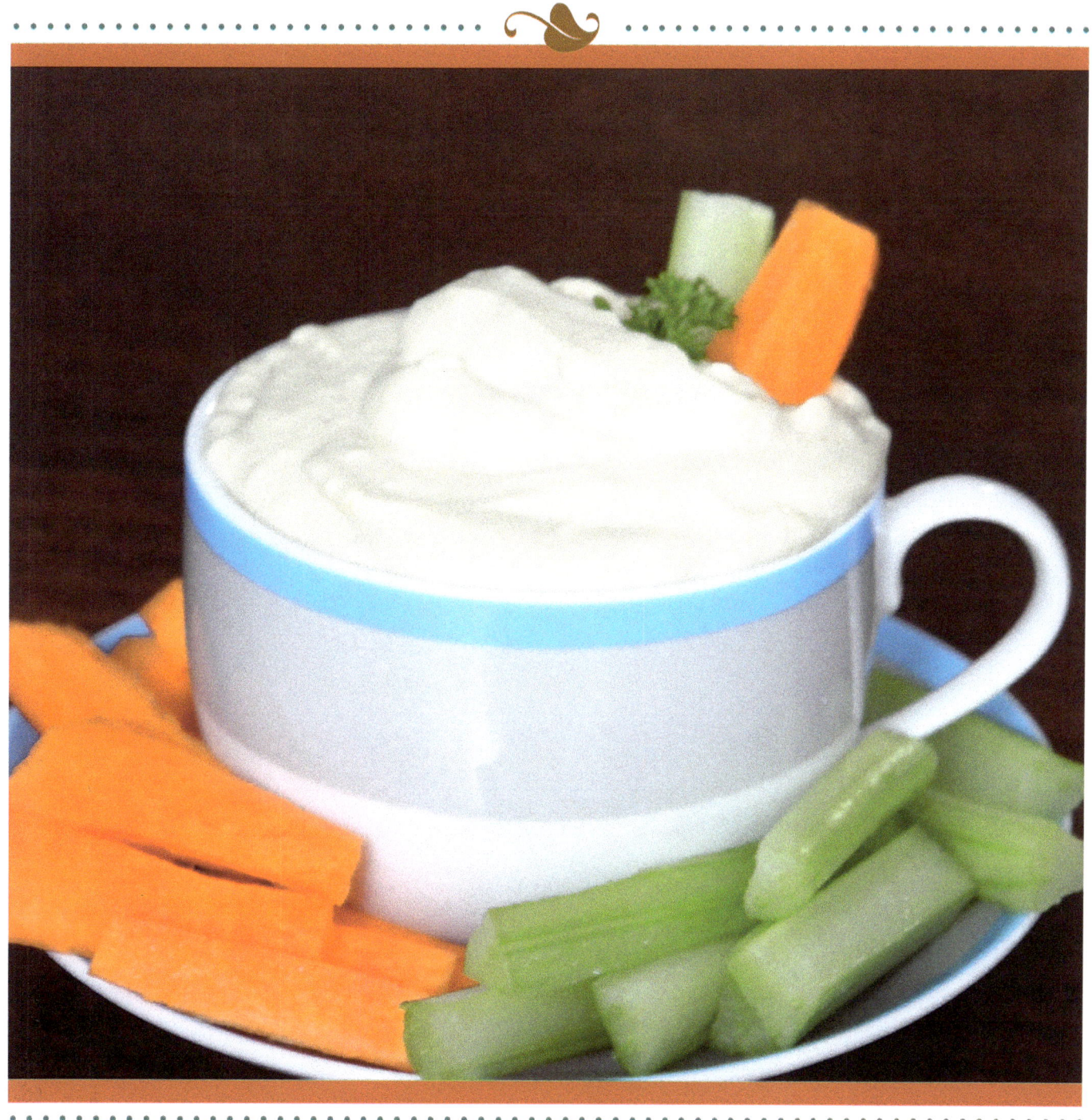

LUNCH & LIGHT MEALS

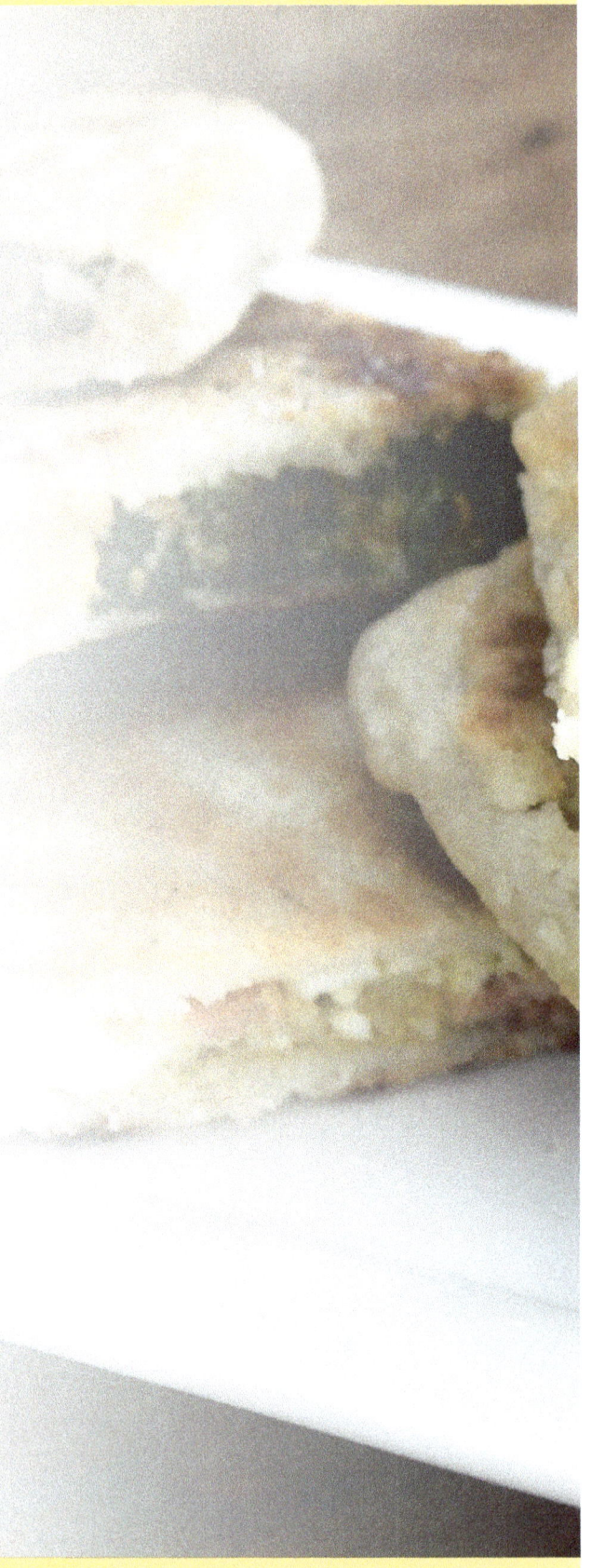

Ham and Asparagus Quiche 138

Chicken and Broccoli Frittata 140

Nachos 142

Mango and Avocado Salad 144

Chicken and Avocado Caesar Salad 146

Curry Pasties 148

Savoury Pancakes 150

Tasty Toasts 152

Pumpkin, Spinach and Feta Toasts 153

Mexican Beef Toasts 153

Egg and Bacon Toasts 153

Paleo Satay Chicken 154

Mini Meat Loaves 156

Hamburger Patties 158

Curried Nut Burgers 160

Creamy Zucchini Noodles 162

Chinese Cauliflower Fried Rice 164

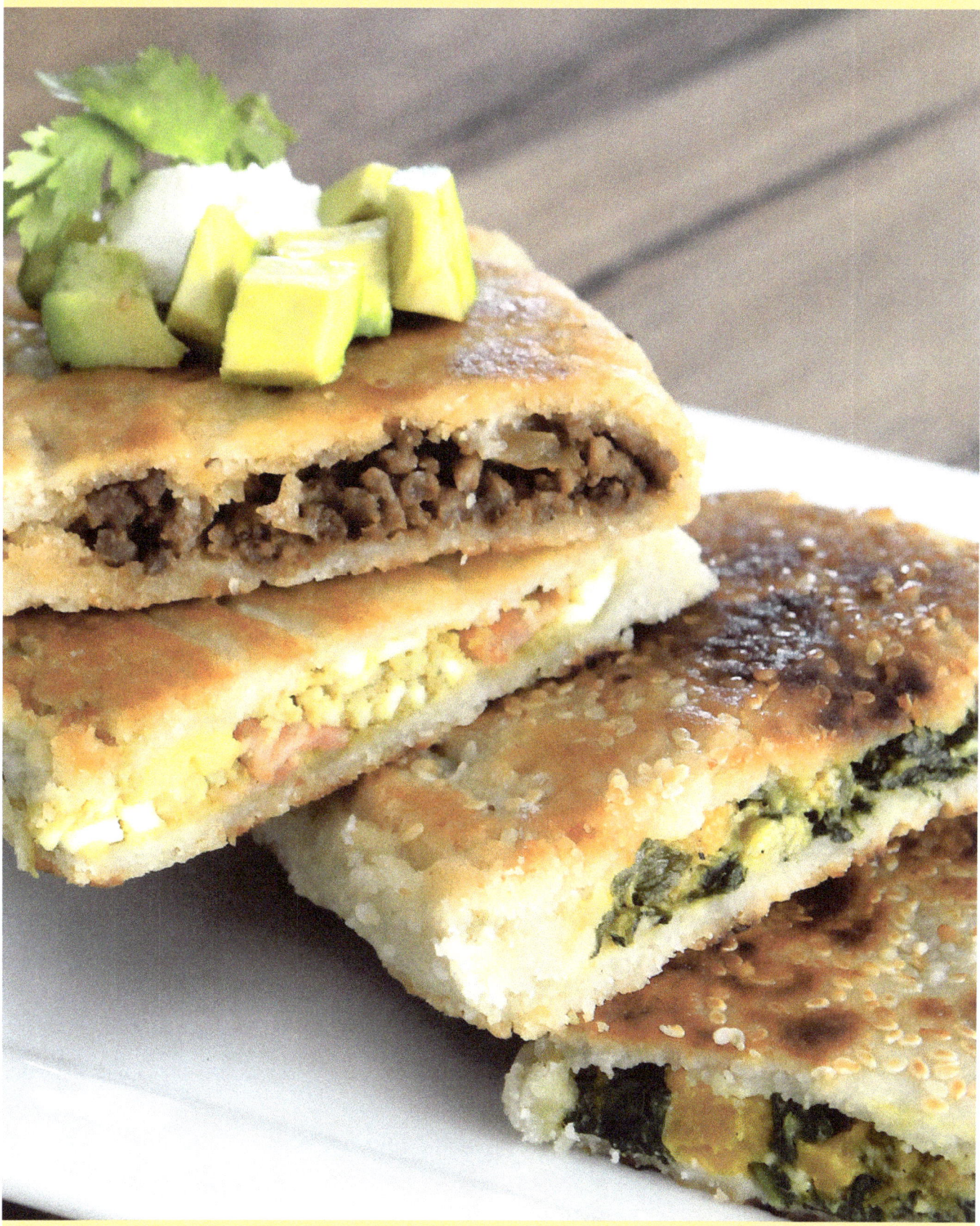

Ham and Asparagus Quiche

This lunch could also be eaten for breakfast or dinner. For a lighter meal or if you are short on time, make this quiche with no crust. Always use free range or organic eggs for optimum nutrition. Eggs provide protein for the body's cells and tissues and for a strong immune system.

Prep time: 15 minutes Cooking time: 35 minutes Serves: 4

Ingredients:

- 1 pre-cooked savoury pie crust page 86 or bake without a crust
- 1 Tbsp ghee
- 1 small onion, finely diced
- 1 bunch fresh asparagus, cut into 4-5cm(2in) pieces
- 1 tsp garlic, minced
- 8 large eggs
- ⅔ cup coconut milk or milk of choice
- ½ cup diced ham, (nitrate free)
- 3 Tbsp Nutritional Yeast Flakes or 1 cup grated mature cheese, if tolerated
- ½ tsp nutmeg
- ¼ tsp fine sea salt
- ¼ tsp white pepper

Method:

Preheat oven to 170c/340f. Have your savoury piecrust pre-baked and cooled or grease a quiche or pie dish with ghee if baking a no crust quiche.

Heat a large frying pan on medium heat. Melt ghee, add onion and cook for 3 minutes. Add cut asparagus and garlic. Cook for a further 5 minutes or until softening. Remove from heat. Add Nutritional Yeast Flakes to the frying pan and stir them through the vegetables.

To a large bowl add eggs and whisk, add coconut milk and stir into the eggs. Add ham, nutmeg, salt and pepper, stir well, then add onion and asparagus mixture and stir through. (If using cheese, add at this point).

Pour into your pie crust or prepared quiche or pie dish.

Bake for 35 minutes or until lightly golden, raised and set in the centre. Cooking time will slightly vary depending on depth of dish or if you are using a crust.

If you find the edges of your crust are browning before the middle is cooked, place a sheet of foil lightly over your quiche.

LUNCH & LIGHT MEALS

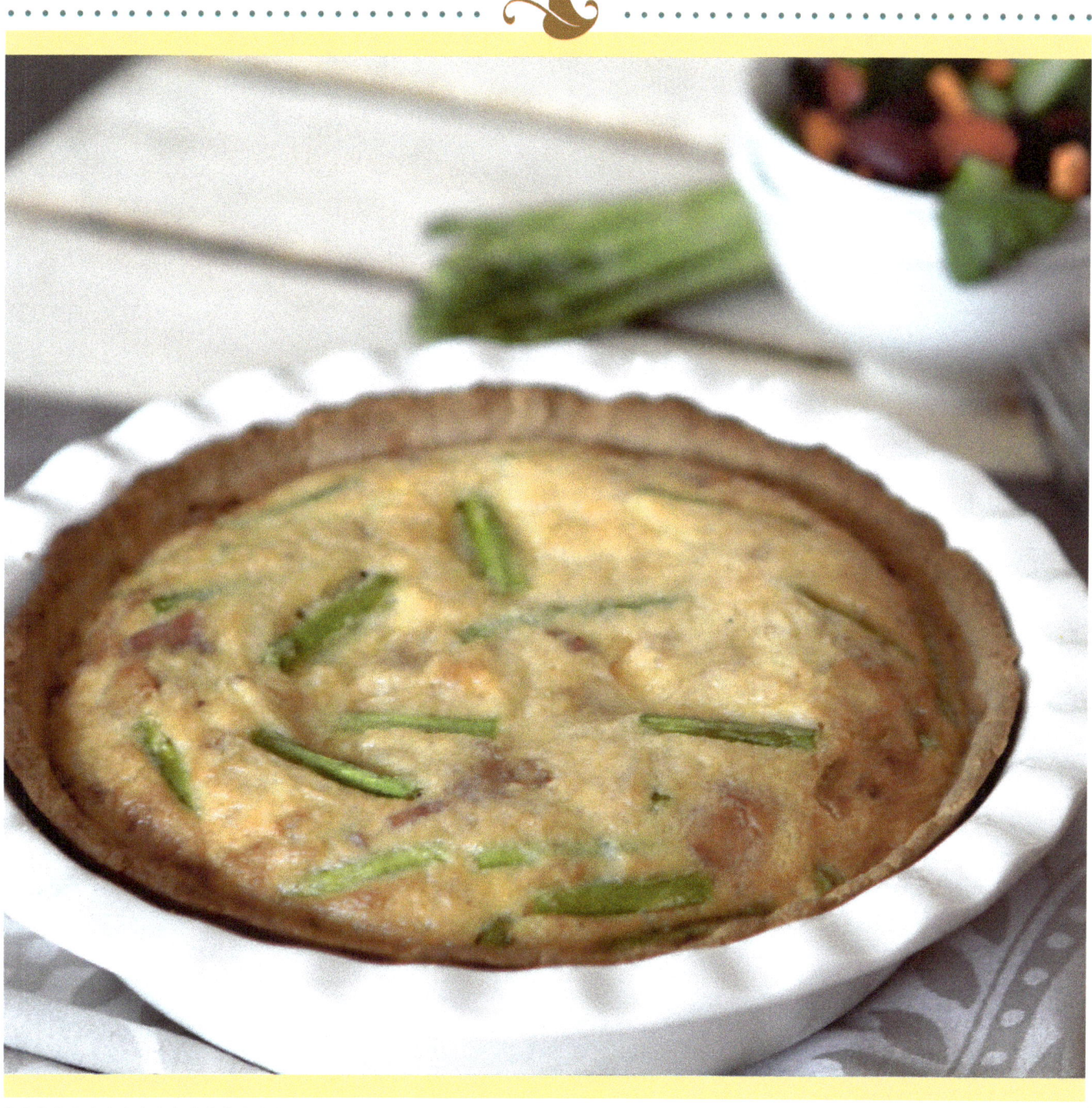

Chicken and Broccoli Frittata

I found baking the sweet potato while I was preparing the other recipe ingredients, produced a better result. Serve warm or at room temperature, great to take on a picnic or to the beach.

Prep time: 20 minutes   Cooking time: 45 minutes   Serves: 4

Ingredients:

- 1 medium sweet potato, sliced thinly
- Sea salt, pepper and ground sage, to season sweet potato
- 2 Tbsp coconut oil
- 1 small onion, diced
- 1 tsp garlic, minced
- ½ large broccoli, florets chopped small
- 1 cup mushrooms, diced
- 2 cups cooked chicken, diced or shredded
- 8 large eggs
- ⅔ cup canned coconut cream
- 10 grape or cherry tomatoes, cut in half
- Extra sea salt and pepper

Method:

Preheat oven to 180c/350f. Grease a 24cm(9.5in) pie dish with coconut oil.

Add 2 layers of sliced sweet potato to the base of dish, making sure to over lap each slice. Sprinkle with sea salt, pepper and ground sage, be generous. Cover pie dish with foil and place in the preheated oven for 20 minutes to partly cook while preparing rest of ingredients.

Heat a large frying pan on medium heat. Melt 1 tablespoon of oil. Add onion and garlic. Cook for 3 minutes.

Add broccoli and remaining oil. Cook stirring frequently for a further 3-4 minutes.

Add mushrooms and cook for 2-3 minutes or until starting to brown. Turn heat off and add chicken, stir to combine.

Add eggs and coconut cream to a bowl and whisk together.

Remove pie dish from oven. Spread vegetable and chicken mixture over sweet potato. Make sure to evenly distribute mixture with broccoli tops showing. Add tomato halves evenly spaced. Sprinkle with sea salt and pepper.

Pour over the egg mixture (if you tolerate dairy you could sprinkle the top with ½ cup of grated matured cheese).

Bake for 30 minutes or until centre is just set. Let sit for 10 minutes before serving.

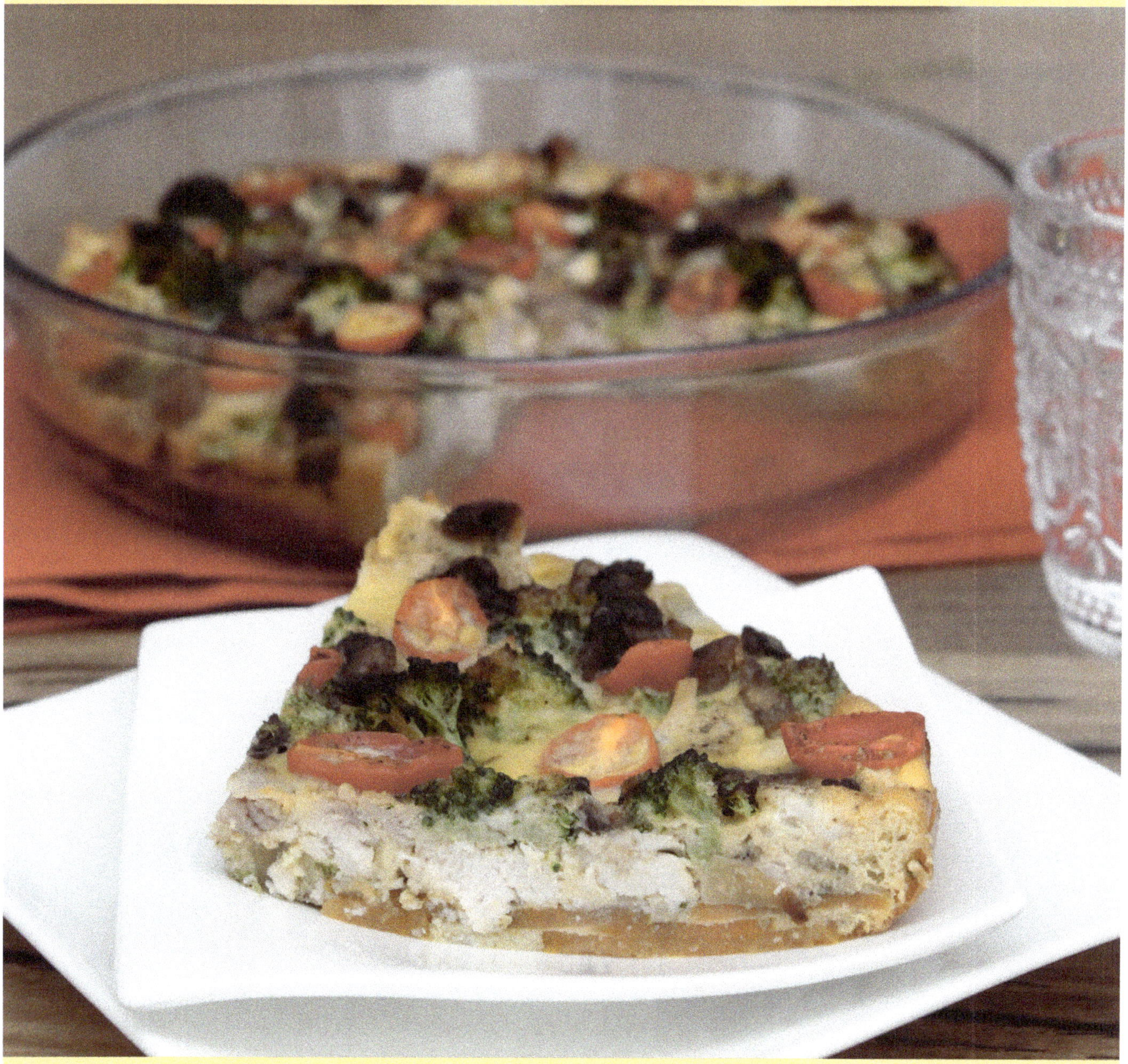

LUNCH & LIGHT MEALS | 141

Nachos

To make your chips, use the Spinach Flat bread recipe on page 78, broken into corn chip size pieces.

Prep time: 20 minutes Cooking time: 20 minutes Serves: 2-3

Ingredients:

Spinach Flat Bread,
broken into pieces, page 78.

MEAT MIXTURE
1 Tbsp ghee or coconut oil
1 small onion, finely diced
1 garlic cloves, finely diced
300g/10.5ozs beef mince
1 tsp ground cumin powder
½ tsp paprika
½ tsp ground coriander
¼ tsp Mexican chili powder or to taste
1 Tbsp tomato paste
1½ cups organic passata or tomato puree
½ tsp of each sea salt and ground pepper

DAIRY FREE CHEEZE SAUCE
1 cup of Nut White Sauce page 211.
1 Tbsp Nutritional Yeast Flakes
⅛ tsp pepper

GUACAMOLE
1 avocado, mashed
½ tsp garlic, minced
1 Tbsp lemon juice
½ tsp sea salt and a pinch of pepper

Method:

Heat a medium size saucepan over medium heat. Melt ghee, add onion and garlic. Cook for 4 minutes or until onions are tender.

Increase heat and add the beef. Cook for 5 minutes, breaking up any lumps. Add the remaining meat mixture ingredients, stir and bring to a boil. Reduce heat to low and simmer for 15 minutes, stirring often.

Meanwhile, prepare the Cheeze sauce. To one cup of Nut White Sauce, add 1 tablespoon of Nutritional Yeast Flakes and pepper. Stir to combine. Set aside.

Prepare guacamole. Add avocado to a small bowl and mash with a fork. Add remaining ingredients and mix well.

To assemble the nachos, place spinach chips around plates leaving centre free. Add meat mixture to centre, pour over Cheeze sauce and top with guacamole. Optional, sprinkle with finely sliced spring onions and a coriander leaf.

LUNCH & LIGHT MEALS | 143

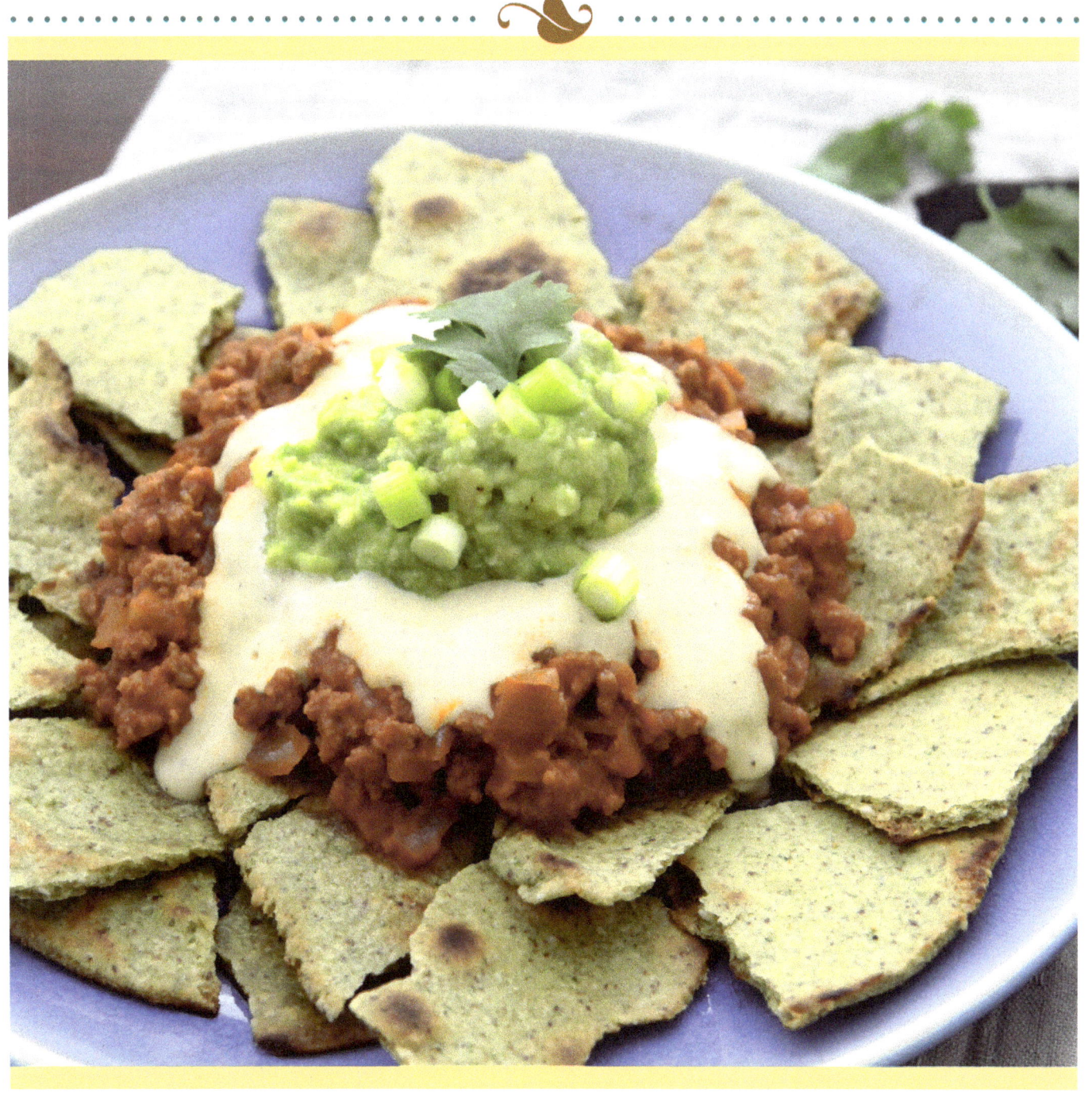

Mango and Avocado Salad

Mangos and walnuts have anti-inflammatory properties. This dish isn't just yummy but very good for you. I've topped the salad with pan-fried chicken but you might like to swap with grilled fish, cooked prawns or use left over roast meat.

Prep time: 15 minutes Cooking time: none Serves: 2

Ingredients:

- 4-6 cups mixed greens, of your choice (rocket, spinach, butter lettuce etc.)
- 1 small carrot, coarsely grated
- 1 mango, sliced thinly
- 1 avocado sliced thinly
- ⅓ cup raw walnuts, roughly chopped
- 200g/7ozs cooked chicken, grilled and sliced
- 2 Tbsp coconut aminos
- 2 Tbsp lemon juice
- 2 Tbsp extra virgin olive oil, mild flavour
- Sea salt and pepper, to taste

Method:

Arrange greens on a serving plate or in a salad bowl. Mix through carrot.

Spread mango and avocado slices on top, mix them around a little, then sprinkle over walnuts.

Top with sliced grilled chicken or fish.

In a small jug whisk together the coconut aminos, lemon juice, oil, salt and pepper.

Drizzle over salad and serve. Optional; you may like to sprinkle with chopped fresh parsley.

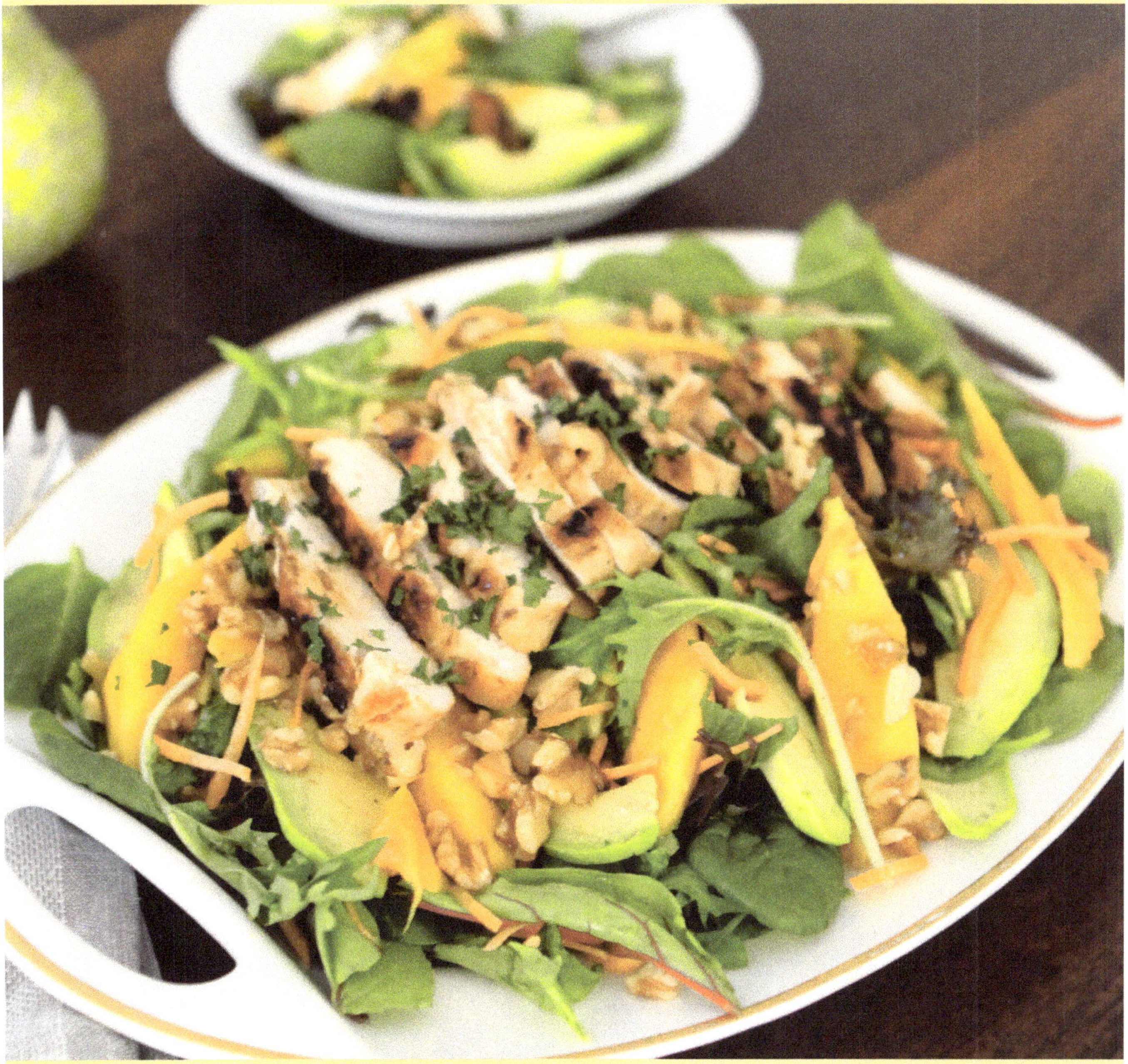

LUNCH & LIGHT MEALS | 145

Chicken and Avocado Caesar Salad

This is perfect for those hot summer days. Great to take on a picnic or just outside under a tree trying to keep cool in the evening. Packed with greens, lots of protein and healthy fats and dressed with a tasty creamy dressing. You will find Caesar salad dressing on page 208.

Prep time: 20 minutes Cooking time: 10 minutes Serves: 4

Ingredients:

- 2-3 baby cos lettuces, depending on size available
- 4 boiled eggs, chopped
- 4 rashes bacon, cooked and diced (nitrate free)
- 500g/1.1lb cold cooked chicken, chopped
- 2 avocados, chopped
- ½ cup Caesar salad dressing, see page 208
- Optional, shaved parmesan cheese, if you tolerate dairy

Method:

Using a platter with sides or a large salad bowl. Combine washed torn lettuce, chopped eggs, bacon, chopped cold cooked chicken and avocado.

Keep a little bacon aside to sprinkle on the top.

Pour over Caesar salad dressing and toss to coat. Top with extra bacon.

Serve immediately after adding dressing.

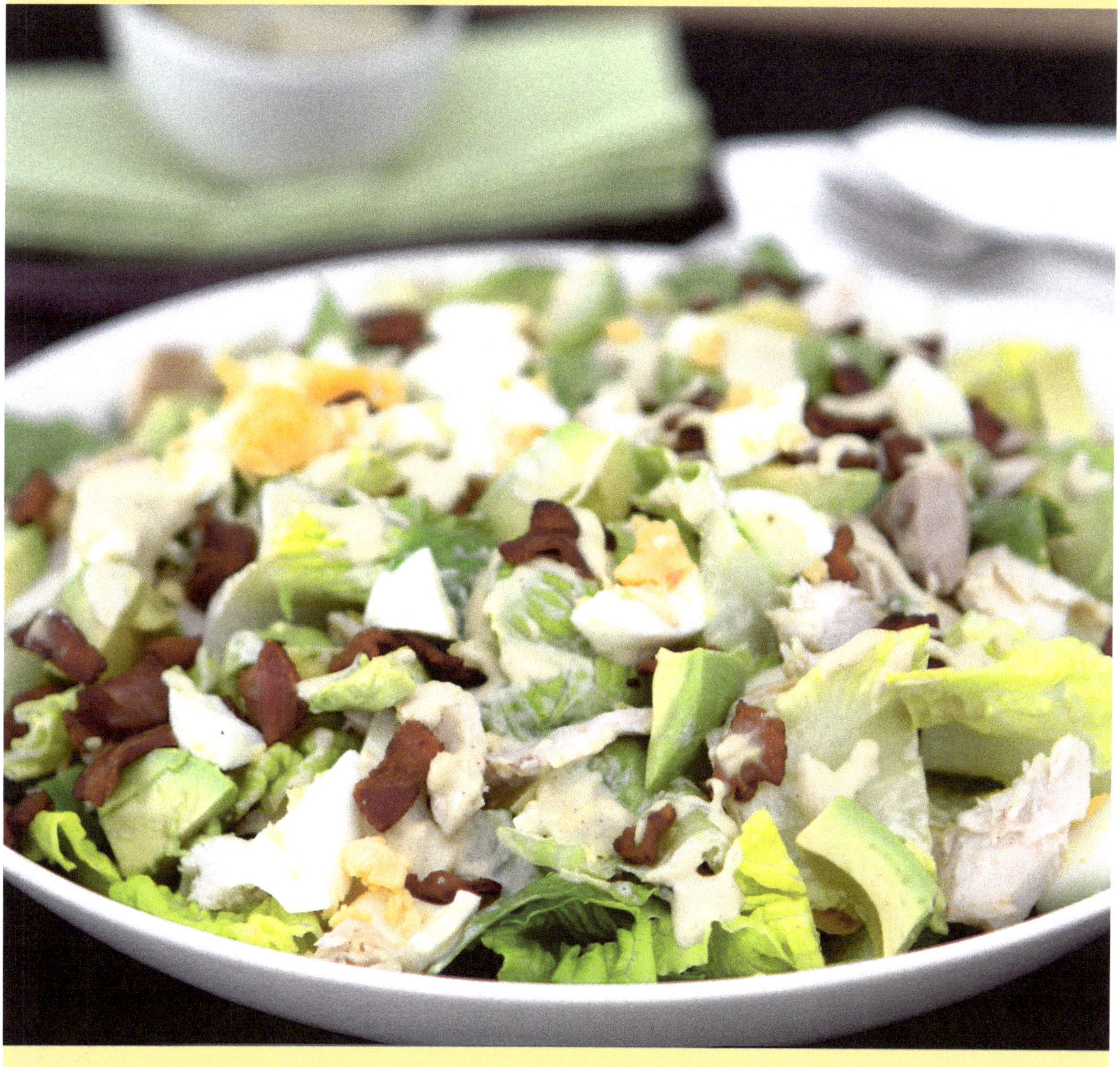

LUNCH & LIGHT MEALS | 147

Curry Pasties

The pastry is partly cooked on the stovetop, then filled and baked in the oven. This produces a lovely light textured grain free pastry. I normally make the curried meat mixture the day before to save on time. You can also make the pasties smaller to use as finger food.

Prep time: 25 minutes Cooking time: 45 minutes Makes: 12

Ingredients:

FILLING
2 Tbsp coconut oil
1 small sweet potato (approximately 300g), diced
1 medium onion, finely diced
2 tsp garlic, minced
1 tsp ginger, minced
2 tsp ground coriander
½ tsp turmeric
½ tsp cinnamon
¼ tsp garam masala
¼ tsp cayenne or to taste
⅓ tsp sea salt
300g/10.5ozs minced beef

PASTRY
1½ cups almond meal/flour
¾ cup arrowroot flour
½ tsp sea salt
1 cup coconut milk
1 cup coconut water or filtered water
2 Tbsp ghee for cooking pastry rounds
1 egg, beaten for egg wash

Method:

Heat a heavy based saucepan on medium heat. Add 1 tablespoon of coconut oil. Add diced sweet potato and fry for 5 minutes.

Add an extra ½ tablespoon of coconut oil. Add onion, garlic and ginger and stir cooking for 3 minutes. Reduce heat and let the sweet potato and onions cook covered for a further 5 minutes.

Add spices and salt, cook stirring for 1 minute or until fragrant. Move vegetables to the sides of saucepan and add minced beef, turning frequently until colour has changed. Mix all cooked ingredients together. Turn off heat and set aside to wait for pastry rounds to be made.

Pastry Rounds:

To a bowl add, almond meal, arrowroot flour, salt, coconut milk and coconut water. Mix well to make a smooth batter.

Preheat oven to 180c/350f. Line 2 baking trays with baking paper.

Heat ½ teaspoon of ghee in a small non-stick frying pan or crepe pan on medium heat (I use 2 fry pans to save time).

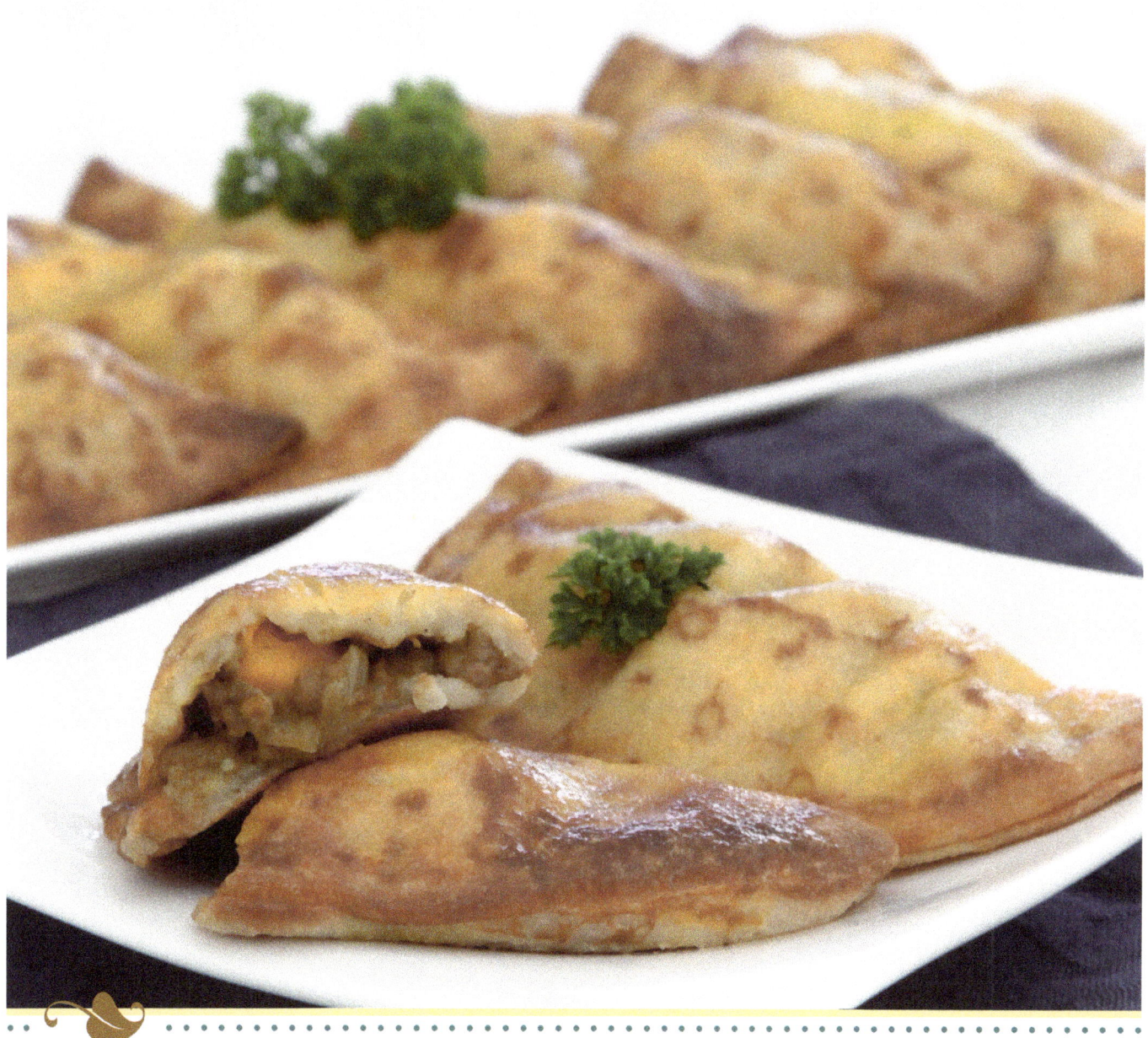

Fill a ¼ measuring cup with batter and ladle into pan to make a round approximately 13cm(5ins) in diameter. Cook pastry until the bottom is slightly cooked, approximately 3 minutes, don't turn over. Uncooked top should have turned from white to cream. You don't want the pastry round crisp, it needs to be soft and flexible to fold. Remove carefully using a thin spatula and place on lined baking tray (keep spatula free of batter, this will prevent sticking to pastry when removing).

Spoon 2 tablespoons of meat mixture onto half of the round, leaving edges free to seal. (Don't over fill.) Use a pastry brush to coat the edges with water or the beaten egg. Fold over carefully so pastry doesn't split. Press the edges together making a pasty.

Line all your pasties up on a baking tray. Brush the tops with egg wash just before placing into the oven. Bake for 25 minutes or until golden and crisp on the outside.

(Using 2 frying pans makes you move fast. While 2 pastry rounds are cooking I fill the previous 2.)

THE JOYFUL TABLE

Savoury Pancakes

These pancakes have a wonderful soft centre due to the moist cabbage but have a very crunchy outside. You could add chopped cooked bacon if you prefer, I wanted them to be just a little different, so I added slices. Great hot or cold. Kids will love them!

Prep time: 15 minutes Cooking time: 25 minutes Makes: 8

Ingredients:

- 1 cup almond meal/flour
- ½ cup arrowroot flour
- ½ tsp baking soda
- ⅓ tsp fine sea salt
- ⅓ tsp ground pepper
- ½ cup chicken broth/stock
- 3 large eggs, lightly beaten
- 2 Tbsp coconut aminos
- 3 spring onions/shallots, finely sliced
- 2 cups Chinese cabbage or savoy cabbage, finely shredded
- 1½ cups fresh bean shoots/sprouts
- 4 slices bacon, cut into 10cm (4in) long pieces (nitrate free)
- 2 Tbsp coconut oil

Method:

To a large bowl add, almond meal, arrowroot flour, baking soda, salt and pepper, mix well. Make a well in the centre.

Pour in chicken broth, eggs and coconut aminos, whisk well to make a smooth batter. Stir in onions, cabbage and bean shoots.

Heat a large non-stick frying pan over medium heat. Add 2 teaspoons of oil and swirl to coat pan. Place 2 pieces of bacon close together in the pan. Add just under ½ cup of batter on top of the bacon pieces. If batter runs away, use a spatula to push back to shape a circle, make sure the vegetables are spread evenly throughout the circle of batter.

Repeat for each pancake. (I can fit 3 in my large 30cm frying pan.) Cook for 3 minutes or until golden brown, turn over carefully. I like to use 2 spatulas when turning as these pancakes have a soft centre.

Add more coconut oil as needed. Cook for a further 3 minutes on second side.

Transfer to a plate and cover to keep warm or place in a warm oven until remaining pancakes are cooked. Serve with bacon side up, add a spoonful of egg mayonnaise and slices of avocado.

LUNCH & LIGHT MEALS | 151

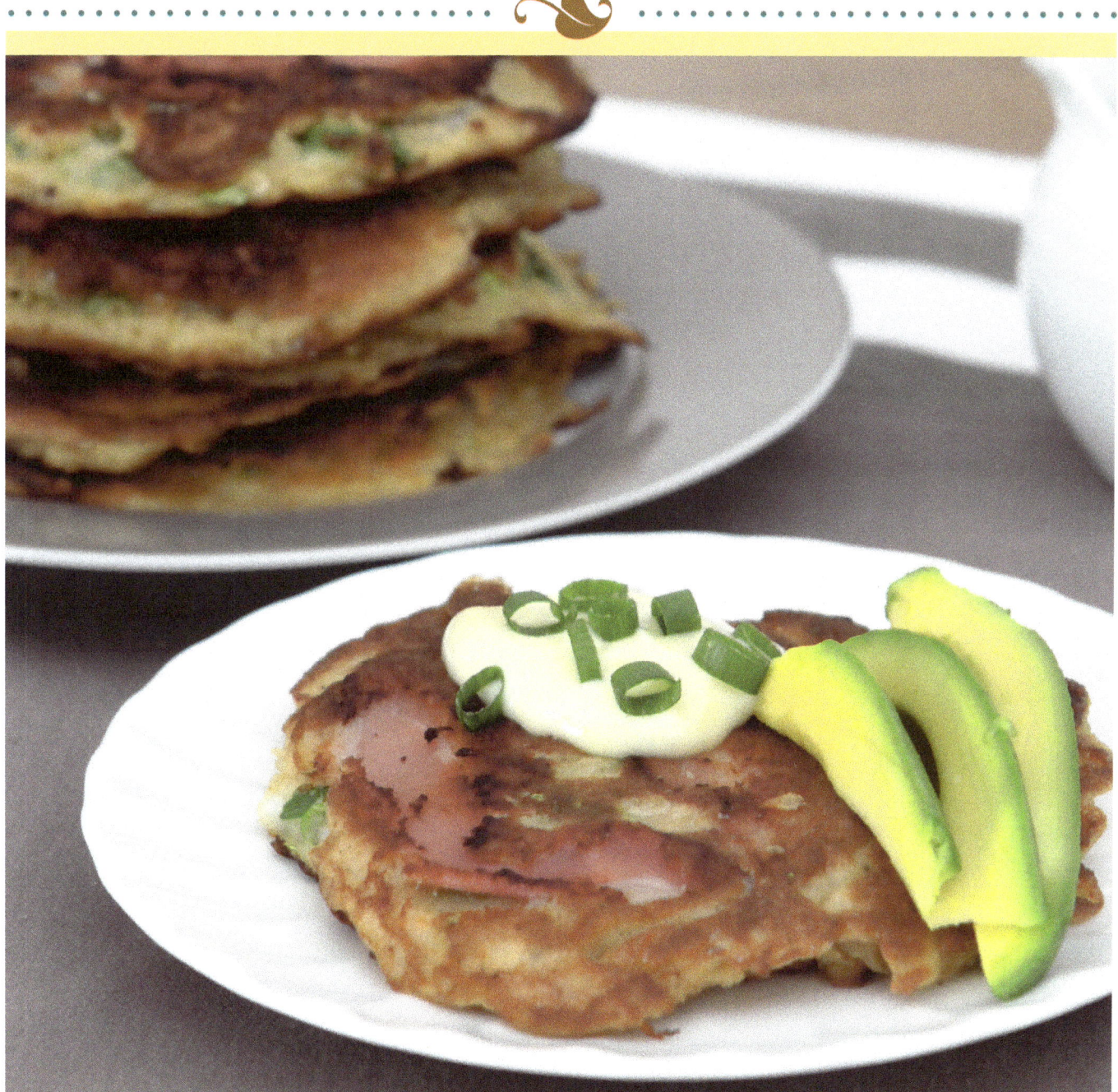

Tasty Toasts

I am so happy with these Toasties, the dough has turned out nice and crispy with a flaky texture. They are based on a Turkish dough called Gozleme. I have included some savoury fillings to get you started but there's no end of ideas to fill them with. A great food for watching a football game. You can also make mini pizza bases with this dough. (Roll out small rounds and fry both sides, add toppings and finish in oven.)

Prep time: 10 minutes Cooking time: 15 minutes
Makes: 4 (quantity for 1 serve included)

Ingredients:

- 3 cups almond meal/flour
- 1¼ cup arrowroot flour
- 1 tsp baking soda
- ½ tsp fine sea salt
- 1 cup natural coconut yoghurt or Greek yoghurt

Single Serve:

- (¾ cup almond meal)
- (⅓ cup arrowroot flour)
- (¼ tsp baking soda)
- (pinch sea salt)
- (¼ cup coconut yoghurt)

Method:

In a bowl, combine flours, baking soda and salt. Mix to combine, breaking up any lumps. Add yoghurt. Mix with a spoon to combine and finish off with hands to knead dough. Mixture should be a soft dough, a little sticky but not overly. Sprinkle some arrowroot flour over dough if your fingers are sticking too much.

Cover bowl and set aside to rest, while you make your filling. When fillings are completed:

Divide dough into four. Use 2 sheets of baking paper for each portion of dough. Dust a little arrowroot flour on bottom sheet. Place one portion on paper, flatten with palm and dust top with a little arrowroot flour. Place second sheet of baking paper on top. Using a rolling pin, roll dough out to a 24cm(10.5in) round. Remove top sheet slowly so dough doesn't stick to it.

Spread ¼ of your filling mixture over half the dough, leaving a 2cm(1in) border. Lift the far end of the baking paper to assist as you fold dough in half, enclosing the filling. Don't over fill. Remove paper slowly.

Press edges together to seal, then roll in sealed edges towards filling. If dough splits, just press together.

Heat a large non stick frying pan on medium heat. Add 1 teaspoon ghee and spread over pan. If dough is easy to handle, slip your hand under to carry and place in frying pan. If a bit fragile, move to pan on the paper and turn over into the pan, then remove paper.

Cook for 3-4 minutes on each side or until brown and crisp. Use a large spatula to flip toasty. Add more ghee as needed so dough crisps up nicely. Use a big enough frying pan so you can cook two at a time. To serve cut in half.

SUSAN JOY

LUNCH & LIGHT MEALS

Pumpkin, Spinach and Feta Toasts

Ingredients:

1 quantity of Tasty Toasts dough (makes 4)
350g/12ozs peeled pumpkin, diced and cooked
120g/4ozs baby spinach leaves, finely shredded
100g/3.5ozs full fat feta, crumbled or finely diced
1½ Tbsp Nutritional Yeast Flakes
Sea salt and pepper to taste
1 Tbsp sesame seeds

Method:

Steam or lightly boil pumpkin until very soft. Combine spinach, feta, Nutritional Yeast Flakes, salt and pepper in a bowl. Add pumpkin while still hot to wilt the spinach and mix. Set aside while rolling dough. After assembling your toasty, sprinkle top with sesame seeds, press lightly into dough. Place sesame side down into pan and sprinkle the up facing side with sesame seeds, press lightly.

Mexican Beef Toasts

Ingredients:

1 quantity of Tasty Toasts dough (makes 4)
1 Tbsp ghee or coconut oil
1 small onion, finely diced
2 tsp garlic, minced
2 tsp ground coriander
2 tsp ground cumin
400g/14ozs beef mince
1½ Tbsp tomato paste
¼ tsp coarse sea salt or to taste

Method:

Heat a saucepan on medium heat. Add ghee, cook onion and garlic for 4 minutes. Add spices, cook and stir for 30 seconds or until fragrant. Add mince, cook stirring to break up lumps for 5 minutes or until browned. Add tomato paste and salt, stir through and cook for a further 2 minutes.

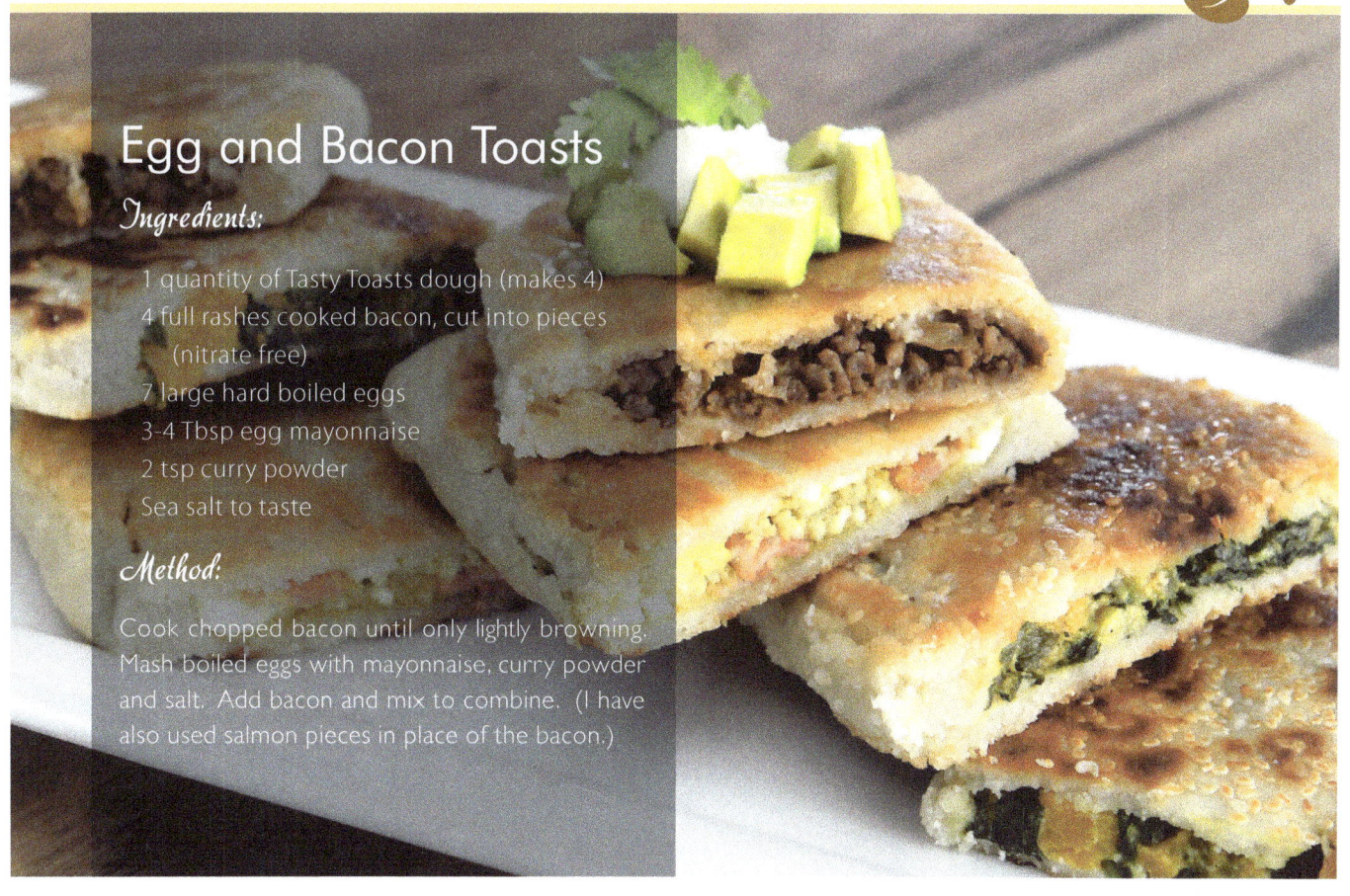

Egg and Bacon Toasts

Ingredients:

1 quantity of Tasty Toasts dough (makes 4)
4 full rashes cooked bacon, cut into pieces (nitrate free)
7 large hard boiled eggs
3-4 Tbsp egg mayonnaise
2 tsp curry powder
Sea salt to taste

Method:

Cook chopped bacon until only lightly browning. Mash boiled eggs with mayonnaise, curry powder and salt. Add bacon and mix to combine. (I have also used salmon pieces in place of the bacon.)

Paleo Satay Chicken

I have used chicken but after you have tried this recipe, go ahead and experiment with beef or lamb. The satay sauce is also an excellent dip for sweet potato fries and crunchy raw vegetables.

Prep time: 20 minutes plus marinating & soaking time
Cooking time: 8 minutes Serves: 4

Ingredients:

- 800g/1.7lbs chicken tenderloins or skinless thigh, cut into 3cm cubes
- ⅓ cup canned coconut milk
- Juice of 1 lime
- 3 Tbsp coconut aminos
- 2 tsp fish sauce
- 3 tsp garlic, minced
- 2 tsp ground ginger
- 2 tsp turmeric
- 1½ tsp ground coriander
- 1 tsp ground cumin
- 1 tsp sea salt
- Coconut oil for cooking
- 12 wooden skewers, soaked in water for 30 minutes before preparing

SATAY SAUCE
- 1 cup raw cashews
- ½ cup raw almonds
- ⅓ tsp sea salt and water for soaking nuts
- ½ cup canned coconut milk
- ¼ cup filtered water
- 3 Tbsp coconut aminos
- 2 tsp curry powder
- 1½ tsp ground ginger
- 1 tsp garlic, minced
- Pinch or 2 of chili powder or to taste
- 2 tsp 100% organic maple syrup
- Juice of ½ lime

Method:

Cut chicken into cubes, set aside. To a bowl add coconut milk, lime juice, coconut aminos, fish sauce, garlic, spices and salt, mix well to combine. Add chicken and coat. Place chicken and marinade in a snap lock bag or sealed container to store in fridge for 4 hours or overnight (I prefer overnight).

To make sauce: Place cashews and almonds in a glass bowl, add salt and cover with hot water, at least 6cm(2.5ins) above nuts. When water has cooled, drain nuts and rinse with clean water, drain well.

Add nuts and remaining sauce ingredients into a high-speed blender or food processor. Blend until nuts have broken down but leave just a little crunch. If you would prefer a thinner sauce add a little water, 1 tablespoon at a time. Makes 2 cups of sauce.

Thread chicken cubes onto skewers, approximately 4 pieces per skewer. Heat a BBQ plate/grill on medium-high heat and grease with coconut oil. Cook for 4 minutes on each side. A large frying pan that skewers will fit into can also be used on the stovetop.

Serve with warmed satay sauce, lime wedges and garnish with coriander leaves.

LUNCH & LIGHT MEALS | 155

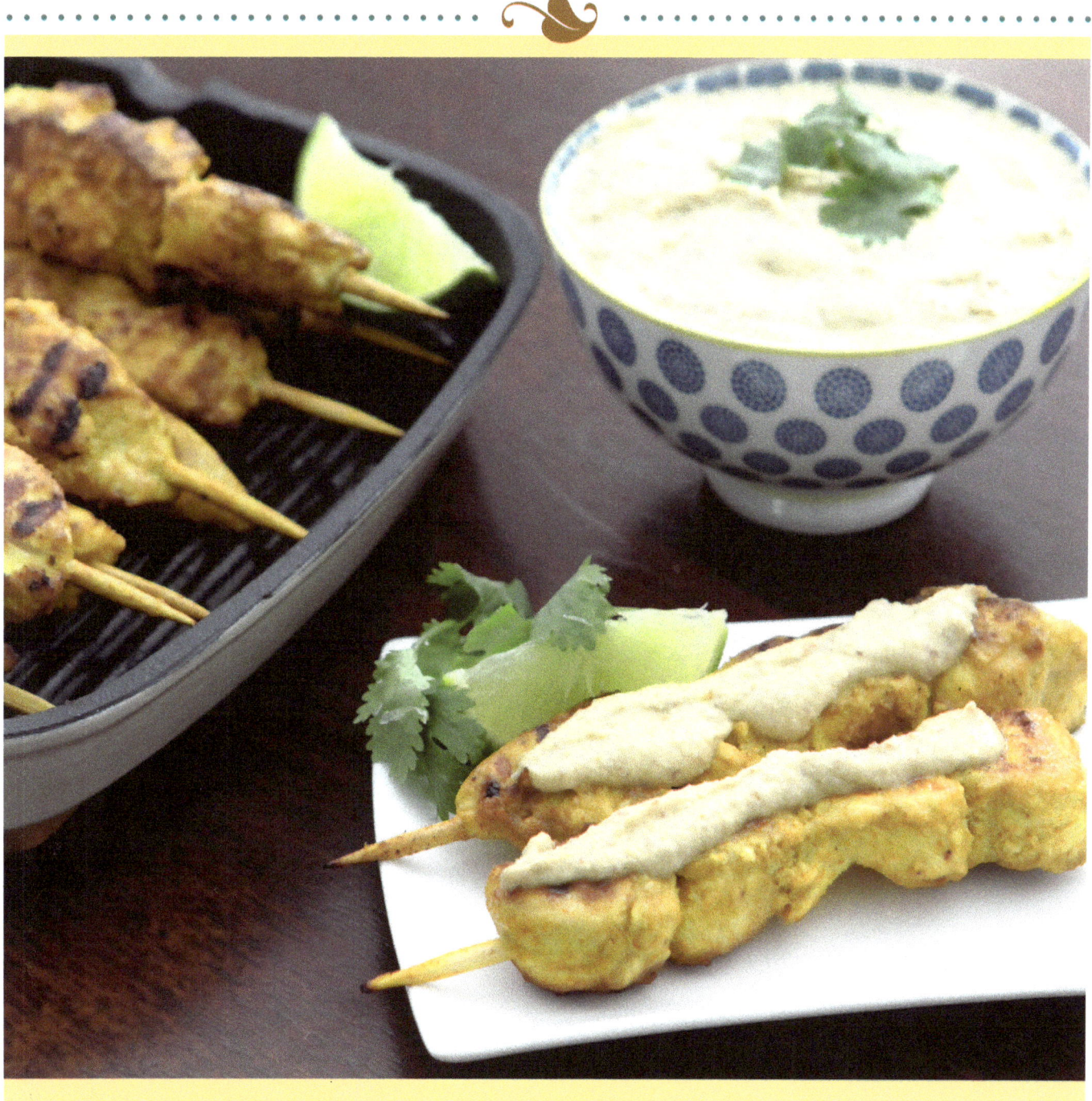

Mini Meat Loaves

I have used this recipe to take to Pot Luck lunches. If you double the recipe, it will feed many and they freeze well. I used square muffin tins but it's just for looks, round ones will do fine. Delicious hot or cold and perfect for picnics.

Prep time: 20 minutes   Cooking time: 40 minutes   Makes: 24

Ingredients:

- 2 cups sweet potato, finely grated (½ large or 1 small)
- 1½ cups mushrooms, finely diced
- 1 onion, finely diced
- 4 eggs, beaten
- 3 Tbsp ground flaxseed
- 3 Tbsp organic maple syrup
- 2 tsp garlic, minced
- ¾ tsp cinnamon
- ½ tsp ground nutmeg
- ½ tsp sea salt
- ⅓ tsp ground pepper
- 600g/1.3lb minced beef
- 300g/10.5ozs minced pork
- 300g/10.5ozs minced lamb
- (or meats of your choice, mixing the meats gives a better flavour)
- Organic tomato sauce/ketchup, to top the meat loaves

Method:

Preheat oven to 190c/375f. Grease muffin tins with coconut oil or ghee.

To a large bowl add all the ingredients, except for the meat. Mix well using a fork.

Add the meats and work them into the vegetable mixture, (using your hands to evenly distribute the ingredients, works best). Make sure you have a well combined mixture.

Fill muffin tins right to the top, pressing down to compact the mixture.

Bake for 25-30 minutes or until meat juices are starting to re-absorb. Remove from oven and coat tops with tomato sauce/ketchup and bake a further 10-15 minutes.

You could substitute pumpkin for the sweet potato, if you prefer.

Eat straight from the oven with salad or vegetables. Keep leftovers to have cold in packed lunches. Place on a platter lined with lettuce leaves to share with friends.

LUNCH & LIGHT MEALS | 157

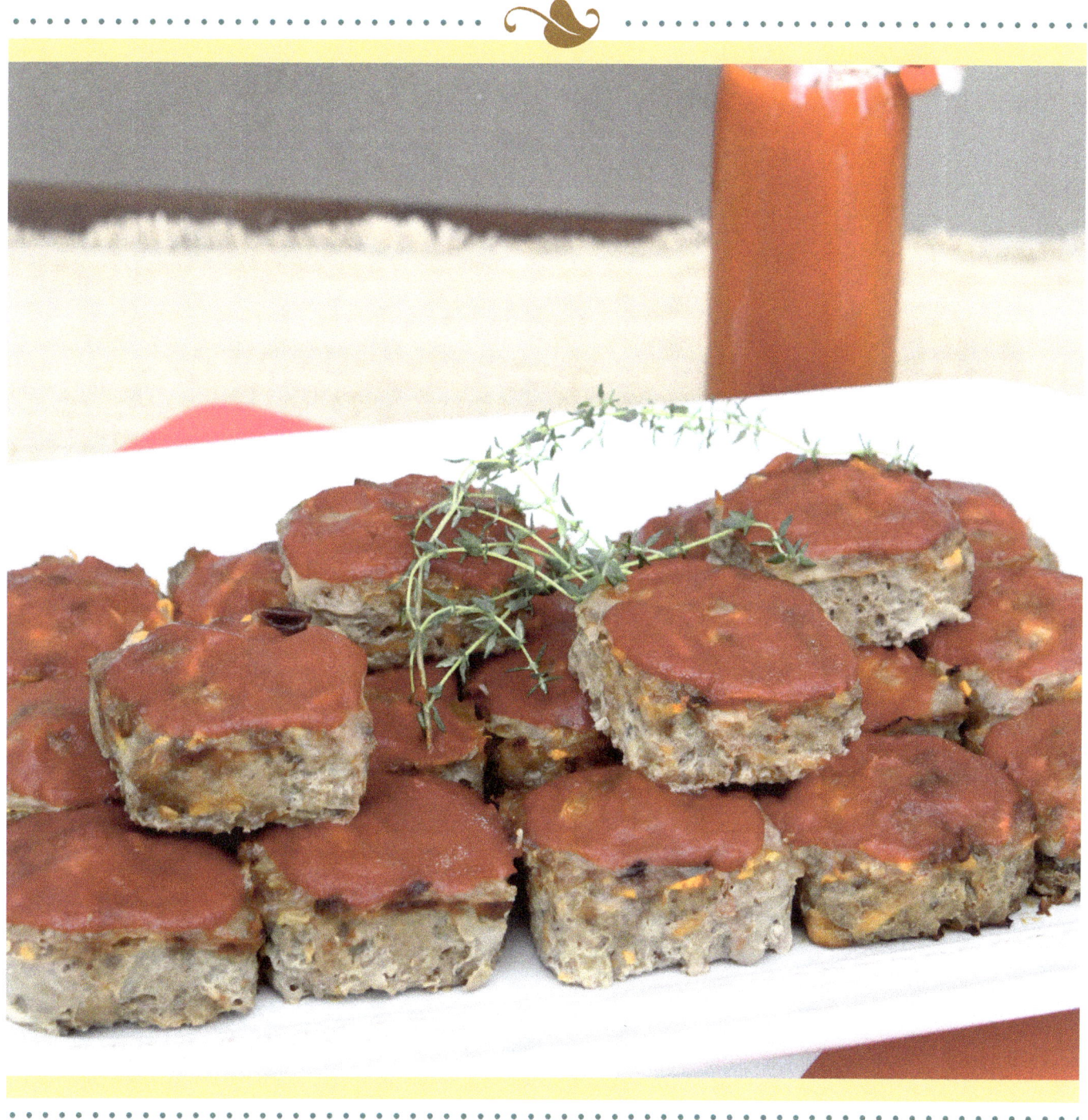

Hamburger Patties

There are unlimited ways to eat your hamburger. You can serve with salad in a Hamburger bun, recipe page 70. Wrapped in a lettuce leaf. Served as rissoles with vegetables or make an Aussie burger "Hamburger with Egg and Beetroot".

Prep time: 10 minutes Cooking time: 9 minutes Makes: 4

Ingredients:

- 1 large egg
- 1 medium onion, finely diced
- 2 tsp garlic, minced
- 1 Tbsp organic Worcestershire sauce
- 1 Tbsp red curry paste, no additives or oil (I use Thai Gourmet)
- ⅓ cup ground sunflower meal or almond meal
- ¾ tsp fine sea salt
- ⅓ tsp ground pepper
- 500g/1.1 lbs beef mince or turkey mince
- 1½ Tbsp coconut oil

Method:

Add egg to a large bowl and whisk. Add all other ingredients except for the beef mince. Combine well with a fork. Add beef, take your time mixing to make a smooth well combined mixture.

Heat a large frying pan on medium-high heat. Add coconut oil.

Divide mixture into four large patties. Cook for 5 minutes. Use a spatula to turn over and cook for a further 4 minutes. Hamburger patties should have caramelized on the outside, making a delicious flavour.

Variation: exchange red curry paste for 1 tablespoon of whole grain mustard.

LUNCH & LIGHT MEALS | 159

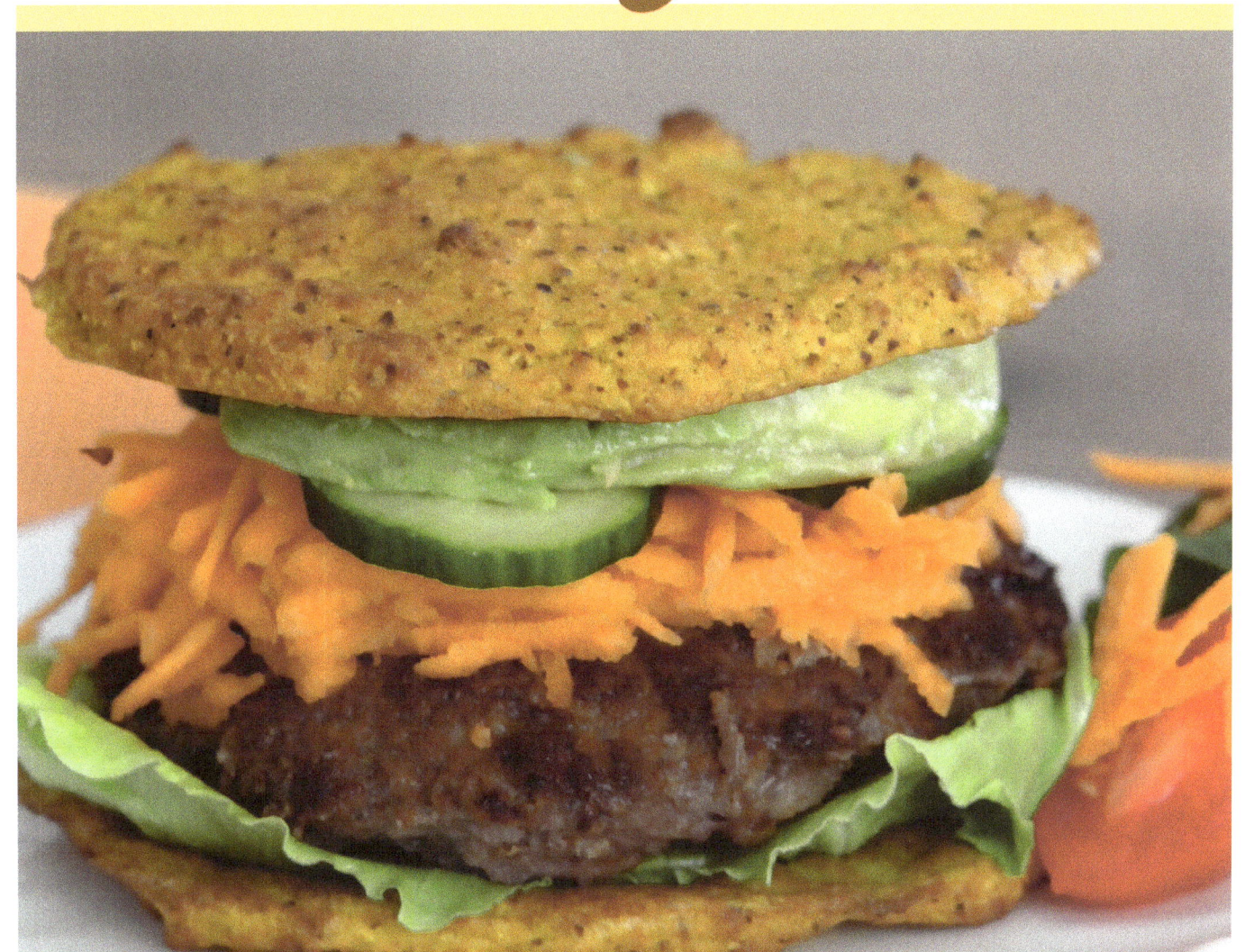

Curried Nut Burgers

These were created from my old Lentil Burger recipe. Swapping to cashews produced a much lighter texture than the heavy lentil version. Soaking your nuts in warm water neutralises enzyme inhibitors, and helps produce beneficial enzymes. It also makes nuts much easier to digest and the nutrients more easily absorbed.

Prep time: 15 minutes plus soaking time   Cooking time: 20 minutes   Makes: 10

Ingredients:

- 2 cups raw cashews
- Hot water plus 1/3 tsp sea salt for soaking nuts
- 3 Tbsp coconut oil, divided
- 4-5 spring onions/shallots, finely sliced
- 2 medium carrots, grated
- 1 large zucchini (approximately 400g), grated
- 2½ Tbsp Red Curry paste (I use Thai Gourmet brand)
- 1/3 cup ground flaxseed
- 3 Tbsp coconut flour
- 1 egg, beaten
- ½ tsp fine sea salt

Method:

Soak cashews in a bowl with hot water and salt. Set aside. When water has dropped to room temperature, drain nuts using a metal sieve. Rinse and drain well.

Add cashews to a high-speed blender. Using the tamper push the nuts onto the blades to produce a nice smooth but thick consistency.

While the nuts soak, heat a large frying pan over medium-high heat. Melt 1 tablespoon of coconut oil. Add spring onions, cook for 1-2 minutes. Add carrots and zucchini, cook stirring for a further 5 minutes or until vegetables are starting to softened. Remove from heat and allow to cool.

In a large bowl add creamed cashews, curry paste, flaxseed, coconut flour, egg and salt. Use a fork to mix well.

Drain the vegetable liquid from pan. Using a slotted spoon, scoop up vegetables a little at a time, squeezing out any extra liquid, by pressing your hand into the spoon. Add to bowl with cashew mixture and incorporate well.

Wipe out frying pan and heat on medium-high. Add 1 tablespoon of coconut oil. Spoon 3 tablespoons of mixture per burger into pan. Use a spoon and fork to shape and flatten mixture into round burger shapes.

Cook first side for 3 minutes or until brown and crunchy. Turn over carefully and cook for a further 2-3 minutes. Add extra oil as needed. Burgers will be soft inside but crunchy and brown on outside. Serve with salad or in a grain free bun.

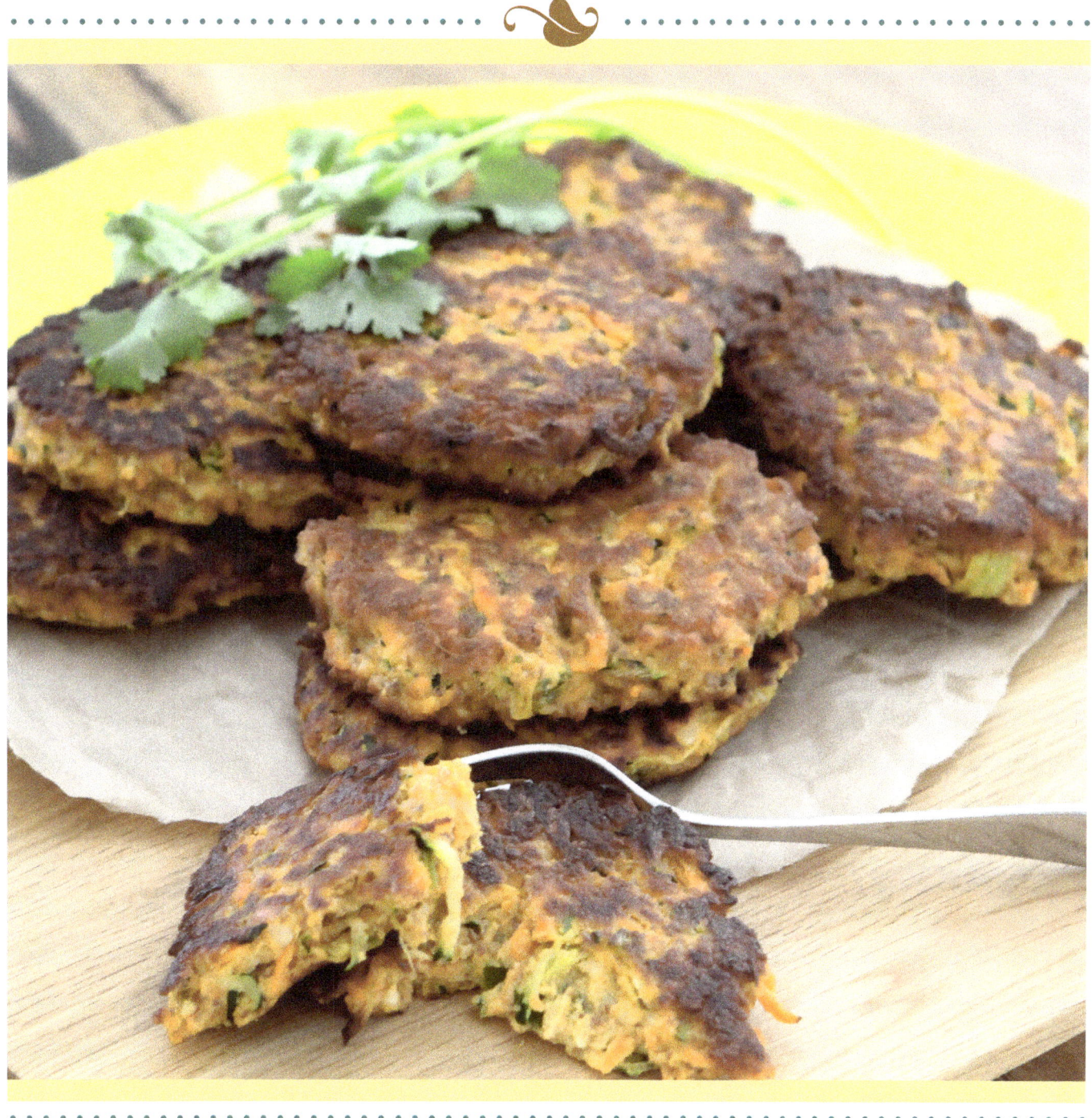

Creamy Zucchini Noodles

This is a lovely fresh tasting dish, just right for the days you only want a light meal. If you don't have a spiral slicer, use a julienne slicer or potato peeler to make the Zucchini noodles.

Prep time: 10 minutes Cooking time: 8 minutes Serves: 3-4

Ingredients:

- 2 large zucchini, unpeeled made into noodles
- 1 Tbsp coconut oil
- 3 spring onions/shallots, sliced
- 1½ tsp garlic, minced
- ¾ tsp ginger, minced or grated
- ¼ cup roughly chopped basil leaves
- 3 cups cauliflower white sauce/puree, recipe page 212 with no added milk
- Juice of 1 lime
- 2 Tbsp Nutritional Yeast Flakes
- ¾ tsp coarse sea salt
- ¼ tsp ground pepper
- 1 large avocado, chopped

Method:

Use a spiral slicer or julienne slicer/peeler to make the noodles. Place in a sieve or colander over the sink, sprinkle a little sea salt through the noodles and let sit for 10 minutes while you make the sauce. This will remove the excess liquid.

Heat a large saucepan over medium heat, melt coconut oil. Add spring onions, garlic and ginger. Cook for 5 minutes or until onion is tender.

Add basil, cauliflower sauce, lime juice, Nutritional Yeast Flakes, salt and pepper. Bring to a light simmer for 1-2 minute.

Add chopped avocado and mix through.

Gently squeeze out any excess liquid in the zucchini and add them to the saucepan. Stir to coat noodles with sauce.

Serve in individual bowls, garnished with basil.

LUNCH & LIGHT MEALS | 163

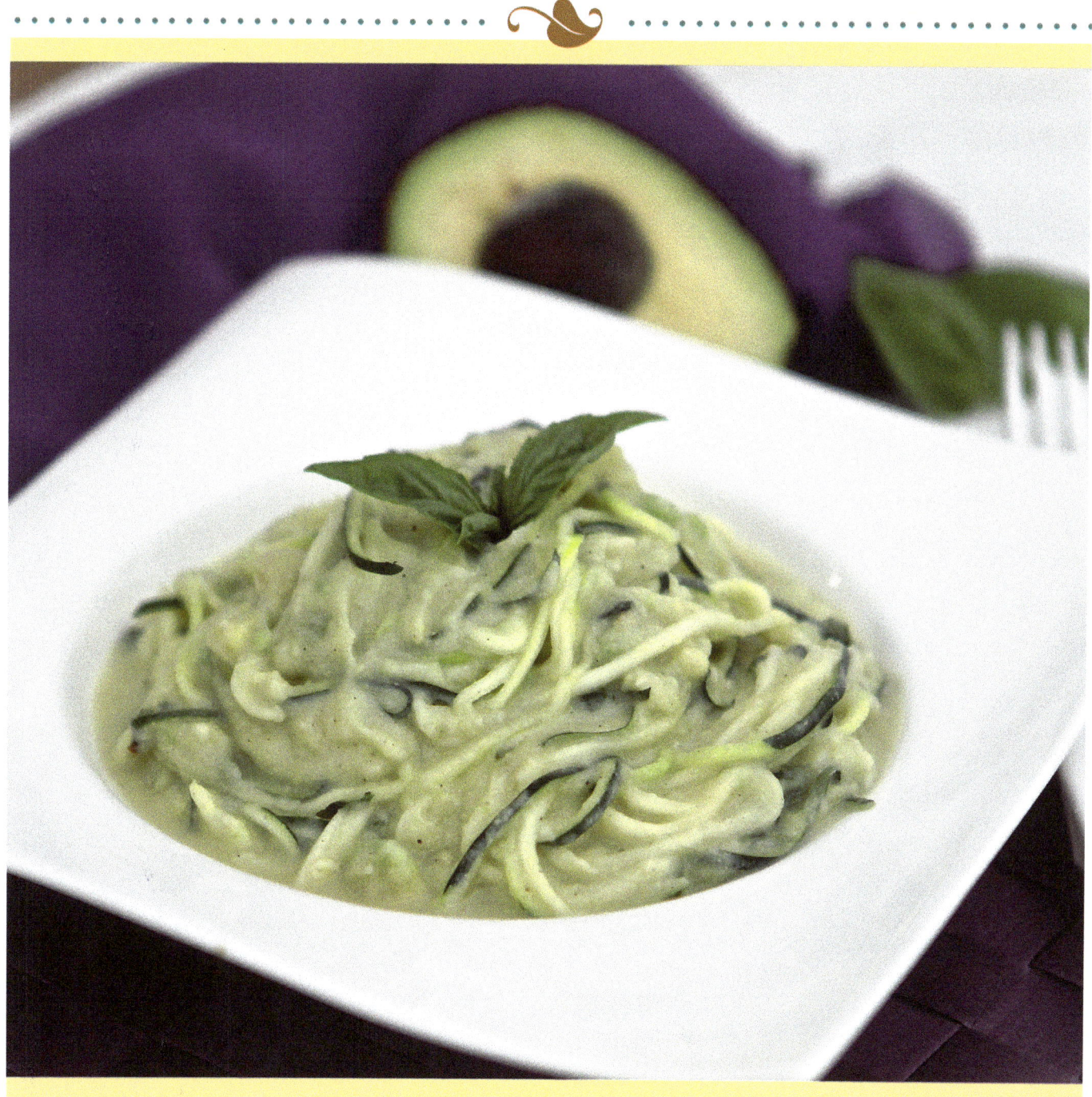

Chinese Cauliflower Fried Rice

Cauliflower has become very popular as a replacement for rice but we may not know just how special cauliflower is. It provides special nutrient support for three systems in our bodies that can help prevent cancer. These three systems are the body's detox system, its antioxidant system, and its inflammatory/anti-inflammatory system. So eat up!

Prep time: 20 minutes Cooking time: 15 minutes Serves: 4

Ingredients:

- 1 head cauliflower, cut in evenly sized pieces
- Coconut oil for frying
- 3 eggs, whisked
- 4 spring onions, sliced
- 2 carrots, diced
- 2 tsp garlic, minced
- 1 tsp ginger, minced
- 4 rashes bacon, diced (nitrate free)
- 1 cup mushrooms, diced
- 1 cup frozen peas, optional
- Sea salt and pepper to taste
- 2 cups cooked prawns, optional
- 2 Tbsp coconut aminos
- 1 tsp fish sauce
- Juice of ½ lemon
- 2 Tbsp fresh chopped parsley
- Add any additional vegetables you like, diced capsicum/peppers, finely chopped broccoli etc.

Method:

To a food processor, add half the cauliflower and pulse until you have rice size pieces. Repeat with remaining half. Set aside.

Heat a large frying pan on medium-high heat and fry bacon. Set aside.

Add the whisked eggs to pan and move pan to spread egg around to form an omelet. When cooked remove to a chopping board and cut into thin pieces.

Add coconut oil to pan and increase heat. Add spring onions, carrot, garlic and ginger, cook stirring for 3-4 minutes. Add peas, salt and pepper and stir.

Add cauliflower rice, toss all ingredients through the cauliflower. Reduce heat to low and cover for 5 minutes until cauliflower has softened, but still firm.

Add prawns, coconut aminos, fish sauce, lemon juice, mix through and heat a further few minutes. Add egg pieces, bacon and parsley, and mix through.

Serve in bowls topped with sliced spring onion.

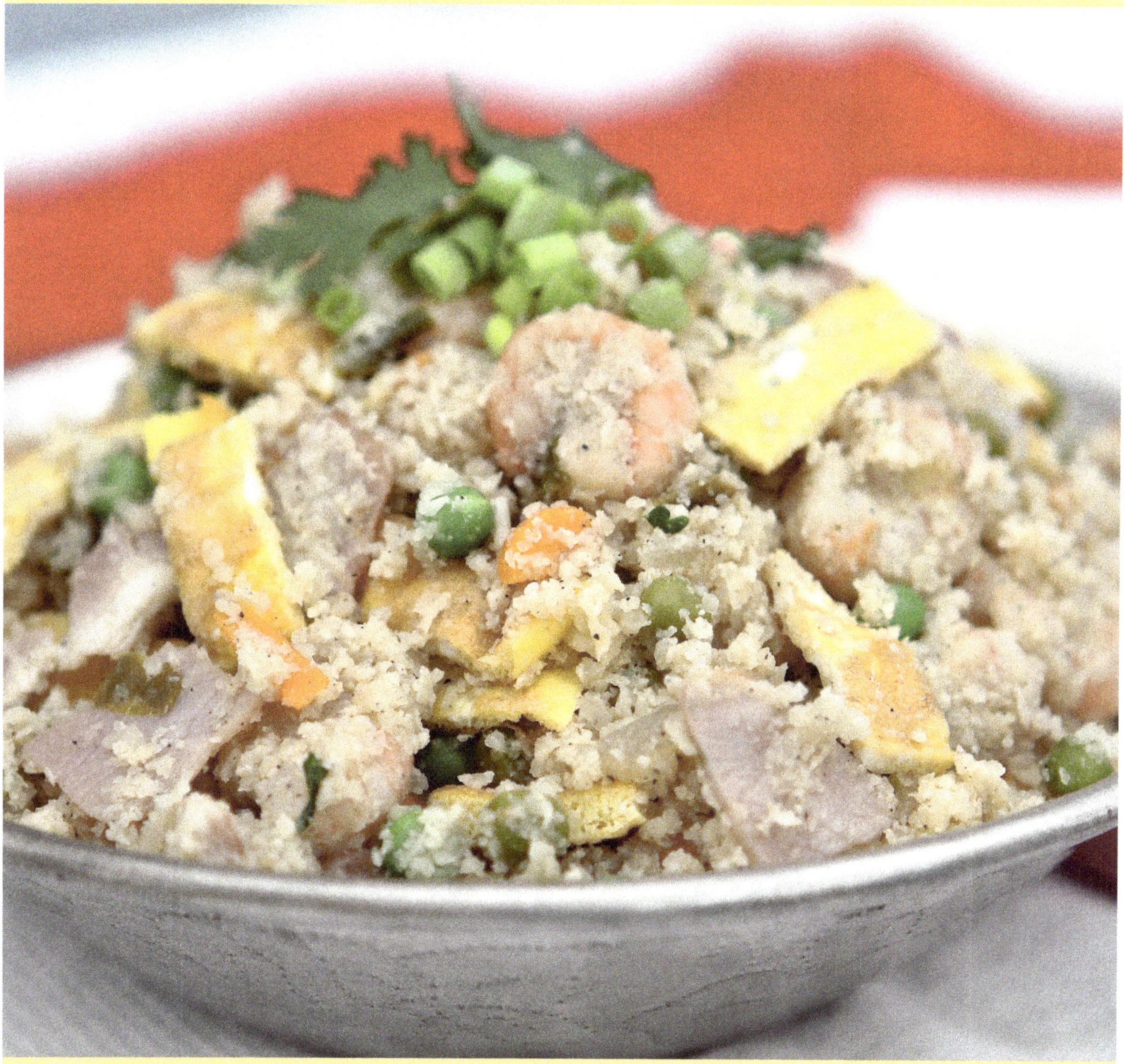

LUNCH & LIGHT MEALS | 165

MAIN MEALS

Beef Stroganoff..168

Bolognese with Sweet Potato Pasta.........................170

Traditional English Meat Loaf.................................172

Cranberry Meatballs...174

Sweet and Sour Meatballs.....................................176

Mexican Shepherd's Pie..178

Corned Silverside (Beef).......................................180

Lamb and Rosemary Pies......................................182

Sue's Irish Stew..184

Chicken and Leek Pie...186

Indian Butter Chicken..188

Green Thai Curry Chicken.....................................190

Crumbed Chicken...192

Turkey Meatloaf..194

Crunchy Nut Fish..196

Battered Fish and Seasoned Fries...........................198

Thai Fish Cakes..200

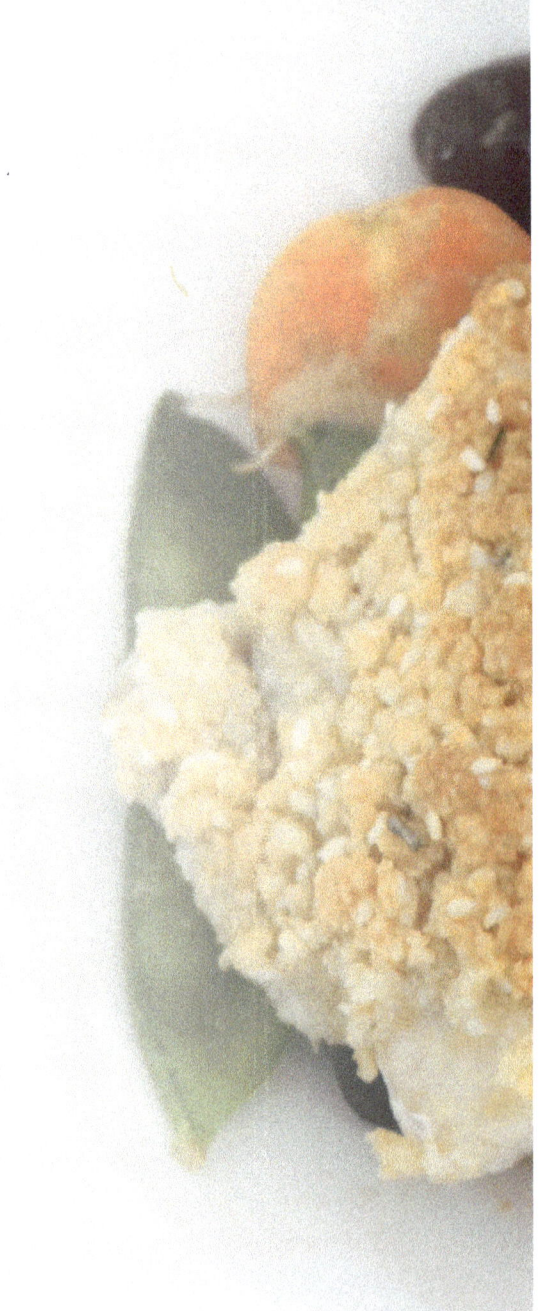

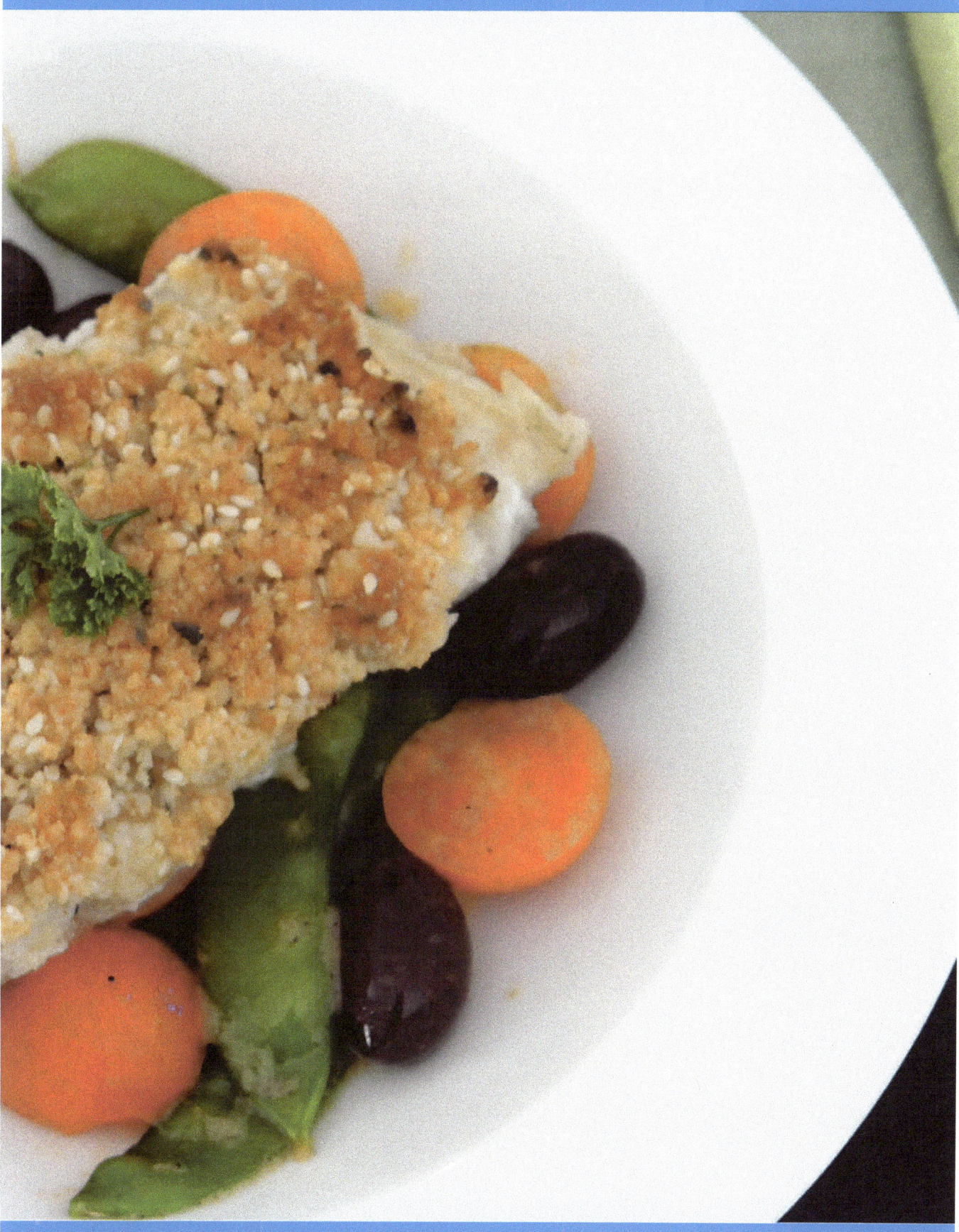

Beef Stroganoff

I have an old recipe file full of family recipes that I have cooked over the years. When I read my old Beef Stroganoff recipe, it reminded me of how we had turned to convenience and missed the nutritional side of cooking. The sauce was a can of "cream of mushroom soup". But now we have a real food Beef Stroganoff. Serve over zucchini noodles or organic Konjac fettuccine, also delicious with mashed cauliflower.

Prep time: 20 minutes Cooking time: 35 minutes Serves: 4

Ingredients:

- 3 Tbsp coconut oil, divided
- 750g/1.6lb beef strips, sirloin steak or stir-frying steak
- 2 onions halved and sliced
- 2 tsp garlic, minced
- 400g/14ozs mushrooms, sliced
- 1 cup beef broth/stock
- 2 Tbsp coconut aminos
- ½ tsp dried thyme leaves
- ½ tsp paprika
- 1½ tsp coarse sea salt
- ½ tsp ground pepper
- 1 cup canned coconut milk
- 1 Tbsp fresh chopped parsley, to garnish

Method:

Heat a large heavy-based frying pan or pot on medium-high heat. Melt 1½ tablespoons of coconut oil.

Cook beef strips in 3 batches. This will prevent meat from being steamed and getting tough. Cook for 2 minutes on each side and set aside for later. Add additional oil as needed.

Cut onions in half, lay on cut side and slice thinly. Add onions to pan. Cook for 5 minutes stirring frequently. Add garlic and mushrooms, continue cooking with onions for a further 5 minutes or until mushrooms start to brown.

Add beef stock, coconut aminos, spices and seasoning. Bring to a boil. Add cooked beef strips and stir through. Reduce to a simmer and cook uncovered for 10 minutes, (if you have a cheaper cut simmer for 20 minutes) or until tender.

Add coconut milk, simmer for a further 4-5 minutes.

Serve over your choice of paleo noodles or mashed cauliflower. Garnish with fresh parsley. Accompanied with lightly sautéed asparagus and green runner beans.

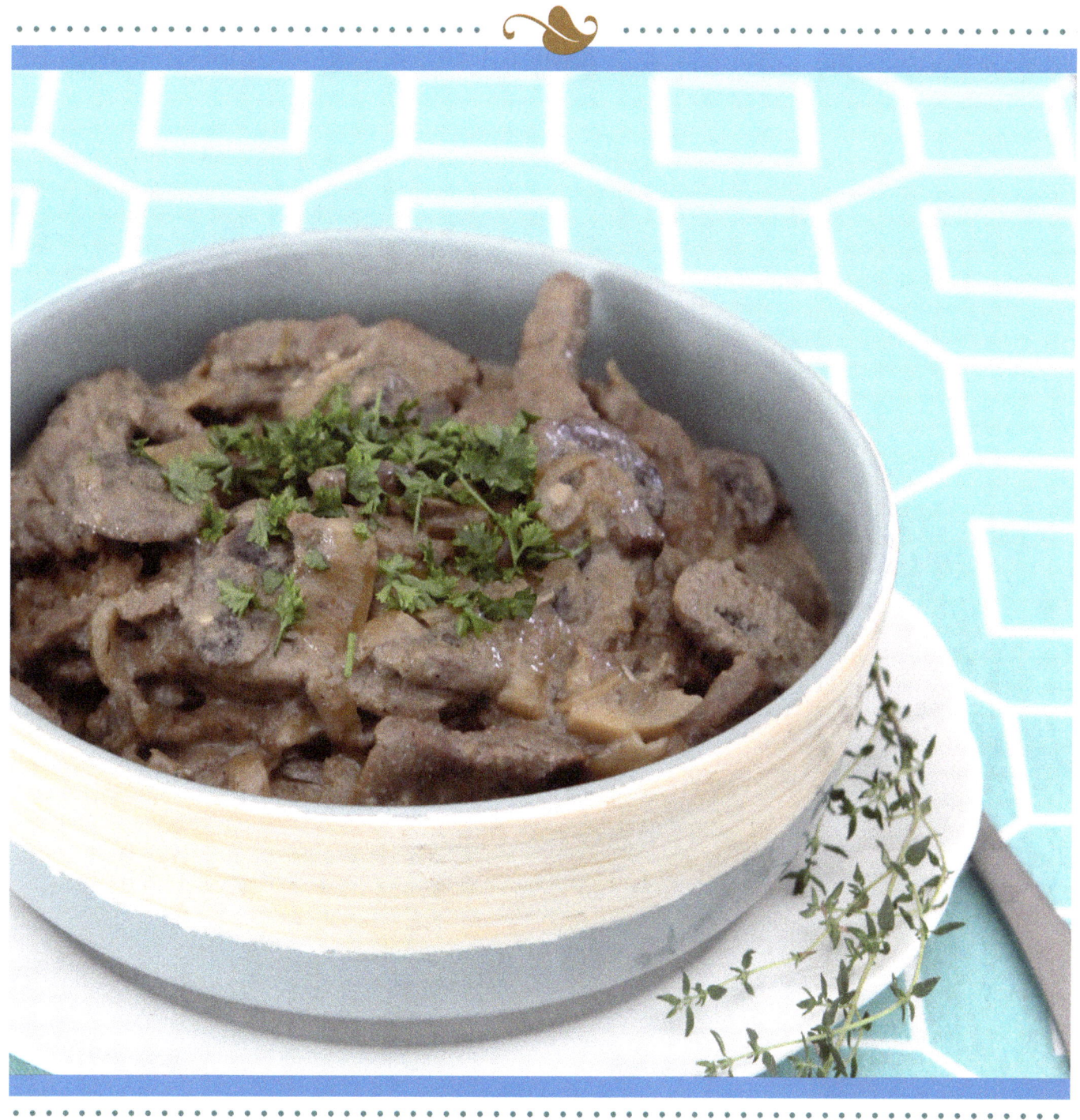

Bolognese with Sweet Potato Pasta

This Bolognese Sauce is flavourful but mild and goes wonderfully with the sweet potato pasta. Delicious for adults adults and kids. If you are wondering why milk is added, it lessens any sharpness of acidity from the tomato and makes for a smoother flavour.

Prep time: 20 minutes Cooking time: 45 minutes Serves: 4

Ingredients:

- 3 Tbsp ghee or coconut oil, divided
- 1 large onion, finely diced
- 3 tsp garlic, minced
- 2 sticks celery, finely diced
- 1 carrot, grated
- 500g/1.1lb beef mince or combination of beef and pork
- 1½ tsp coarse sea salt
- ½ cup almond milk or milk of choice
- 120g/½ cup organic tomato paste
- 1 cup beef broth or a mix of broth and red wine
- 2 cups bottled organic passata or tomato puree
- 2 Tbsp Apple Cider vinegar
- 1 Tbsp coconut sugar
- 3 bay leaves
- 2 tsp dried Italian herbs
- 1 tsp ground cinnamon
- ⅓ tsp ground pepper
- 1.2 kg/2.6lbs sweet potato, peeled, plus coconut oil for cooking
- Handful of fresh basil leaves, roughly chopped

Method:

Heat a large heavy based saucepan over low-medium heat. Melt half the oil. Add onion, garlic, celery and carrot. Cook for 5 minutes or until onion is soft. Transfer to a bowl and set aside. Add remaining oil to pan. Increase heat to high. Add beef and cook, breaking up until browned. Season with sea salt.

Reduce heat to medium. Add milk and cook, stirring occasionally for 5-6 minutes. Milk will reduce.

Add tomato paste and cook, stirring for 3 minutes. Add beef broth, passata, vinegar, sugar, bay leaves, Italian herbs, cinnamon, pepper and the cooked vegetables. Bring slowly to a boil. Reduce heat to low and simmer gently, uncovered, stirring occasionally for 35 minutes. Turn off the heat and remove the bay leaves and then toss through the chopped basil.

Meanwhile, prepare sweet potato pasta. Cut any large potatoes in half before spiraling. Use a spiral slicer or julienne slicer/peeler to make your pasta.

Heat a large non-stick frying pan on high and add 1 tablespoon of coconut oil. Add sweet potato pasta in batches. Cook, tossing to just soften the noodles for 2-3 minutes, you want the noodles al dente.

Serve pasta topped with Bolognese sauce and a leaf or two of fresh basil.

MAIN MEALS | 171

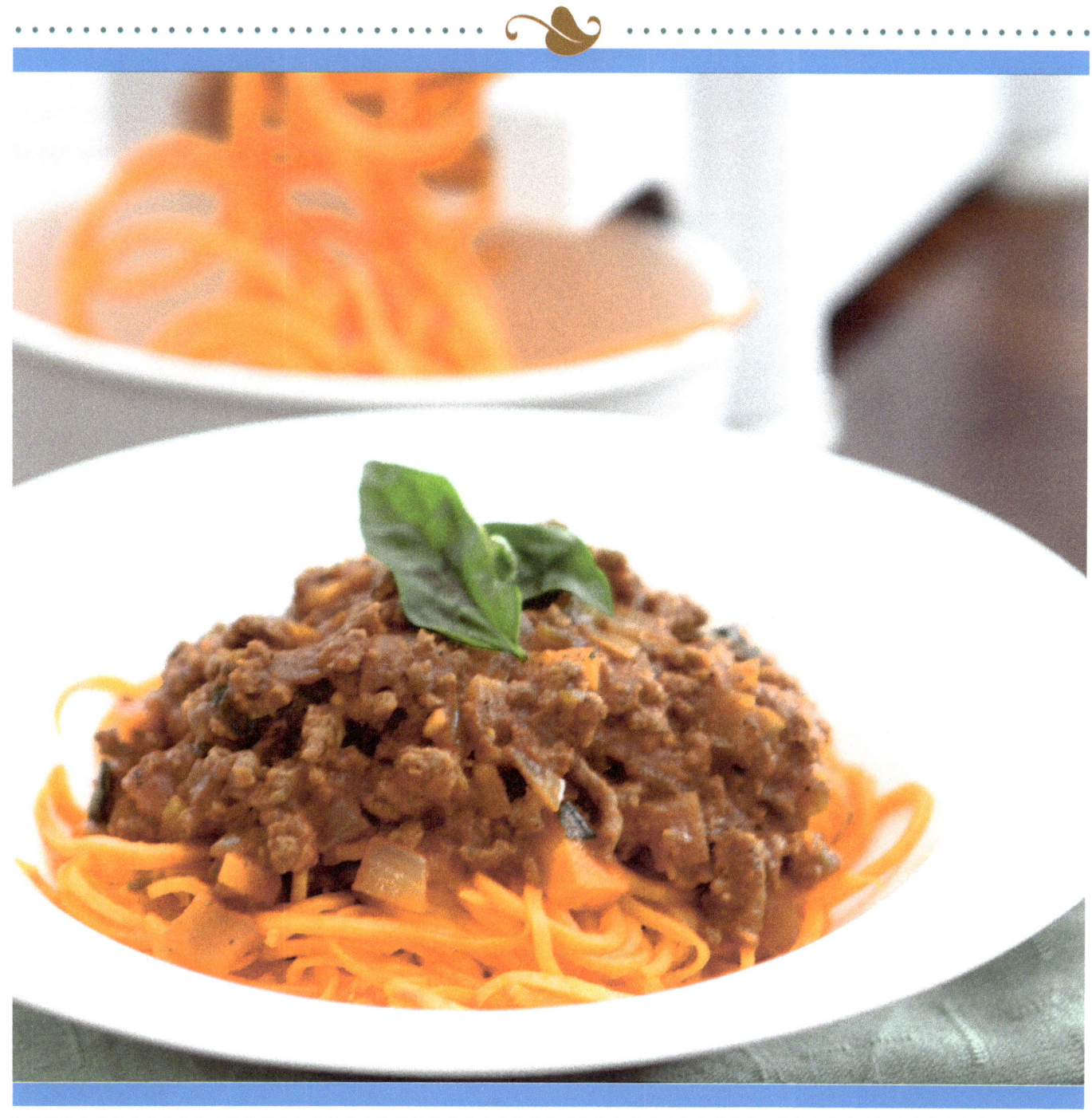

Traditional English Meat Loaf

This old traditional recipe has had its breadcrumbs removed and replaced with almond meal. For a nut free version, use sunflower meal. Make sure you use organic Worcestershire sauce so you avoid the gluten and additives. If possible find yourself a specialty Delicatessen that sells organic or grass fed nitrate free bacon.

Prep time: 15 minutes Cooking time: 55 minutes Serves: 6

Ingredients:

- 1½ Tbsp ghee
- 2 large or 3 small onions, finely diced
- ½ tsp coarse sea salt
- 1kg/2.2lb beef mince
- 1 large egg, beaten
- 2½ Tbsp organic Worcestershire sauce
- 1 cup almond meal
- ⅓ tsp sea salt
- ⅓ tsp pepper
- 4 hard boiled eggs
- 200g/7ozs streaky bacon (nitrate free)

Method:

Preheat oven to 180c/350f.

Heat a saucepan over medium heat and melt ghee. Add onions, cook for 2 minutes then sprinkle ½ teaspoon of sea salt into pan. This will bring out the liquid and prevent browning. Cook until tender. Set aside.

To a large bowl add beef mince, egg, Worcestershire sauce, almond meal, salt and pepper. Mix well with your hands, making sure all ingredients combine well. Add cooked onions and mix through.

Grease the bottom of a baking pan or tray. Take half of your mixture and place on the baking pan, make a rectangle, press mixture firmly together. Make an indent along your meat to place your hard-boiled eggs in.

Place the remaining half of the mixture on top of the eggs, molding top and bottom together. Press firmly to ensure the mixture comes together in a log shape with eggs hidden inside and the ends sealed.

Take bacon strips and wrap around the 2 ends first, then lay the remaining strips neatly across the top of the meat loaf, touching each other. Insert a toothpick on each end of the bacon strips, leaving just a little sticking out. This will keep the bacon in place while cooking.

Cook for 55 minutes or until juices have started to dry up in bottom of pan. Let stand for 10 minutes before slicing, remove toothpicks.

Serve with seasonal vegetables, tomato sauce/ketchup or gravy page 204.

MAIN MEALS | 173

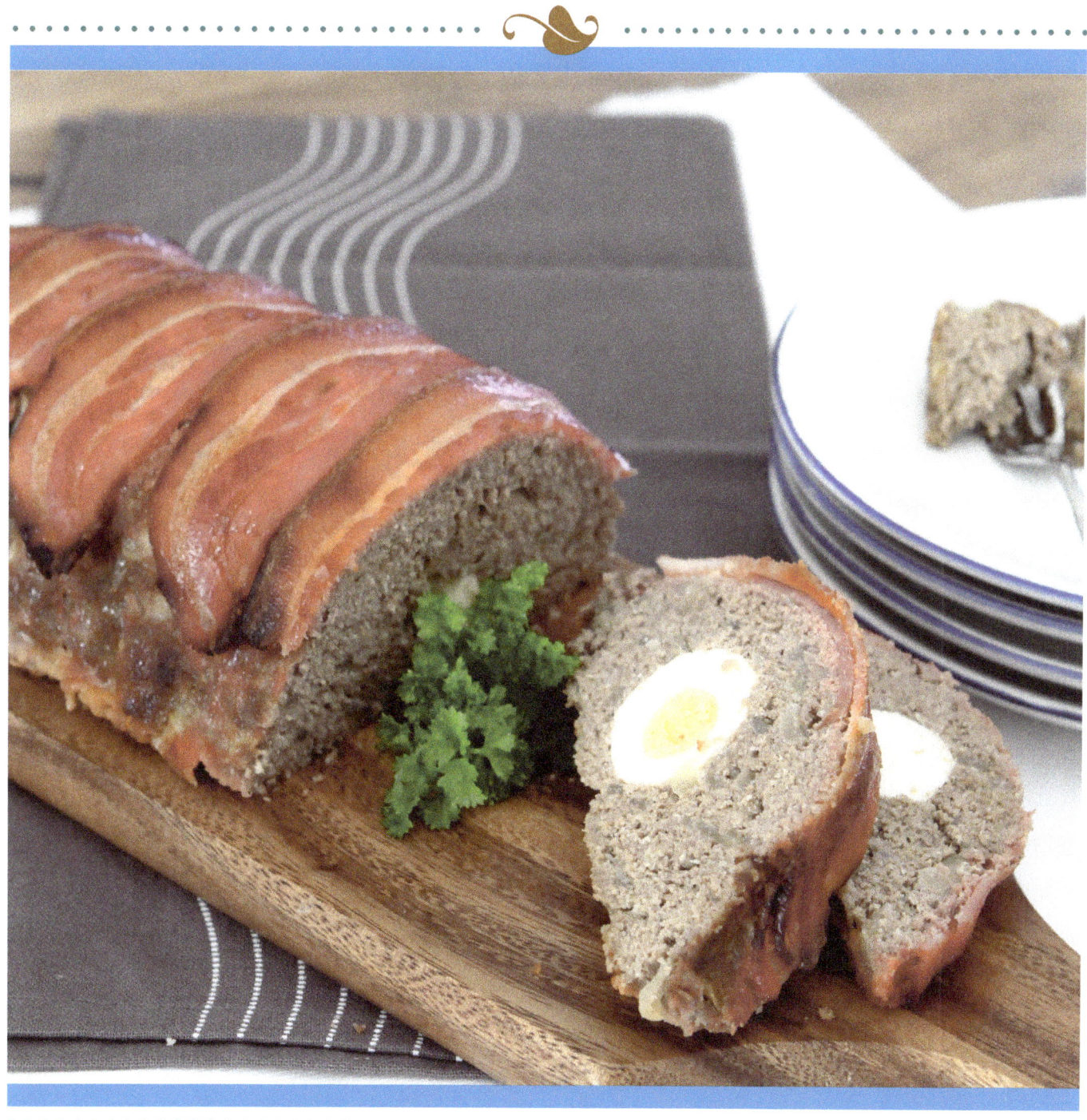

Cranberry Meatballs

This is a great party recipe, you can stick toothpicks into the meatballs so people can help themselves. I love the fragrant smell of the kitchen while the meatballs are cooking. The celery seeds have anti-inflammatory and anti-bacterial properties, while caraway is known for its anti-oxidant and digestive properties. Cardamom is an exotic spice that has anti-oxidant and disease preventing properties too.

Prep time: 30 minutes   Cooking time: 45 minutes   Makes: 30 meatballs

Ingredients:

SAUCE
- 113g/4oz Organic Dried Cranberries (I use Eden Organic)
- ¾ cup filtered water, to simmer cranberries
- 185ml/¾ cup Organic Sweet Chili Sauce
- 500ml/2 cups organic passata or tomato puree
- 2 Tbsp Apple Cider vinegar
- ¼ cup organic coconut sugar
- ⅓ cup filtered water
- 2 tsp beef bone broth powder (I use Nutra Organics brand)
- ¾ tsp sea salt

MEATBALLS
- 2 tsp caraway seeds
- 1½ Tbsp celery seeds
- ¾ tsp cardamom seeds
- 1 onion, finely diced
- 1 cup almond meal/flour or sunflower meal
- 1½ tsp fine sea salt
- 2 eggs, beaten
- 1kg/2.2lb beef mince

Method:

In a medium saucepan add dried cranberries and water. Simmer for 15 minutes or until they become plump, stir often. Add the remaining sauce ingredients. Bring to a boil and reduce to a simmer for a further 15 minutes, stirring often.

Preheat oven to 180c/350f. Line 2 large baking trays with baking paper.

To a blender add caraway, celery and cardamom seeds and whiz for a few seconds to break up seeds.

To a large bowl add, onion, almond meal, ground spices, salt and eggs. Use a fork to combined well.

Add beef mince to bowl, use hands to combine meatball mixture together.

Shape mixture into balls about the size of golf balls and place on baking trays. Makes approximately 30 meatballs. Bake for 25-30 minutes or until just turning brown.

Place meatballs into a large pot with a lid, pour over sauce. Simmer covered on the stovetop for 10-15 minutes for the meatballs to absorb some sauce.

Tip: For large gatherings double the recipe and serve from a slow cooker to keep them warm.

MAIN MEALS | 175

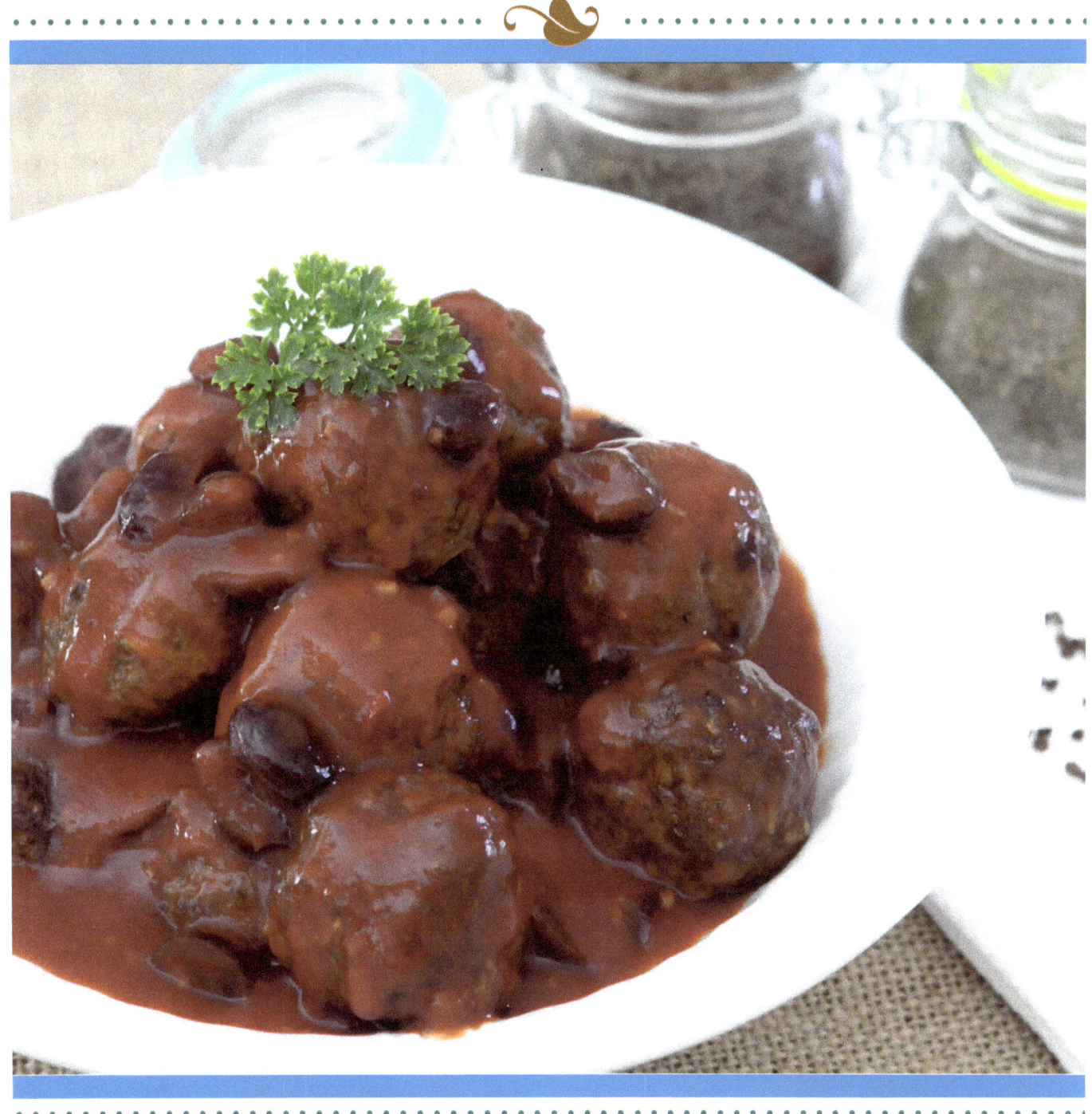

Sweet and Sour Meatballs

Fresh pineapple pureed into the meatball sauce gives it a depth of flavour. Serve this dish over cauliflower mash; the white sets off the deep colour of the sauce. Make a small well in the centre of each serve of cauliflower mash to place the meatballs and sauce in. You may like to garnish with a sprinkling of chopped parsley and a few pieces of pineapple.

Prep time: 30 minutes Cooking time: 35 minutes Serves: 6 (makes 30 meatballs)

Ingredients:

MEATBALLS
- 1 large onion, cut into quarters
- 2 cloves garlic
- 2 tsp ginger, chopped or minced
- ¼ cup coconut flour
- 1 tsp coarse sea salt
- ¾ tsp ground paprika
- 2 eggs
- 500g/1.1lb minced beef
- 500g/1.1lb minced pork

SAUCE
- 1½ cups fresh pineapple, diced (¼ small pineapple) or 440g can unsweetened pineapple, drained
- 3 Tbsp water to add to blender with pineapple
- 1 Tbsp ghee for frying
- 1 onion, diced finely
- 2 tsp garlic, minced
- 1 tsp ginger, minced
- ¼ cup coconut sugar
- 1 Tbsp organic molasses, unsulphured
- 700ml/13.5oz jar organic passata or tomato puree
- ⅓ cup coconut aminos
- ¼ cup Apple Cider vinegar
- 1 tsp Dijon mustard
- 1½ tsp coarse sea salt
- ¼ tsp pepper

Method:

Preheat oven to 180c/350f. Line 2 baking trays with baking paper.

To a food processor, add onion, garlic and ginger, pulse until onion is finely minced.

Add coconut flour, salt and paprika. Give one or two quick pulses. Add the eggs and meat, blend until all ingredients are combined.

Form meat mixture into balls. Mixture will be quite soft, so use your hands to pat into a ball shape. Place meatballs on trays and bake for 30-35 minutes or until starting to brown. (Makes 30 meatballs). While the meatballs are cooking make your sauce.

Remove skin and eyes from pineapple and dice. Puree pineapple with 3 tablespoons of water in a blender (should produce approximately 1 cup of thick juice). Set aside.

In a large heavy based pot over medium-low heat, melt ghee. Add onion, garlic and ginger. Cook for 4-5 minutes or until onion is soft and transparent. Add coconut sugar and molasses stirring to incorporate with onion. Add pureed pineapple and remaining sauce ingredients. Bring to a boil, reduce and let simmer for 20 minutes.

Place cooked meatballs into sauce and continue to simmer for a further 10 minutes, for meatballs to absorb a little sauce. (If making ahead of time, leave adding meatballs until 10 minutes before serving).

Serve over cauliflower mash page 116 and sprinkle with chopped fresh parsley.

MAIN MEALS | 177

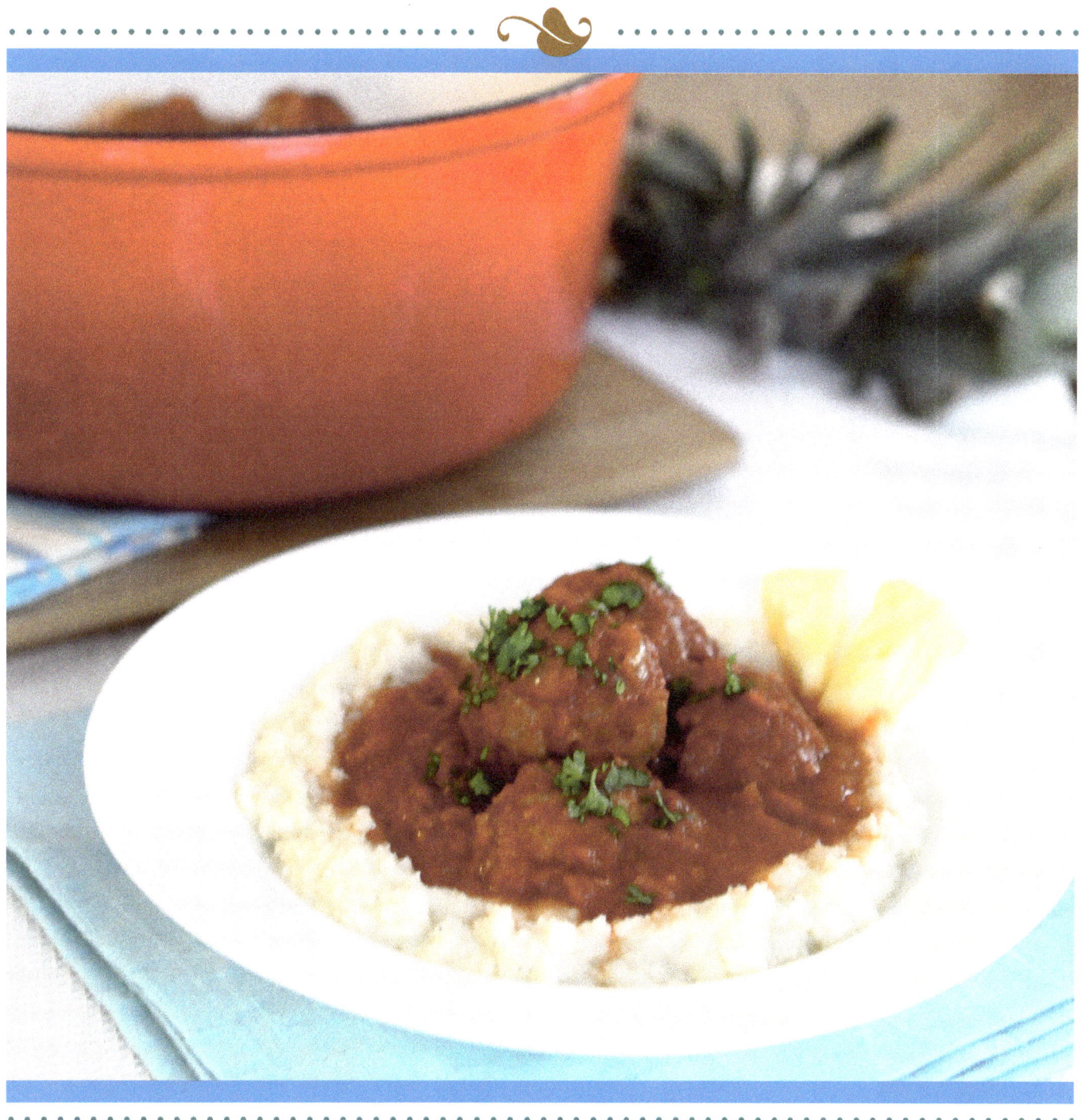

Mexican Shepherd's Pie

This is a twist on the regular Shepherd's Pie recipe. I have topped the pie with mashed sweet potato but mashed cauliflower would work too.

Prep time: 20 minutes Cooking time: 40 minutes Serves: 4-6

Ingredients:

- 1½ Tbsp ghee or coconut oil
- 1 large onion, diced
- 2 carrots, finely diced
- 2 tsp garlic, minced
- 2 Tbsp ground cumin
- 2 tsp dried oregano
- ½ tsp chili powder or to taste
- ½ tsp paprika
- 700g/1.5lb minced beef
- 1 cup organic passata or tomato puree
- ½ cup filtered water or broth
- 2 Tbsp organic Worcestershire sauce
- 1 tsp coarse sea salt
- ¼ tsp ground pepper
- 1 cup frozen green peas, optional

TOPPING
- 1.3kg/2.8lb sweet potato, peeled and cubed
- 1½-2 Tbsp ghee
- Sea salt and pepper to taste

Method:

Grease an ovenproof dish that holds approximately 10 cups (I use a 23cm square dish).

In a large heavy based saucepan on medium heat, melt 1 tablespoon of oil. Add onion, carrot and garlic. Cook for 5 minutes or until vegetables have softened, stirring frequently.

Add dried spices with the remaining ½ tablespoon oil and mix them through the vegetables and cook for 1 minute, until fragrant.

Push vegetable mixture to outer sides of saucepan and add minced beef. Break up any lumps of meat and once it changes colour mix through the vegetables.

Add passata, water, Worcestershire sauce, salt and pepper. Bring to a boil. Then reduce to a simmer and cook uncovered for 20 minutes, stirring occasionally.

Add peas during the last 5 minutes.

Preheat oven to 180c/350f.

To make the topping, boil the sweet potatoes until soft. Drain and place back in saucepan, add ghee, salt and pepper. Mash to a smooth consistency, if you feel the potato needs milk add a little at a time. You want the potato smooth and creamy with no lumps, but not sloppy.

Spoon beef mixture evenly into the ovenproof dish. Spoon sweet potato topping over mixture. Smooth over with a spatula. Use a fork to run decorative lines over the topping or use a spatula to make swirling marks.

Place in preheated oven under top element or grill for approximately 10 minutes or until topping is lightly browned. Watch closely to prevent burning.

MAIN MEALS | 179

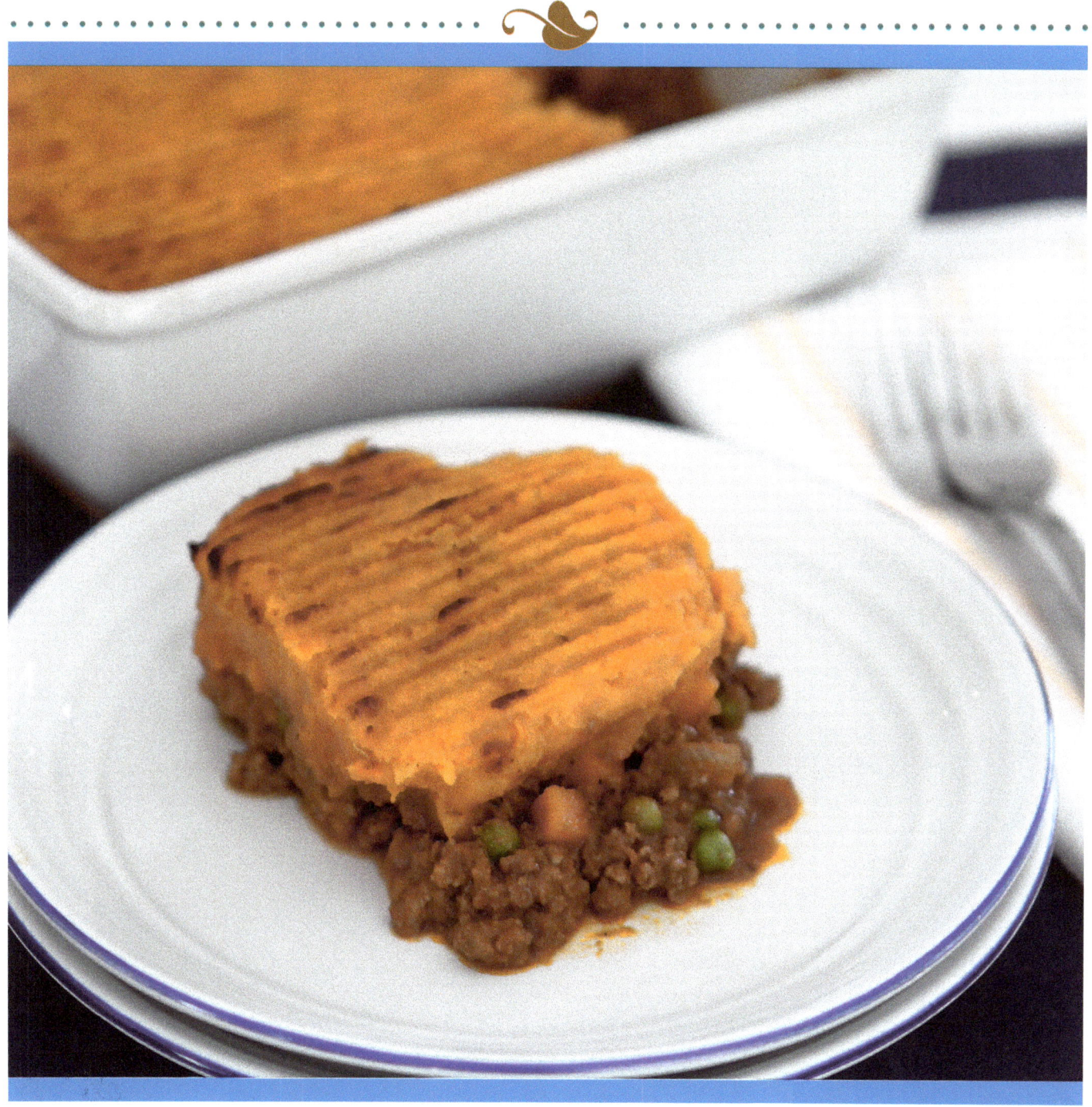

Corned Silverside (Beef)

"Corned" refers to the large grains of salt traditionally used to preserve meat. This is one of the oldest ways meat was preserved or pickled, I have added spices to the salt and sugar. Regular corned beef is prepared with added nitrites and chemicals. Excessive consumption of nitrites has been linked to various health problems. The meat in this recipe won't be as red, it will be a more greyish colour as no chemicals have been added. The flavour is so delicious you won't miss the colour.

Prep time: 5 minutes Cooking time: 4 hrs on high or 8 hrs on low Serves: 6

Ingredients:

- 1.5kg/3.3lb whole piece grass fed Beef Gerrelo (or use Virginia silverside trimmed lean)
- ¼ cup fine sea salt
- 2 tsp coconut sugar
- 1 Tbsp cinnamon
- 1 tsp ground cloves
- 1 tsp mustard powder
- ½ tsp ground nutmeg
- ½ tsp ground ginger

TO COOK
- Filtered water
- ⅓ cup Apple Cider vinegar
- 2 Tbsp 100% maple syrup
- Assorted vegetables (choose from swede, parsnip, carrot, sweet potato, baby onions, cabbage)

Method:

Use a tray with sides. Place your piece of beef on tray and pierce several times with a skewer.

To a small bowl add, salt, sugar and spices, mix to combined. Rub spice mixture all over the meat, pressing in well. Any spice mix that falls away, rub back into the meat. Cover and store in fridge for 36 hours.

Remove tray somewhere between 12-18 hours and drain off blood that has been draw out of meat. Re-cover and place back in fridge for the duration of pickling time.

After 36 hours, rinse meat under filtered water, washing off all the salt and spice mix. Turn your slow cooker to high. Add meat and fill with water up to ¾ level of the meat. Add Apple Cider vinegar and maple syrup and cover. When water has heated turn to low if cooking for 8 hours.

When cooking on high, at the 2 hour mark, add chopped vegetables of choice. If cooking on low, add vegetables at the 4 hour mark.

Before removing cooked meat and vegetables, check if they are tender or leave a further 30 minutes.

To serve, slice meat and serve with drained vegetables. Condiments that you may like to use; mustard, tomato sauce/ketchup or White Cauliflower sauce on page 212 or all of them.

MAIN MEALS | 181

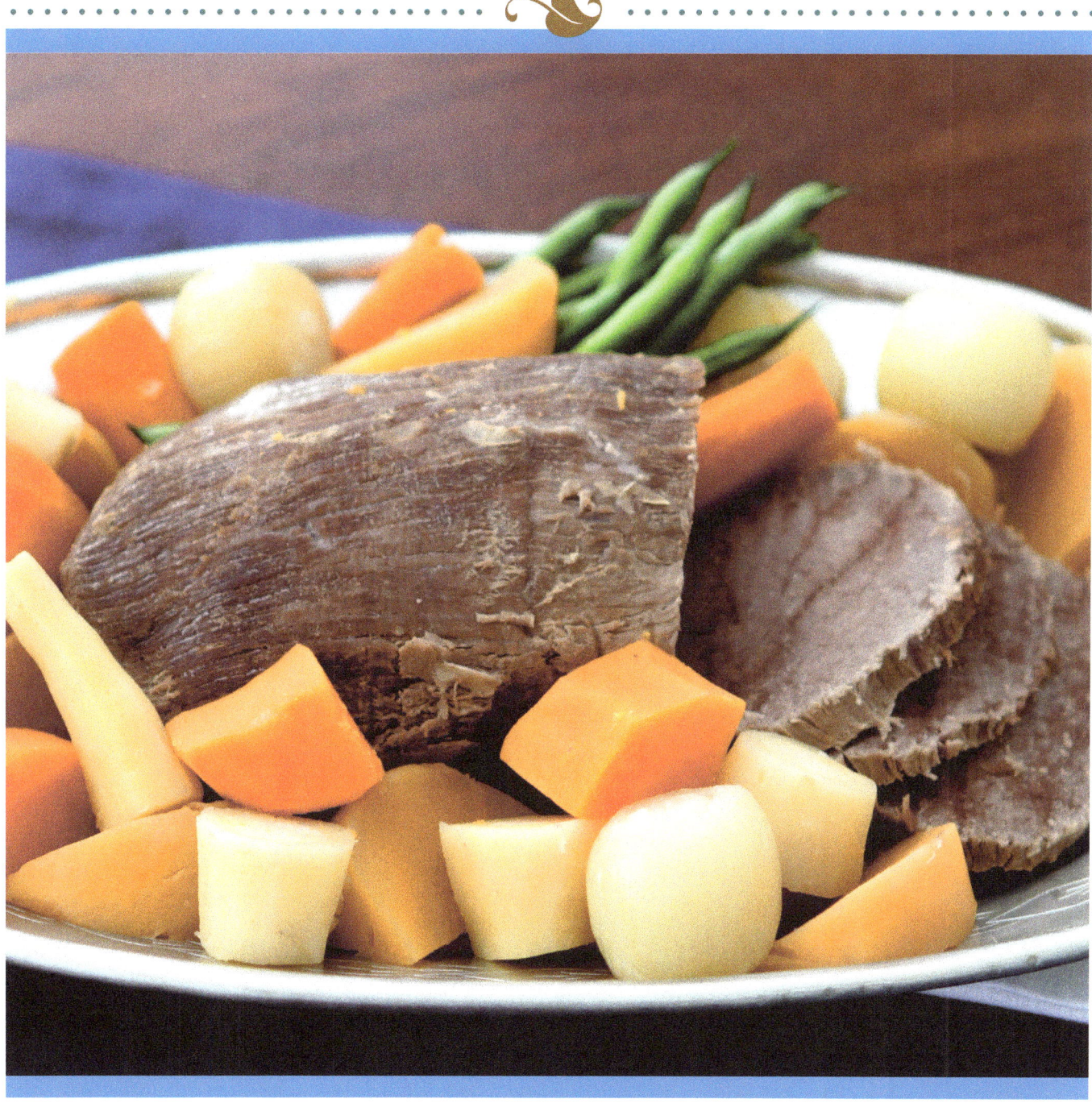

Lamb and Rosemary Pies

I've made individual pies but you can make one large pie if you prefer. I have blended some of the vegetables from the pot to produce a flavoursome gravy without thickeners.

Prep time: 30 minutes Cooking time: 50 minutes Serves: 6

Ingredients:

- 3 Tbsp ghee, divided
- 850g/1.9lb lamb steak or boneless shoulder, diced
- 1 large onion, diced
- 2 large carrots, diced
- 2 sticks celery, finely chopped
- 1 tsp garlic, minced
- 2 cups beef broth/stock
- 2 Tbsp organic Worcestershire sauce
- 2 Tbsp organic tomato passata or puree
- 1½ Tbsp fresh chopped rosemary leaves
- 1 tsp coarse sea salt
- ⅛ tsp ground pepper

PASTRY
- 3 cups almond meal/flour
- 1 Tbsp coconut flour
- 1 Tbsp arrowroot flour
- 1 tsp Herbamare seasoned salt
- ¾ tsp baking soda
- ⅓ cup macadamia oil
- 2 Tbsp water
- 1 egg, beaten for egg wash

Method:

Heat a large saucepan on medium-high heat. Melt 1½ tablespoons of ghee. Brown lamb in small batches, 1-2 minutes per side, keep heat high so lamb doesn't steam and become tough. Set lamb aside.

Reduce heat to medium. Melt remaining ghee and add onion, carrot, celery and garlic, cook for 5 minutes, stirring often.

Add lamb back to the pot, add broth, Worcestershire sauce, tomato passata, rosemary, salt and pepper. Bring to a boil, then reduce to a simmer. Simmer for 30 minutes.

Meanwhile, make your pastry. To a food processor add, almond meal, coconut flour, arrowroot flour, herbamare seasoned salt and baking soda. Pulse a couple of times to combine. Add oil and water. Process until everything comes together into a ball.

Divide pastry into 6 equal portions, cover and place in fridge.

Preheat oven to 160c/320f. Grease 6 individual 10cm(4in) pie dishes.

Transfer 2½ cups of vegetables and liquid from saucepan to a blender. Blend for a couple of seconds to just break up vegetables to make a thick gravy. Add back to saucepan and mix through.

Fill each pie dish with meat and vegetable filling.

Remove pastry portions one at a time from fridge. Place between 2 sheets of baking paper. Use a rolling pin to roll a circle with a diameter of 11cm(4.5in). Remove top sheet and carefully lift with your hand under baking paper and flip over on top of the filled pie dish. Trim edges and press pastry to the dish rim. Carefully poke a fork into the top of pastry to releasing steam while cooking. Repeat for each pie.

Using a pastry brush, egg wash the pies immediately before placing in oven. Bake for 20 minutes or until pastry is light brown and crisp. Serve with Cauliflower mash, page 116 and steamed broccoli.

MAIN MEALS | 183

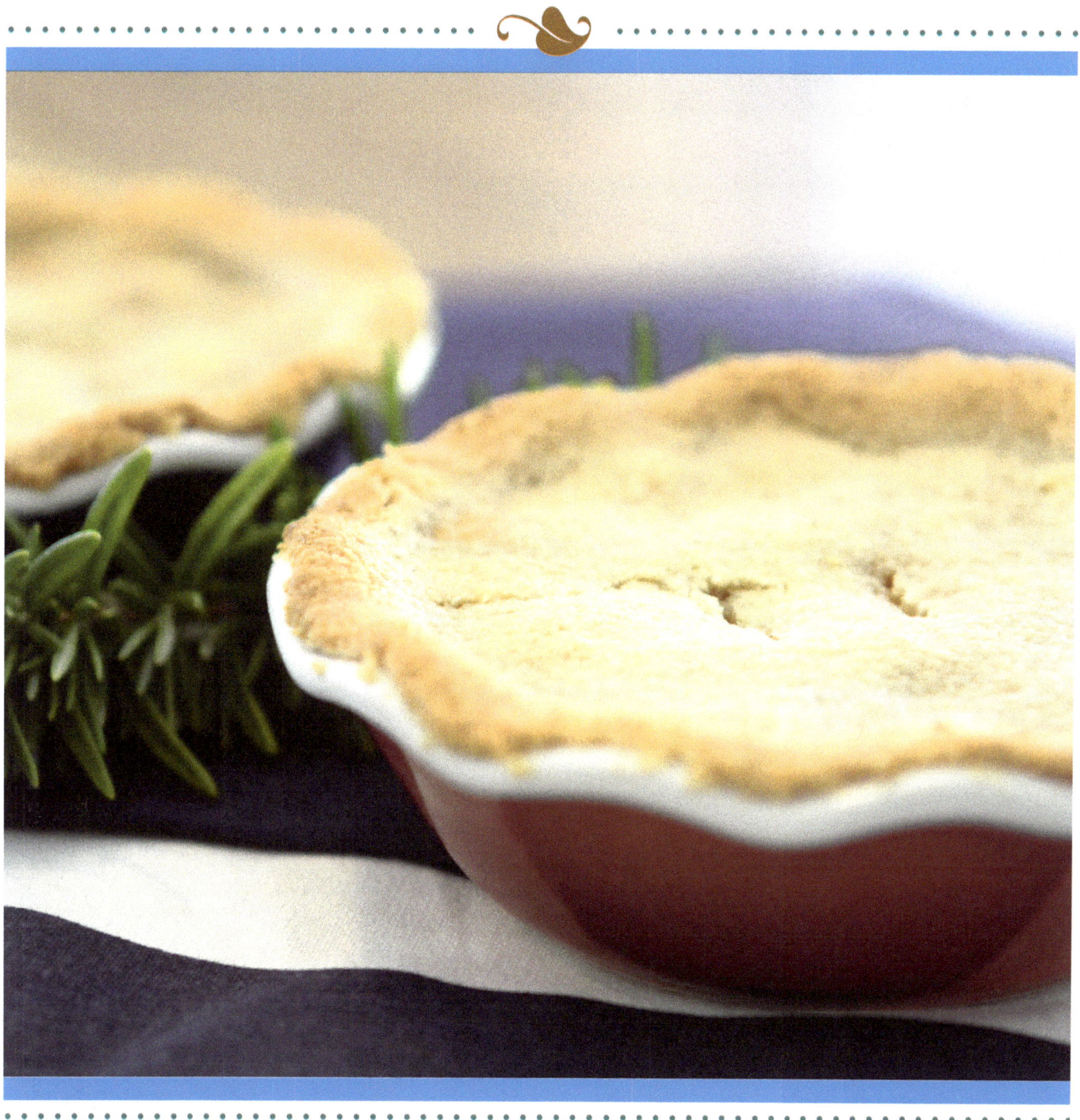

Sue's Irish Stew

Traditional Irish Stew is nothing more than mutton, onions and potatoes. No potatoes in this recipe, I have substituted with swede, celeriac and carrots. Other vegetables that would work are turnips or parsnips. The most important aspect of this recipe is that it becomes a bone broth within a Stew. Make sure to purchase lamb on the bone instead of just lamb meat, the bones will simmer for a couple of hours allowing the gelatin and nutrients from the bones to go into your stew.

Prep time: 15 minutes Cooking time: 2 hours Serves: 4-5

Ingredients:

- 1 Tbsp ghee or coconut oil
- 1kg-1.3kg/2.2-2.8lb lamb chops, depends on the amount of fat to remove (I use forequarter or loin chops)
- 2 large onions, roughly diced
- 3 cups beef broth/stock, or enough to cover meat by 3cm
- 2 Tbsp organic Worcestershire sauce
- 1 Tbsp Apple Cider vinegar
- 3 swede, in chunks
- 1 celeriac, in chunks
- 3 carrots, in chunks
- 1½ tsp coarse sea salt
- ½ tsp ground pepper
- 1 cup frozen peas, optional
- 3 Tbsp arrowroot flour with a little water to make a slurry

Method:

Trim lamb chops of fat. Cut some meat off the bones, so some meat breaks up in the stew to help make a rich gravy.

Heat a large stock/soup pot on medium-high heat. Melt ghee and brown meat in batches to seal, 1-2 minutes per side. Set aside.

Add onions to pot and cook for 3 minutes in the meat juices. Return meat to pot with onions.

Add broth/stock, Worcestershire sauce and Apple Cider vinegar and bring to a boil, reduce and simmer for 1¼ hours.

Add swede and celeriac, cook for 15 minutes. Then add carrots, sea salt and pepper. Continue to simmer until all vegetables are tender and meat should be falling off the bones. 10 minutes before serving, add frozen peas.

Make a slurry with arrowroot flour and a little water, add to pot, stir until gravy thickens. Add extra stock if more gravy is required. Avoid strong boiling after adding arrowroot slurry.

Remove some of the bones that meat has fallen off before serving. Serve with grain free bread or plain scones to dip into the gravy.

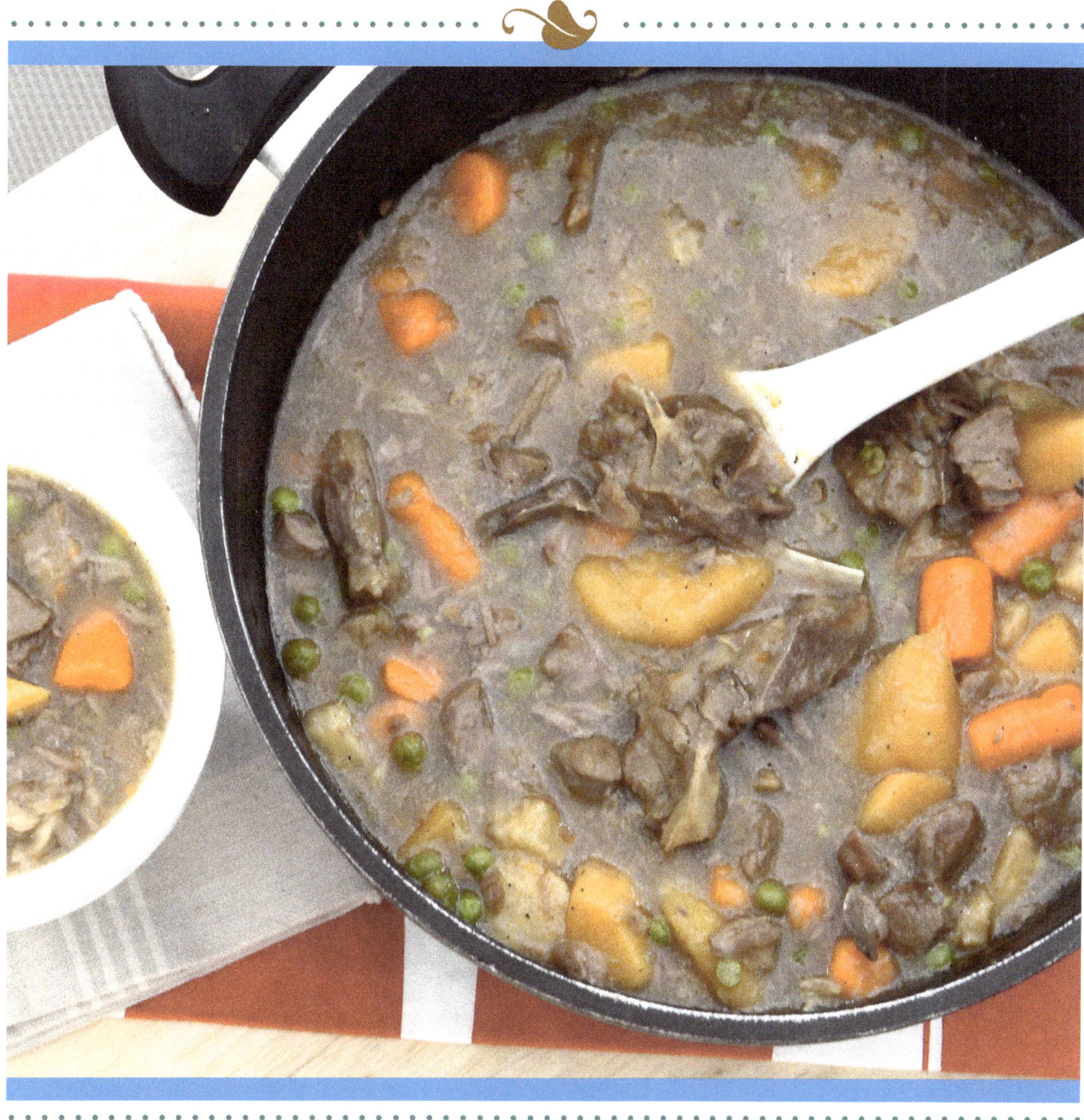

Chicken and Leek Pie

You would normally use shortcrust pastry for this recipe. I am hoping you will be pleasantly surprised with my version. The leek imparts a mellow, sweet onion flavour to this pie.

Prep time: 35 minutes   Cooking time: 50 minutes   Serves: 4

Ingredients:

FILLING
- 1½ Tbsp coconut oil plus extra to grease baking dish
- 1 onion, finely diced
- 1 large leek, finely sliced
- 800g/1.7lb skinless chicken breast or thigh, diced
- 3 tsp coconut flour
- 1 cup coconut milk
- 2 Tbsp Dijon mustard
- 1 tsp sea salt
- ⅓ tsp ground pepper

PASTRY
- 1 Tbsp flaxseed meal
- 2 Tbsp water to soak flaxseed
- 1½ cups almond meal/flour
- 2 Tbsp arrowroot flour
- ½ tsp Herbamare seasoned salt or fine sea salt
- ¼ tsp baking soda
- 2 Tbsp macadamia oil
- 2 tsp filtered water
- 1 egg, beaten for egg wash

Method:

Heat a large frying pan over medium heat. Melt oil, add onion and leek. Cook for 7-8 minutes stirring often, or until softened.

Increase heat, add chicken and cook for 9-10 minutes or until just cooked through. Sprinkle the coconut flour over the chicken mixture in pan and mix through well.

Reduce the heat and pour the coconut milk into the pan. Stir until it simmers. Add mustard, salt and pepper. Stir through to combine and simmer for a further 5 minutes.

Spoon mixture into a greased 6 cup capacity baking dish. Set aside to cool slightly, while you make pastry.

To make pastry: Preheat oven to 180c/350f. Add flaxseed and water to a small jug and mix. Let sit for 5 minutes before using.

To a food processor add, almond meal, arrowroot flour, herbed salt and baking soda. Pulse 3-4 times to mix dry ingredients. Add macadamia oil, water and flaxseed mix. Blend until the dough comes together and forms a ball.

Roll pastry between two sheets of baking paper similar to the shape of your baking dish but a little larger. Don't roll it too thin or it will be hard to handle. Remove top sheet of paper and slide your hand under bottom sheet, turnover so pastry lands over the dish. Trim overhang with a knife. If any cracks appear, press together, pastry may break but it's easy to repair.

Re-roll trimmings and cut into thin strips to place around the rim of your dish to make a double layer. Pinch with your fingers to make a decorative edge. Using a sharp knife, cut a cross in the middle of your pie to let out any steam. Use a pastry brush to egg wash pie and edges.

Place straight into the oven. Bake for 25 minutes or until pastry is golden. Serve with a garden salad.

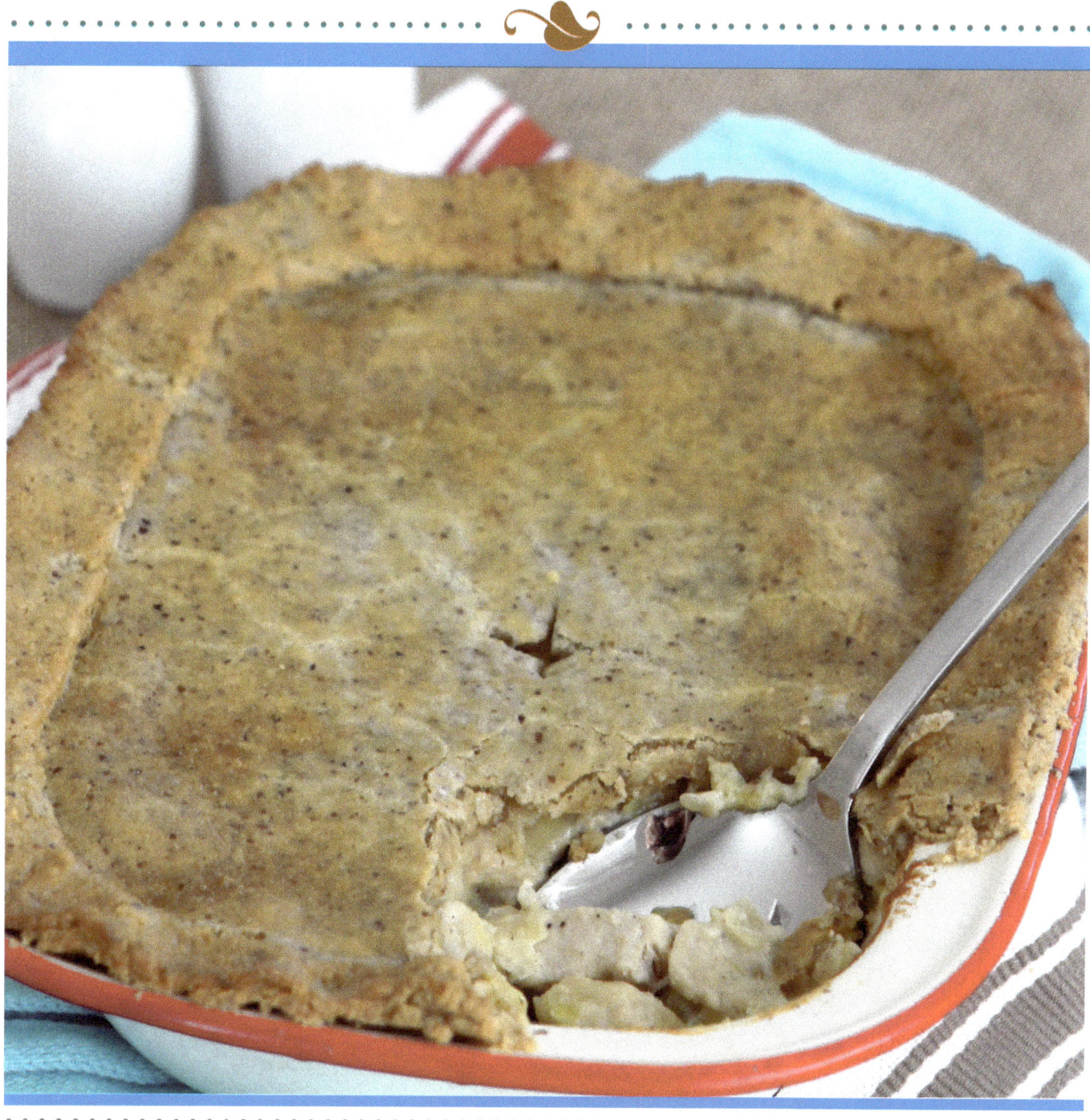

Indian Butter Chicken

This Indian specialty is so delicious. Adjust the spices to suit your own taste buds. Enjoy the Naan bread on page 74 to dip into the butter chicken sauce.

Prep time: 15 minutes plus marinating time
Cooking time: 40 minutes Serves: 5-6

Ingredients:

1kg/2.2lb skinless chicken breast, tenderloins or thigh, cubed

MARINADE
½ cup canned coconut cream, room temperature
Juice of 1 lime
½ tsp ground turmeric
½ tsp ground cumin
¼ tsp paprika
¼ tsp ground coriander
¼ tsp Garam Masala
¼ tsp of sea salt and ground pepper

BUTTER CHICKEN SAUCE
1½ Tbsp coconut oil
1 large onion, diced
4 tsp garlic, minced
2 tsp ginger, minced
1 tsp ground coriander
½ tsp Garam Masala
½ tsp cayenne pepper
500ml/2 cups organic passata or tomato puree
1½ cups canned coconut milk
2 cups diced pumpkin
¾ tsp sea salt or to taste

Method:

Add chicken and marinade ingredients to a sealed glass container. Mix well to combine. Refrigerate for 1-2 hours, before cooking the sauce.

Heat a large heavy based saucepan on medium heat, add coconut oil. Cook onion, garlic and ginger for 5 minutes or until soft.

Add coriander, garam masala and cayenne pepper. Mix through the onion mixture for 30 seconds or until fragrant.

Increase heat and add chicken and marinade to pot. Stir often until chicken changes colour.

Add passata, coconut milk, pumpkin and salt. Bring to a boil, then reduce to a simmer. Cook uncovered for 35 minutes or until chicken and pumpkin are tender.

Serve with Naan bread page 74, natural coconut or Greek yoghurt, diced cucumber and lime wedges. Then garnish with fresh coriander.

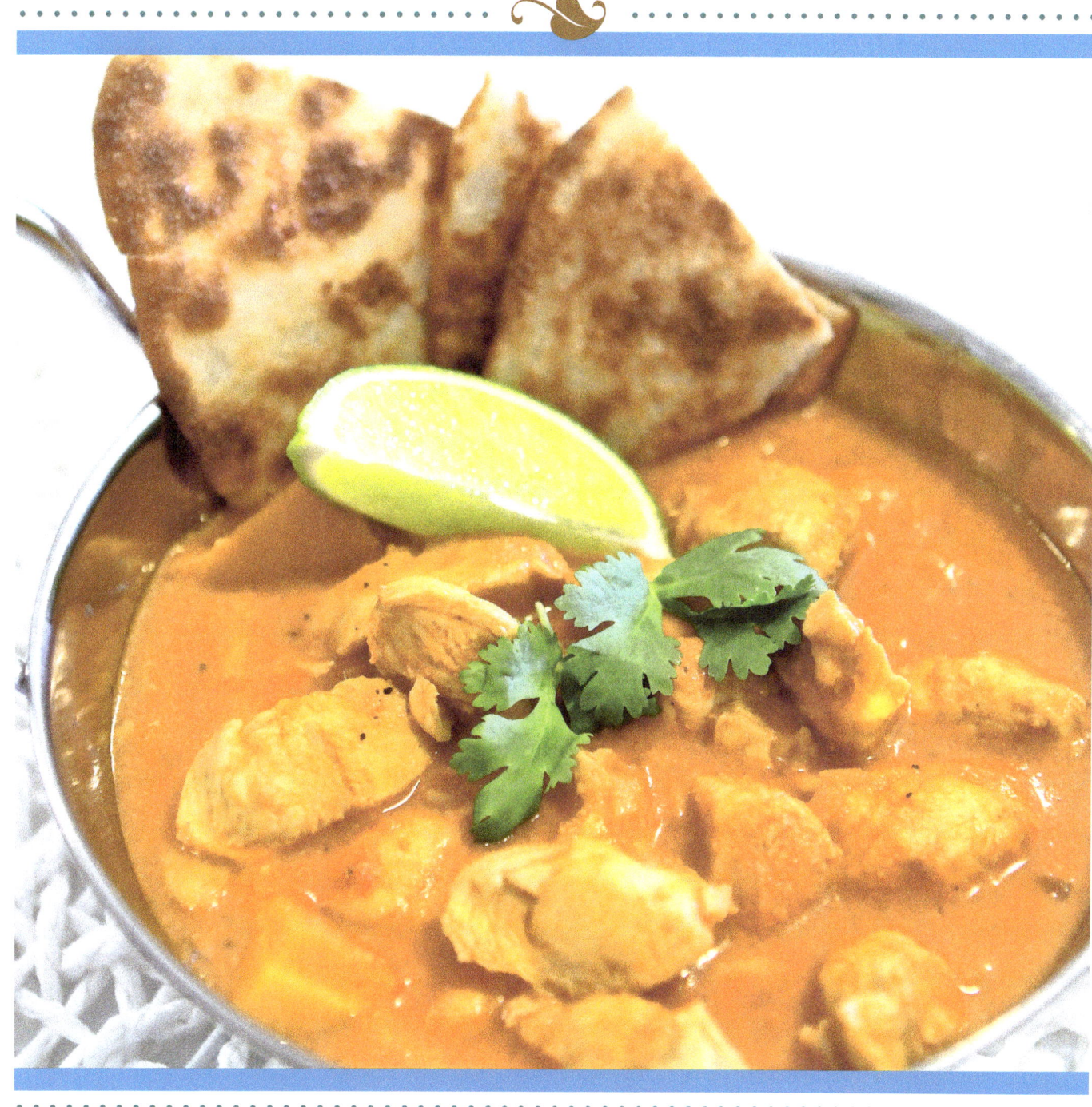

Green Thai Curry Chicken

This is a quick weekday meal, sneak as many vegetables as you like into the coconut green Thai sauce. My husband always asks me to add extra coconut cream. He loves lots of sauce left at the bottom of his bowl to eat like a soup.

Prep time: 15 minutes Cooking time: 25 minutes Serves: 4

Ingredients:

- 2 Tbsp coconut oil
- 600g chicken tenderloins or skinless breast, cut into small chunks
- 1 large onion, diced
- 1 carrot, julienne style
- 2 tsp garlic, minced
- 1 tsp ginger, minced
- 1½-2 Tbsp green curry paste, or to taste (I use Thai Gourmet brand)
- 1½ cups canned coconut cream (extra if you like a lot of sauce)
- ½ head broccoli, floret sliced
- ¼ head cauliflower, florets cut small
- 12 snow peas, cut diagonally in half
- ¾-1 tsp coarse sea salt
- ⅓ tsp ground pepper

Method:

Heat a large heavy based frying pan on medium-hot heat. Add 1 tablespoon coconut oil. Add chicken in two batches. Cook for 2 minutes on each side to seal the chicken. Set aside.

Add remaining coconut oil. Reduce heat to medium. Add onion and carrot, cook for 4-5 minutes. Add garlic, ginger and green curry paste, cook for 3 minutes, stirring often.

Return chicken to pan and stir through. Cook for 5 minutes. Add coconut cream and bring to a simmer.

Add broccoli and cauliflower, let simmer in the sauce for 4-5 minutes. Stir in snow peas, salt and pepper, heat through. Taste and adjust green curry paste and seasonings if needed.

Serve alone or over cauliflower rice.

MAIN MEALS | 191

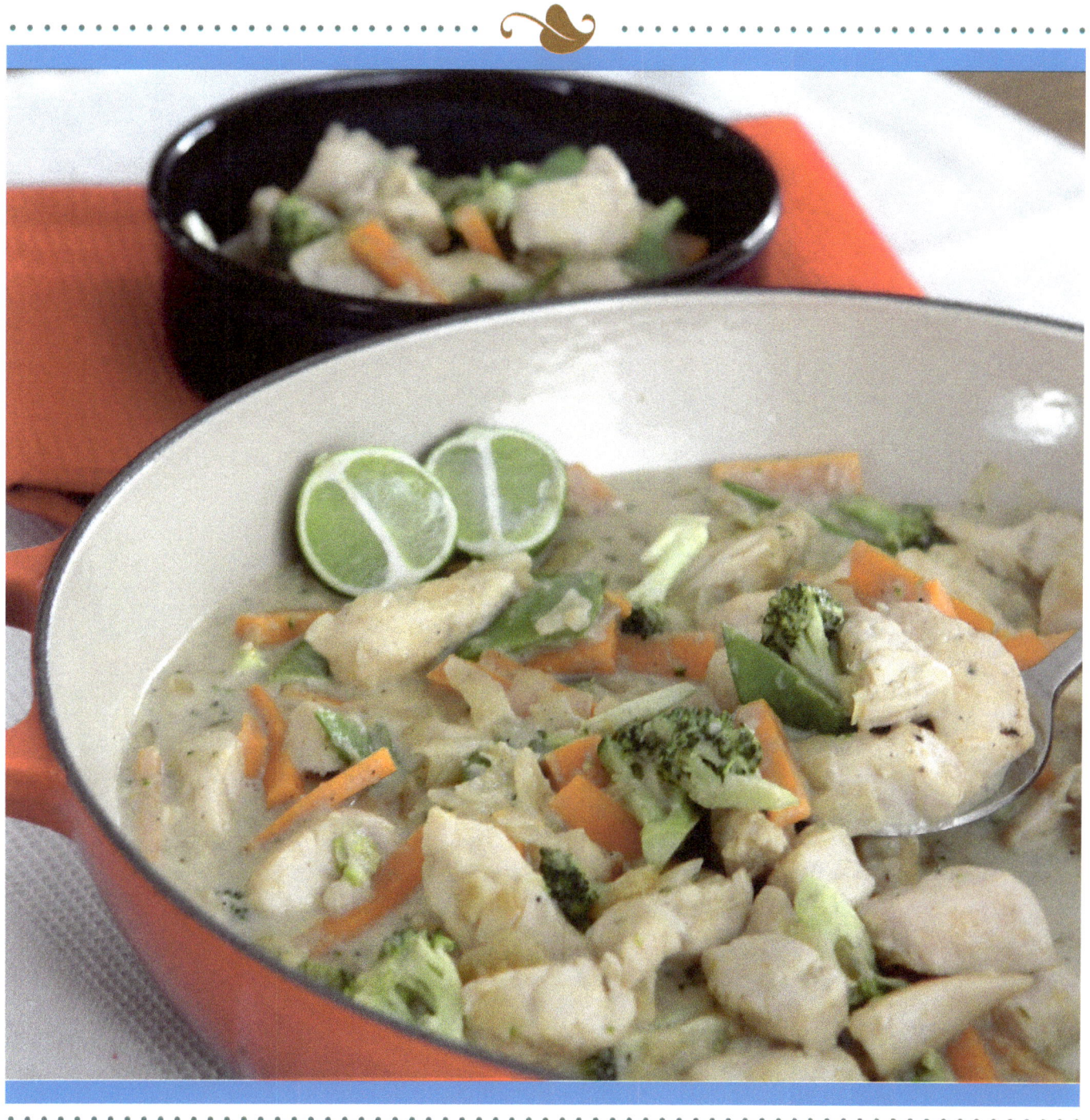

Crumbed Chicken

This is an easy dish to prepare, but tasty enough for a dinner party. It's my good old trusty go to meal when I am not sure what guests like to eat. I make my Mango and Apple Chutney page 213 to accompany it and to add a bit of spice.

Prep time: 10 minutes Cooking time: 25 minutes Serves: 4

Ingredients:

- 500g/1.1lb chicken tenderloins
- 1 cup almond meal/flour
- ½ cup grated Romano cheese or 2 Tbsp Nutritional Yeast Flakes
- ½ tsp fine sea salt
- ¼ tsp ground pepper
- 1 egg, beaten
- 2-3 Tbsp coconut oil

Method:

Line a baking tray with baking paper. To a shallow bowl, add almond meal, cheese or Nutritional Yeast Flakes, salt and pepper. Mix well to combine.

Add egg to a bowl and whisk. Place 2 chicken tenderloins at a time into the bowl with egg. Use a fork to turn and coat.

Add egg-dipped chicken into the almond meal mixture, pressing down firmly to coat each side. Place on tray. Repeat until all chicken is coated well. Let sit for 10-15 minutes for the coating to settle to the chicken.

Just before browning chicken, preheat oven to 150c/300f. This will finish off the cooking and keep chicken warm while preparing vegetables and salad.

Heat a large non-stick frying pan on medium heat. Add 1 tablespoon coconut oil. Add the crumbed chicken, cook for 5 minutes or until light golden. Flip and cook other side for 3-4 minutes. Add extra oil when needed.

Place lightly browned chicken on a freshly lined baking tray. Repeat with remaining chicken.

If you are cooking for guests, skip preheating the oven for the time being. Set aside the chicken and just before arrival time, place in oven to heat and finish off the last bit of cooking.

Serve with Mixed Steamed Vegetables, with Lemon dressing on page 111 or Spinach and Sweet Potato salad on page 101. Accompany with Mango and Apple chutney page 213.

MAIN MEALS | 193

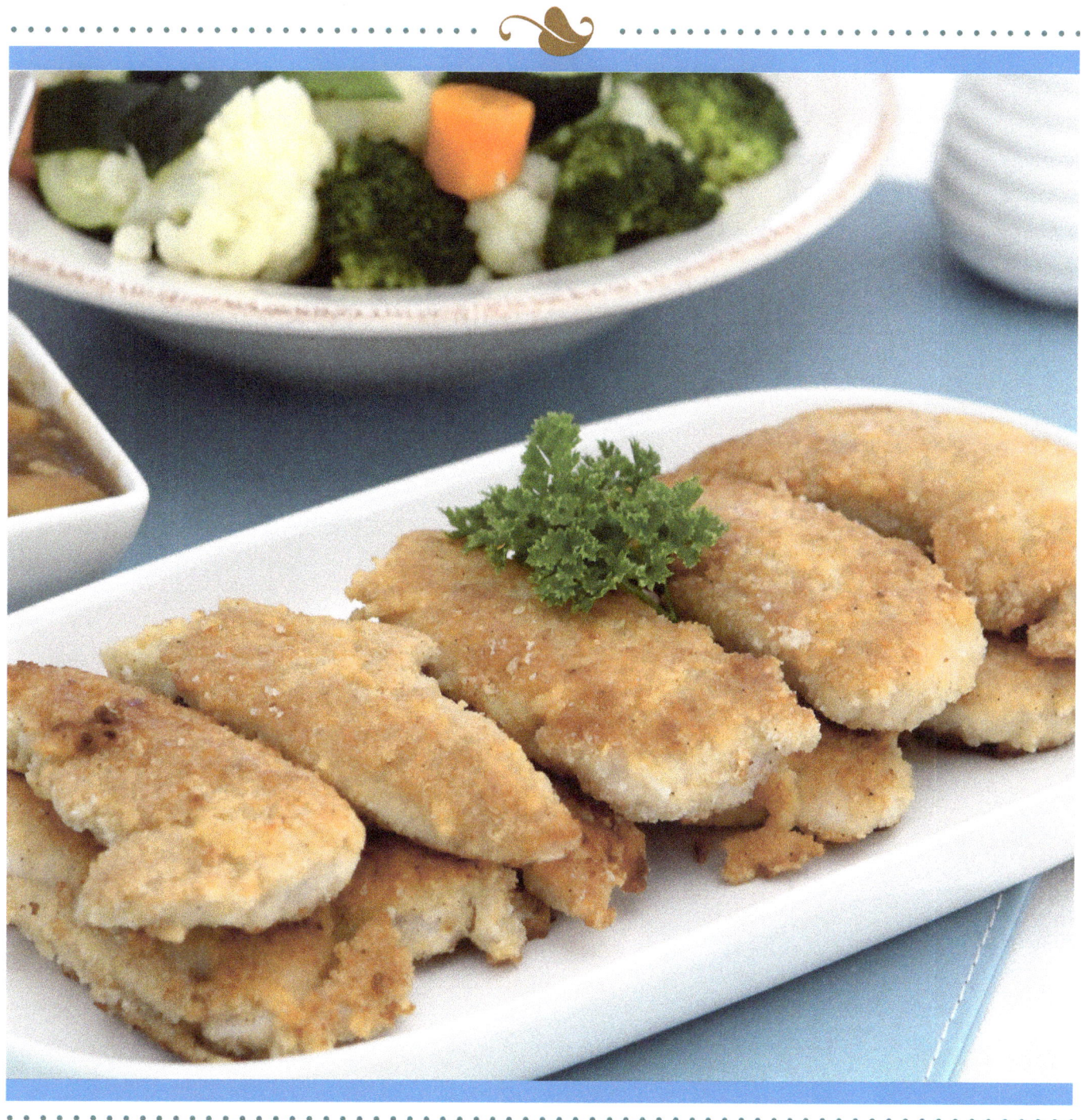

Turkey Meatloaf

Such a quick dinner, only 15 minutes is needed to chop, grate and mix together this tasty meatloaf. Then pop into the oven and don't bother about it for an hour. Keep leftovers to go with eggs for breakfast, packed lunches or cold with salad. Turkey is a rich source of protein, iron, zinc, potassium and phosphorus. It also contains vitamin B6 and niacin, which are both essential for the body's energy production.

Prep time: 15 Cooking time: 1 hour Serves: 6

Ingredients:

- 2 large eggs
- 1 medium onion, finely diced
- ½ cup grated zucchini (skin on and firmly packed)
- 1½ tsp garlic, minced
- 1 Tbsp organic Worcestershire sauce
- 1 Tbsp whole grain mustard
- 1 Tbsp Nutritional Yeast Flakes, optional
- 1 tsp sea salt
- ⅓ tsp pepper
- ½ teaspoon mixed herbs (dried)
- ¼ cup finely chopped fresh parsley
- ¾ cup almond meal
- 600g/1.3lb free range turkey mince

TOPPING

- ¼ cup organic tomato sauce/ketchup

Method:

Preheat oven 180c/350f. Grease a medium-large loaf tin and line base with baking paper.

In a large mixing bowl, whisk eggs. Add all other ingredients except for turkey mince. Mix well to combine.

Add turkey mince. Using clean hands, mix all ingredients together well.

Press mixture firmly into loaf pan, smooth top and pour tomato sauce evenly over the top.

Bake for 1 hour. It will be ready when juices have stopped coming to the top.

Let cool in tin for 10 minutes, loosen sides with a knife. Slice and serve hot with vegetables or cold with salad.

MAIN MEALS | 195

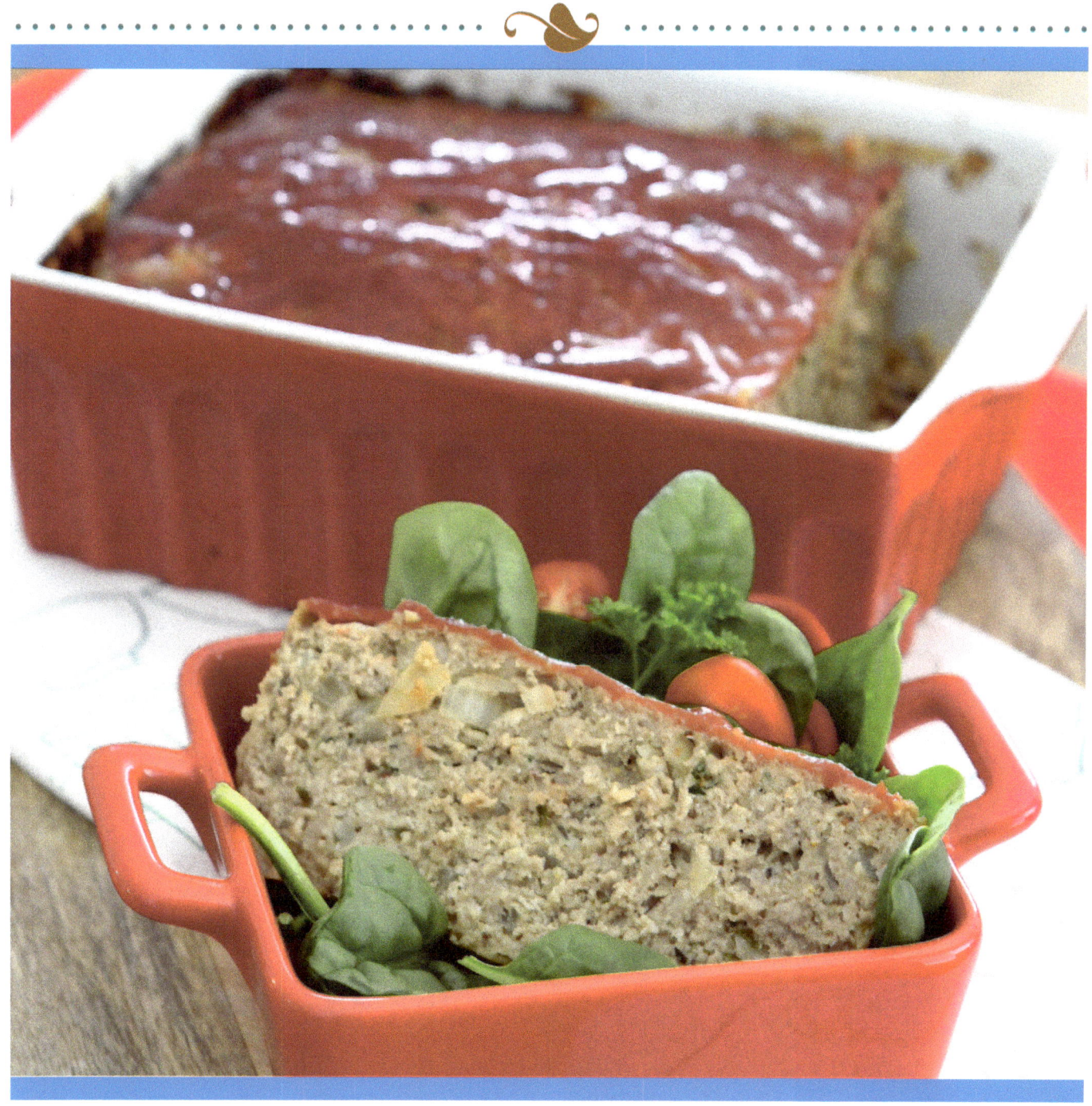

Crunchy Nut Fish

This crunchy nut topped fish, sits on a bed of lightly cooked snow peas, cherry tomatoes and olives, in a lemon tahini cooking sauce. If you soak your fish in milk before cooking, it removes the fishy smell. In addition to having odor free cooking, it will also help to keep the fish moist and whiter.

Prep time: 10 minutes plus soaking time Cooking time: 15 minutes Serves: 2

Ingredients:

- 2 x 180–200g/16.5ozs cod portions or fish of choice
- 1 cup almond milk
- ⅓ cup macadamia nuts
- 1 Tbsp almond meal/flour
- 1 Tbsp coconut flour
- 2 tsp sesame seeds
- ¼ tsp fine sea salt
- ¼ tsp ground coriander
- ¼ tsp ground cumin
- ¼ tsp dried oregano
- 1 Tbsp coconut oil, melted
- Pinch sea salt and pepper to sprinkle over fish

Method:

Place the fish in a bowl with almond milk. Let sit at room temperature for 20 minutes.

Preheat oven to 200c/400f. Line a baking tray with baking paper.

Add macadamia nuts, almond meal and coconut flour to a blender. Using a low speed, blend for a second to just break up the nuts. Add sesame seeds and blend for a further second or two. You want crushed or fine nuts but not a nut-meal.

Transfer to a small bowl, add salt and spices, mix to combine. Add coconut oil, stir until all the mixture comes together in a clump.

Drain fish and pat dry with paper towels. Sprinkle both sides of fish with salt and pepper. Place flat side of fish down on the tray. Bake for 5 minutes. Remove from oven and turn fish over. Press nut mixture onto the flat side of fish that's now turned up. Pressing down so it sticks well.

Return to oven and bake for an additional 9-10 minutes. Very thick pieces may need 12 minutes, or until the nut topping has browned. While the fish is baking, prepare vegetables and sauce to serve the fish on.

Snow Pea, tomato and olives cooked in Lemon Tahini sauce:

- 2 Tbsp olive oil
- Juice of ½ lemon
- 1 tsp tahini
- Sea salt and pepper to taste
- Pinch chili powder
- 20 small snow peas
- 10 kalamarta olives, pitted
- 6 cherry tomatoes, halved

Heat a small frying pan on medium. Add oil, lemon juice, tahini, salt and pepper. Stir while heating.

Add snow peas and toss to coat and cook for 2 minutes. Add olives and tomatoes, stir through to warm them.

To serve, add vegetables and cooking sauce to shallow bowls. Top with fish and garnish with parsley.

MAIN MEALS | 197

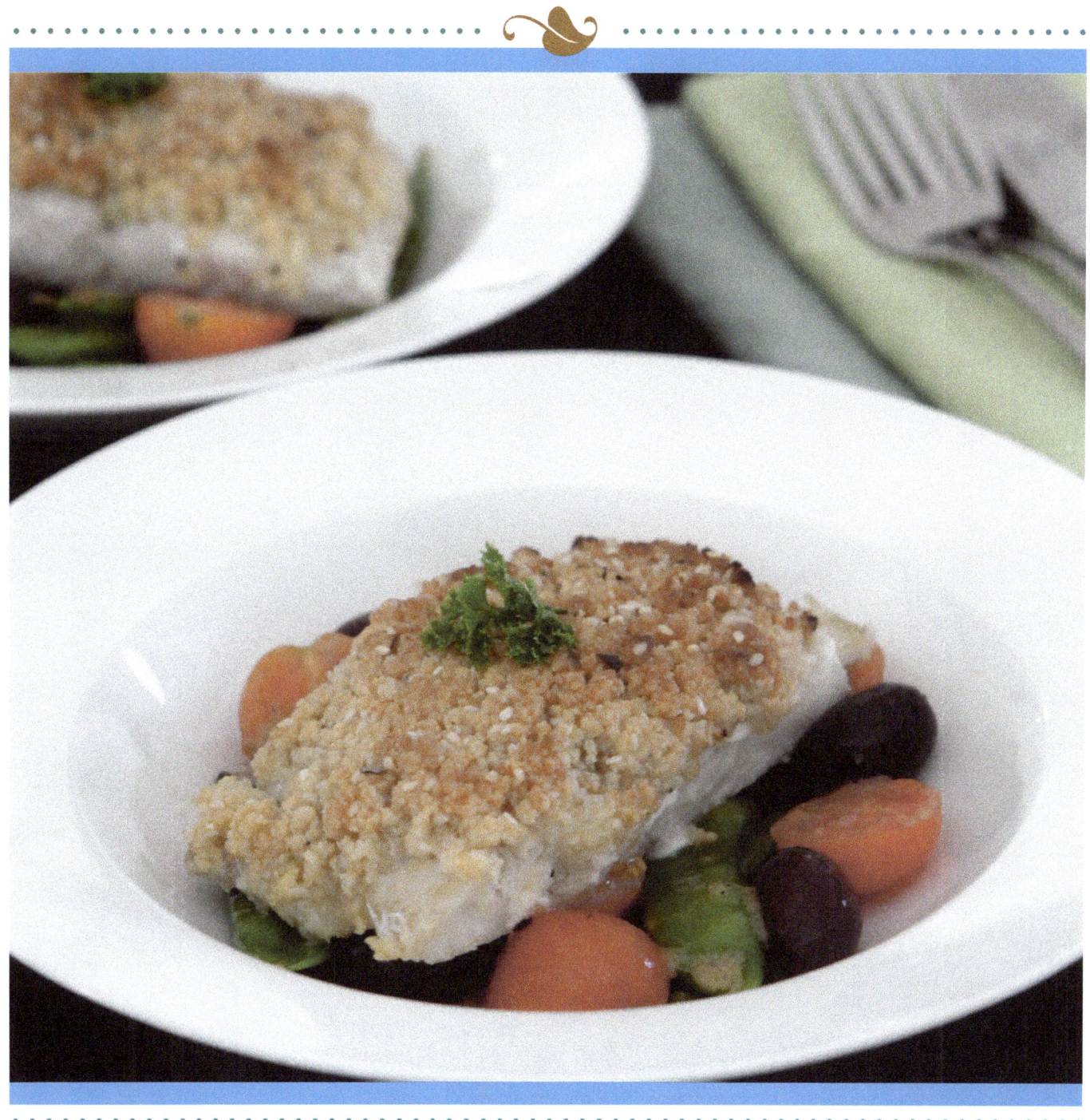

Battered Fish and Seasoned Fries

One of my daughters in law, requested a battered fish and if I mastered it she wanted it in my book. Good news, she loves it. I have seasoned and coated the fries, which has helped them to have some crunch.

Prep time: 15 minutes Cooking time: 8 minutes fish, 30 minutes fries Serves: 4

Ingredients:

SEASONED FRIES
- 1kg/2.2lb sweet potato, cut into thin sticks
- ⅓ cup macadamia nuts
- 3 tsp sesame seeds, divided
- 1½ tsp fine sea salt
- ½ tsp ground cumin
- ¼ tsp ground coriander
- ¼ tsp dried oregano
- 1½ Tbsp arrowroot flour
- ¼ cup coconut oil, melted

FISH
- 4 fish fillets (I use haddock, it's best to use a thin fillet), plus almond milk for soaking
- ⅓ cup arrowroot flour
- ⅓ cup almond meal/flour
- 1 large egg
- ¼ cup almond milk or milk of choice
- ¼ tsp fine sea salt
- ¼ cup arrowroot flour extra, to coat fish
- 3-4 Tbsp coconut oil for frying

Method:

Prepare fries before cooking fish. Preheat oven to 190c/375f and line 3 oven trays with baking paper.

Add macadamia nuts to a blender for a couple of seconds, to crush. Add 2 teaspoons of sesame seeds and spices, pulse for 2-3 seconds to combine.

Transfer nut mix to a large bowl, add arrowroot flour and remaining teaspoon of sesame seeds. Add melted coconut oil, mix well.

Add cut potato sticks and coat using your hands, mix for 1 minute. The heat from your hands will help the coating to stick.

Line up on the oven trays, leaving space between fries. Bake for 30 minutes. Turn over after 15 minutes to brown both sides.

Place fresh fish into a container with 1 cup of almond milk for 20 minutes, turn fish over while soaking. Then drain and pat dry with paper towels.

In a bowl beat together arrowroot flour, almond meal, egg, almond milk and salt, to make a smooth batter. Let it sit for 8-9 minutes before coating fish; batter will thicken a little.

Heat a large frying pan on medium-high heat and add coconut oil. Place the ¼ cup of arrowroot flour on a plate. Lightly coat one piece of fish at a time with flour, dust off excess. Dip into batter and let the excess drip off. Place in heated oil. Repeat for remaining fish fillets. Add extra oil when needed.

Cook for 4-5 minutes on each side or until fish is cooked through and batter is golden. Use a spatula to carefully turn fish.

Serve with Seasoned fries, lemon wedges and a salad on the side.

MAIN MEALS | 199

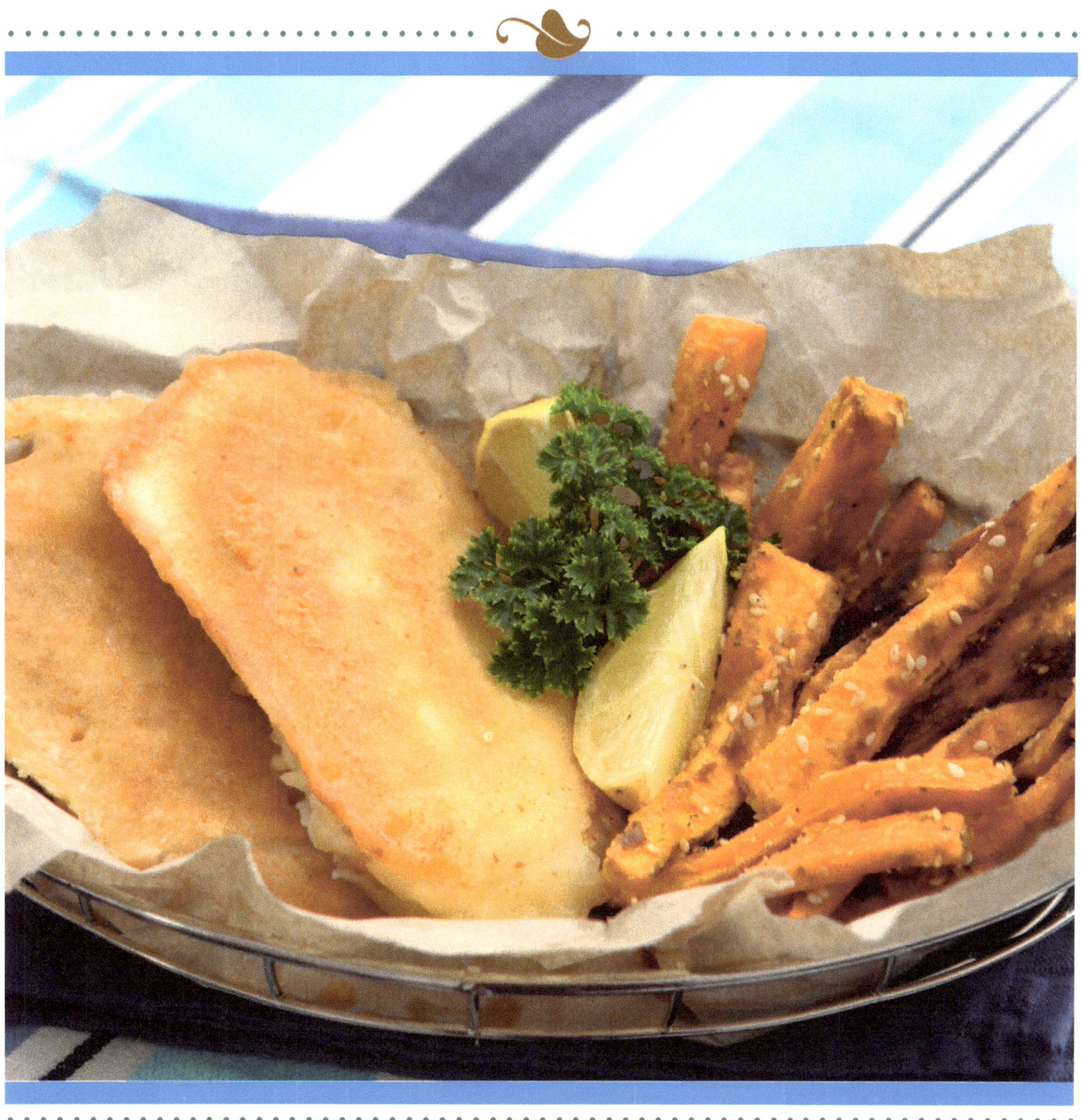

Thai Fish Cakes

My husband loves these fish cakes and adds extra chili sauce on the side to spice them up. If you are using thawed fish, squeeze gently and remove excess water.

Prep time: 10 minutes Cooking time: 10 minutes Serves: 4

Ingredients:

500g/1.1lb white fish fillets, roughly chopped (I use cod or haddock, wild caught)
½ cup fresh coriander leaves
¼ cup almond meal or sunflower meal
1 Tbsp coconut flour
2 Tbsp fish sauce
2 Tbsp organic sweet chili sauce or to taste
1 egg
2 spring onions/shallots plus some green tops, finely sliced
¼ cup coconut oil for frying
Lime wedges, to serve

Method:

Place the fish in a food processor and process until smooth. Scrape down the sides of bowl. Add the coriander, almond meal, coconut flour, fish sauce, sweet chili sauce and egg. Process until well combined.

Transfer the fish mixture to a bowl. Add the spring onions and stir until well combined.

Heat ½ the coconut oil in a large frying pan over medium heat.

Divide the fish mixture into 8 equal portions. Shape into round patties. As mixture is soft I use the back of a spoon to pat into shape and flatten in the palm of my hand.

Cook for 5 minutes on each side or until golden brown, take care when turning. Add oil as needed.

Transfer to a plate lined with paper towel. Repeat with the remaining fish mixture. Keep warm in oven until ready to serve.

Serve fish cakes with salad, wedges of lime, and chili sauce on the side.

MAIN MEALS | 201

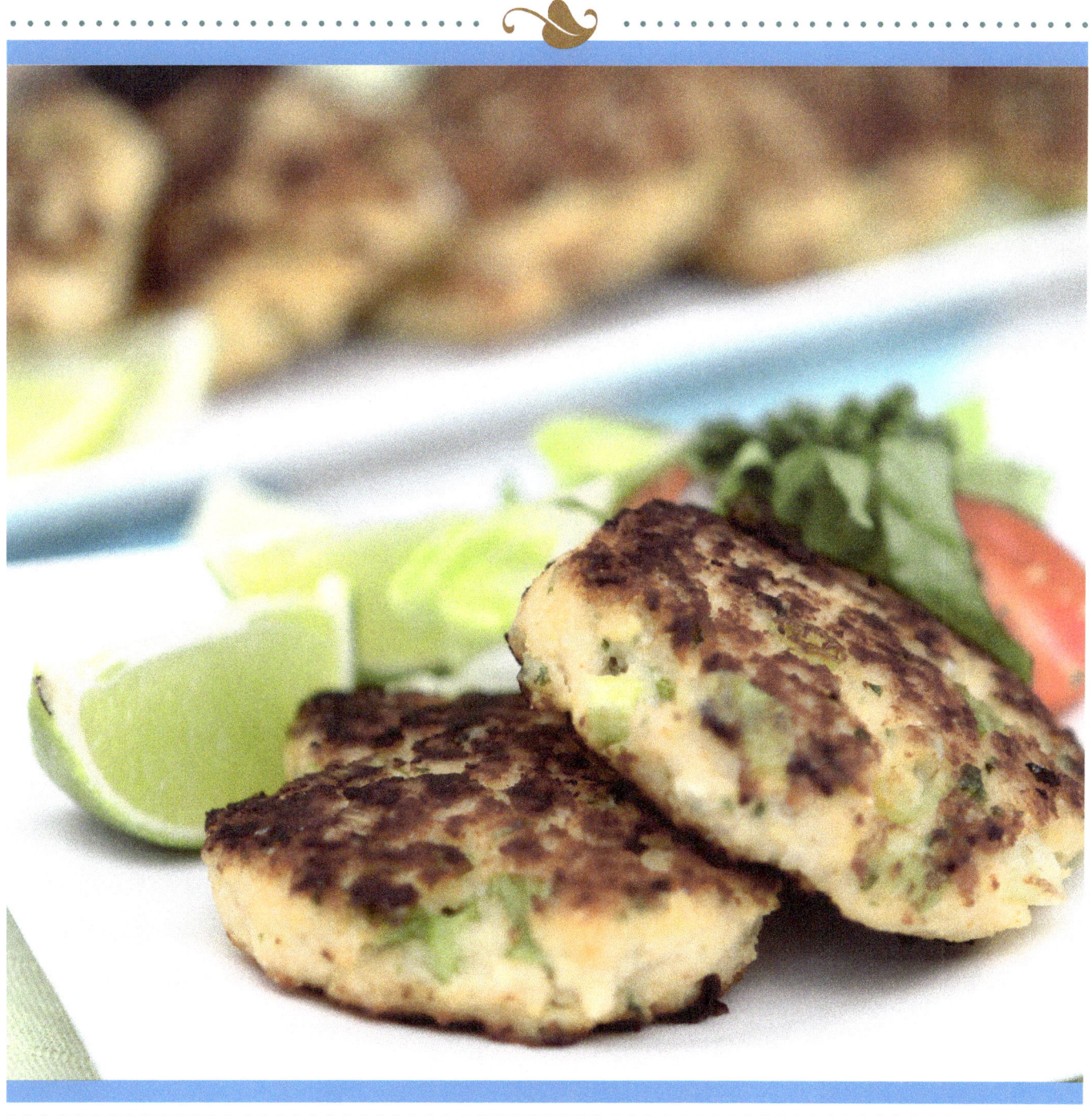

GRAVY, SAUCES AND DRESSINGS

Gravy (Beef and Chicken) 204

Mushroom Gravy 206

Egg Mayonnaise 207

Caesar Dressing 208

Tahini Vinaigrette 209

Spicy Guacamole Salsa 210

White (Nut) Sauce 211

White (Cauliflower) Sauce 212

Apple and Mango Chutney 213

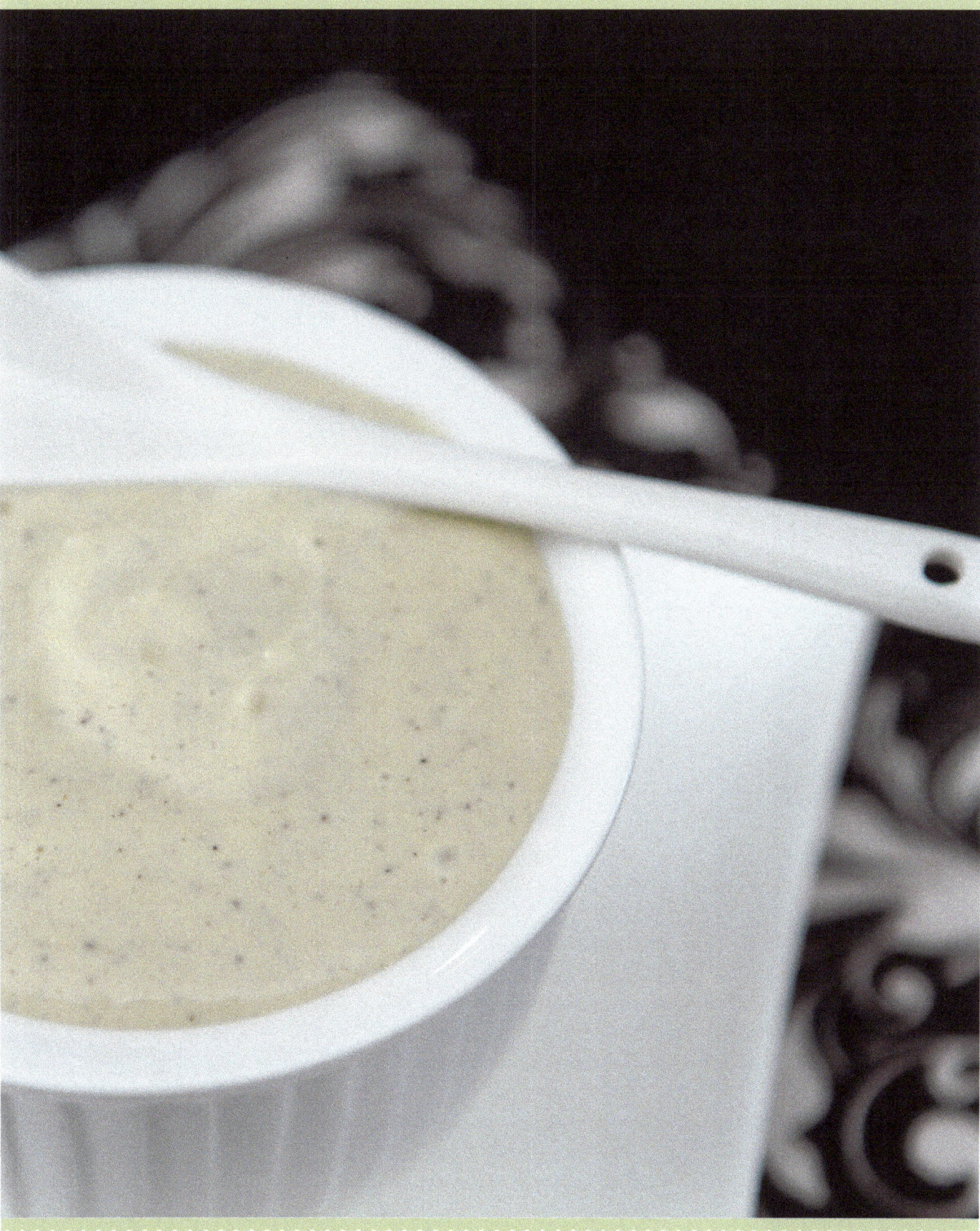

Gravy (Beef and Chicken)

This is a very flavoursome gravy thickened with vegetables instead of flour. When I started thickening my stews by blending some of the vegetables from the pot, it gave me the idea to make gravy this way. Make sure to brown the vegetables well, this will help to colour the gravy. Change broth/stock and herbs depending if you are cooking beef or chicken.

Prep time: 5 minutes Cooking time: 20 minutes Makes: approximately 2 cups

Ingredients:

- 1 Tbsp ghee
- ⅓ cup pumpkin, diced
- ⅓ cup carrot, diced
- 1 medium onion, chopped
- 1 clove garlic, chopped
- 375ml/1½ cups beef or chicken broth/stock
- 2 Tbsp coconut aminos
- 1-2 tsp organic Worcestershire sauce
- Sea salt and ground pepper, to taste
- 1 sprig of rosemary if making gravy for beef or lamb
- ½ Tbsp fresh thyme, chopped if making gravy for chicken

Method:

In a small saucepan over medium-high heat, melt ghee. Add pumpkin, carrots, onion and garlic. Fry vegetables until brown, approximately 6 minutes. Stir often and add extra ghee if needed. (The browner the nicer the gravy, but watch it doesn't burn.)

Add broth, coconut aminos, Worcestershire sauce, salt, pepper and herbs. Bring to a boil then reduce to a simmer. Simmer uncovered for 10-15 minutes.

If you are using rosemary remove sprig from broth, but leave any leaves that have come off. Pour the contents of the saucepan into a blender (be careful not to burn yourself). Blend on a low-medium speed making gravy come together and thicken.

If the gravy is not thick enough for your purpose, make a slurry with arrowroot flour and a small amount of water. Return gravy to pan, stir slurry into the gravy over low heat until it thickens.

Gravy can be made ahead of time and warmed in a saucepan just before serving.

Pour into a gravy jug and serve over roast meat and vegetables.

GRAVY, SAUCES AND DRESSINGS | 205

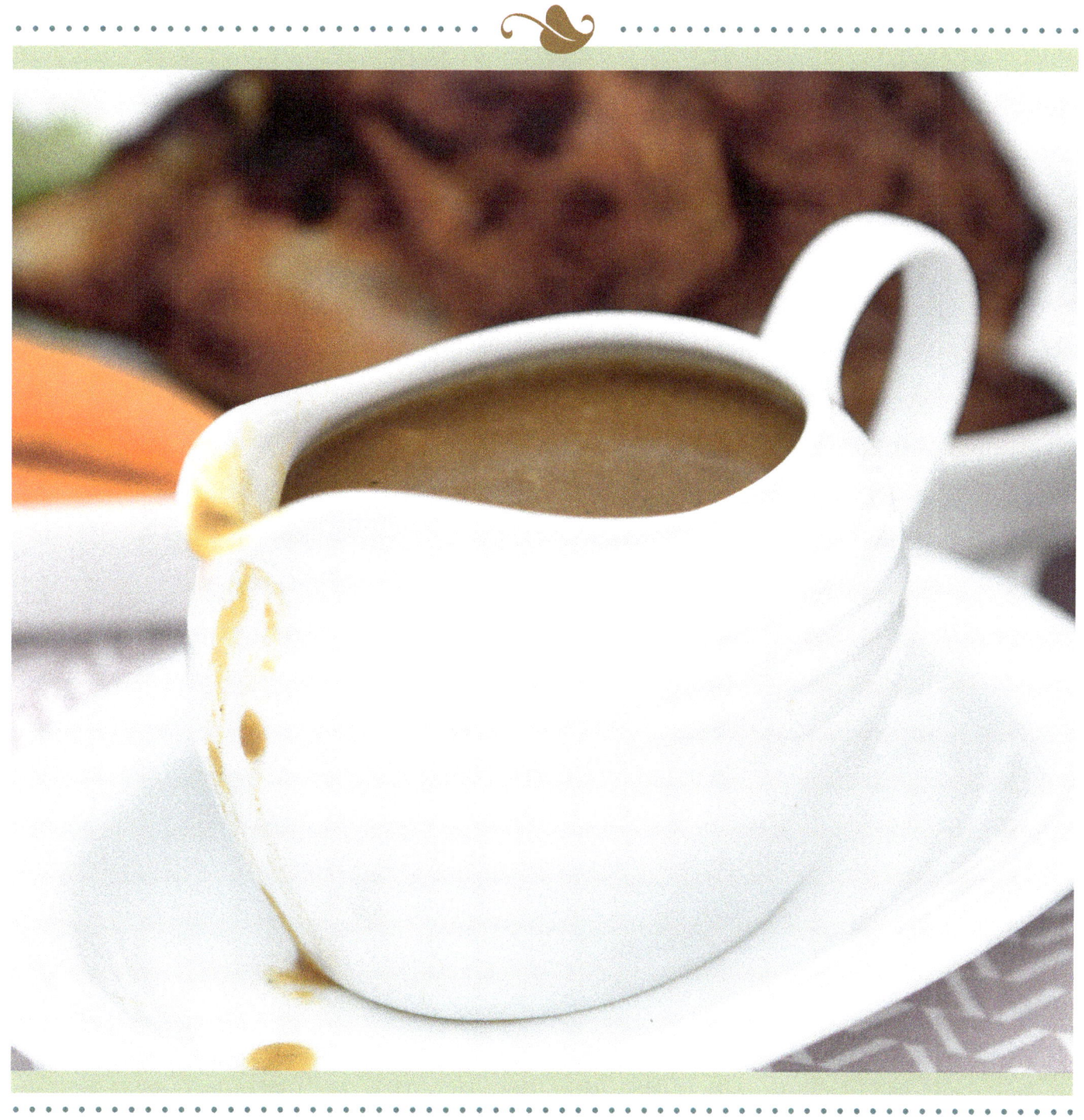

Mushroom Gravy

This gravy is really delicious, but best of all it's very good for you. Mushrooms are good sources of B vitamins, selenium, iron, and other minerals. Mushrooms are also quite good at neutralizing free radicals. The plain old white button mushroom beats even colourful veggies like green capsicum/peppers, carrots, green beans, and tomatoes! Best of all, mushrooms contain antioxidants that are not deactivated or destroyed by cooking.

Prep time: 8 minute Cooking time: 20 minutes Makes: 2½ cups

Ingredients:

- 1 Tbsp ghee
- 1 onion, finely diced
- 1 clove garlic, minced
- 2½ cups mushrooms, finely diced (button or field mushrooms)
- ¾ tsp dried thyme leaves
- ½ tsp sea salt
- ¼ tsp pepper
- 2 cups beef or chicken broth/stock
- 1 Tbsp coconut aminos
- ¼ cup canned coconut cream
- 1½ Tbsp arrowroot flour

Method:

Heat a medium saucepan over medium-high heat, melt ghee. Add onion, cook for 4-5 minutes until browned, this will add colour to the gravy.

Add garlic, mushrooms, thyme, salt and pepper. Cook stirring for a further 4 minutes.

Add broth and coconut aminos, leave a little broth aside to make a slurry with the arrowroot flour. Bring to the boil, then simmer on low for 10 minutes.

Add coconut cream and stir in the arrowroot flour slurry. Let simmer gently for a further couple of minutes.

Serve over steak or your favourite meat pie.

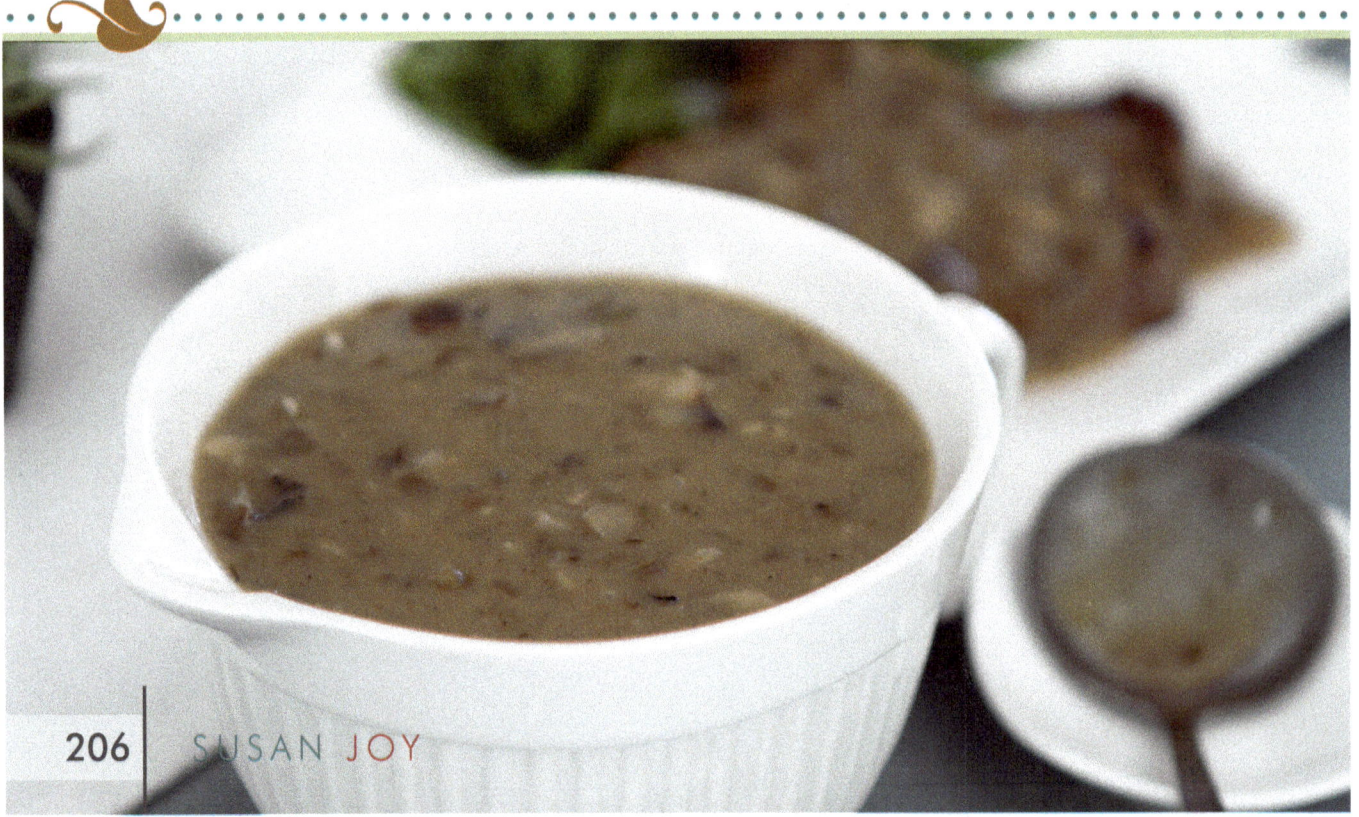

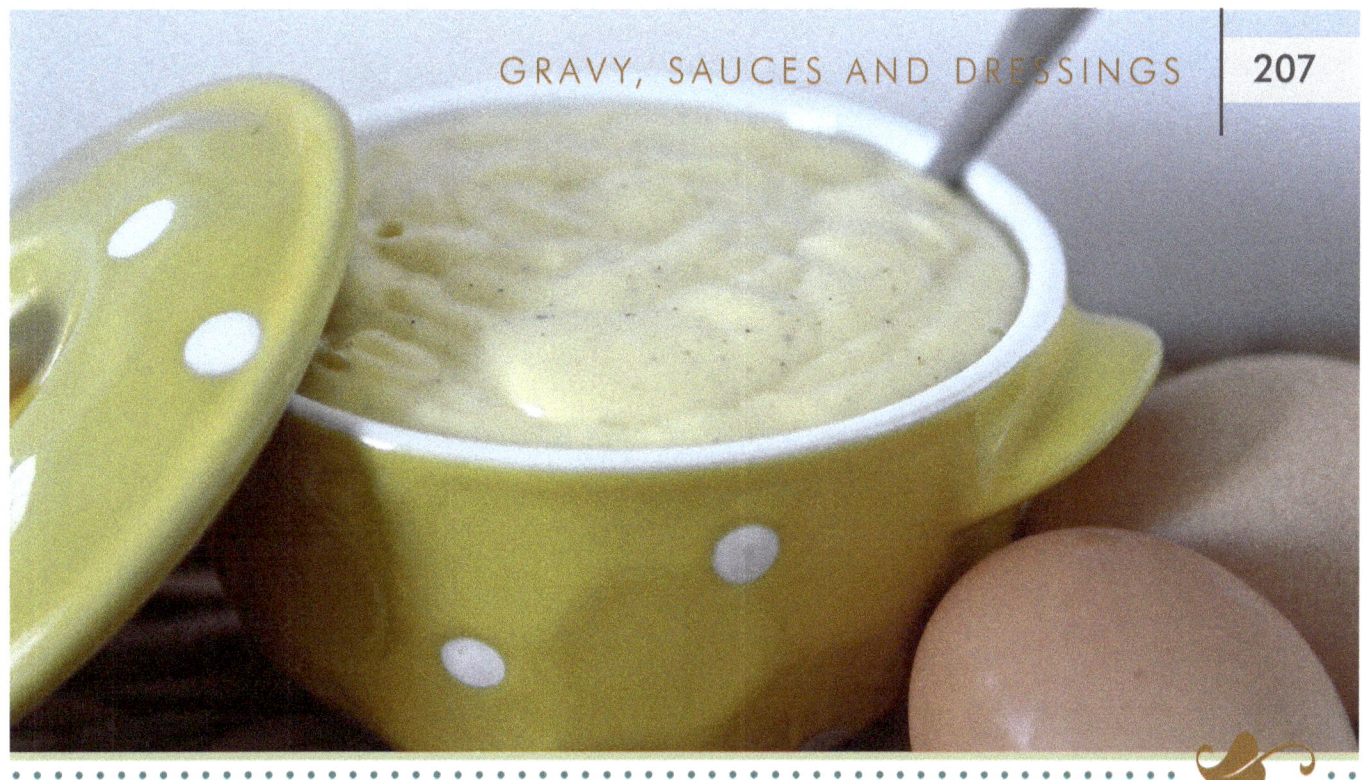

Egg Mayonnaise

This is a basic mayonnaise recipe that you can use to make other sauces and dressings from. Supermarket mayonnaise has so many additives hidden amongst the hydrogenated vegetable oils. I have found that even the organic mayo's don't always come in good quality oils and are so expensive. Most importantly; use a very mild flavoured olive oil, as the flavour can be very overpowering.

Prep time: 10 minutes Cooking time: none Makes: 1½ cups

Ingredients:

- 1 egg, room temperature
- 1 egg yolk, room temperature
- 1 Tbsp fresh lemon juice, room temperature
- 1 Tbsp white wine vinegar
- 1 tsp Dijon mustard
- ½ tsp honey
- ¾ tsp fine sea salt
- ⅛ tsp pepper
- 1 cup mild flavoured olive oil or almond oil
- 2 Tbsp coconut oil, melted

Method:

Add to a blender, egg, yolk, lemon juice, vinegar, mustard, honey, salt and pepper. Blend for 5 seconds on low to combine.

Remove the small cap in the blender lid. With the blender running at a medium speed, add the olive oil in a very, very, slow drizzle, or by tablespoon. You are waiting for the mixture to come together and emulsify into a creamy consistency. (I place my oil into a small jug to help with controlling the flow.) Once this happens you can add the rest of the oil in a slow steady stream. Usually after the first ⅓ cup it should have emulsified and you will hear a difference in the blender. Add the coconut oil, in a steady stream while blender is running. Adjust seasoning if required.

Store in a covered airtight glass container in the fridge for up to 7 days. If you used freshly laid eggs it will keep up to 14 days. It is best to cool in the fridge before serving for the flavours to come out.

GRAVY, SAUCES AND DRESSINGS

Caesar Dressing

Sorry, no anchovies in this dressing, I've used fish sauce. Not a great fan of anchovies but I am very happy for you to add them in yourself (use 3 or 4 anchovy and omit the fish sauce).

Prep time: 10 minutes Cooking time: none Makes 1 cup

Ingredients:

- 1 egg, room temperature
- 1 Tbsp fresh lemon juice
- 2 tsp Dijon mustard
- 2 tsp Apple Cider vinegar
- 1 tsp fish sauce
- 1 tsp organic Worcestershire sauce
- 1 tsp 100% maple syrup, or to taste
- 1 tsp garlic, minced
- ¼ tsp black pepper, ground
- ½ cup olive oil, mild flavoured
- 2 Tbsp coconut oil, melted, optional (can replace with olive oil)

Method:

Add to a blender, egg, lemon juice, mustard, vinegar, fish sauce, Worcestershire sauce, maple syrup, garlic and pepper. Blend for 15 seconds to combine.

Remove the small cap in the blender lid. With the blender running at a low-medium speed, add the oil in a very, very, slow drizzle, or by tablespoon. You are waiting for the mixture to come together and emulsify into a creamy consistency. (I place my oil into a small jug to help with controlling the flow.) Once this happens you can add the remaining olive oil and coconut oil in a slow steady stream.

Store in an airtight glass container in the fridge for up to 7 days. It's best to leave to cool in fridge for several hours before using, for the flavours to come out.

Use this recipe for Chicken Avocado Caesar Salad page 146.

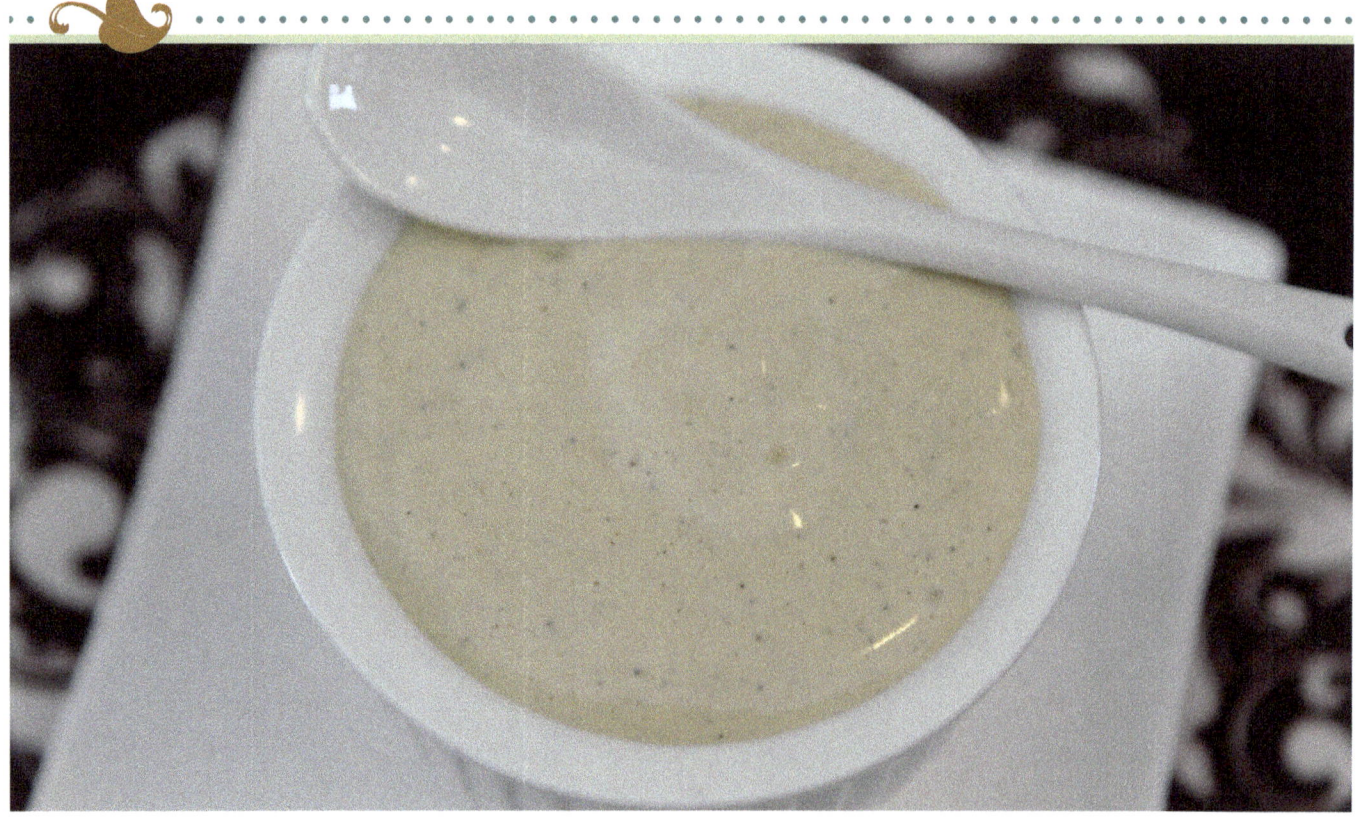

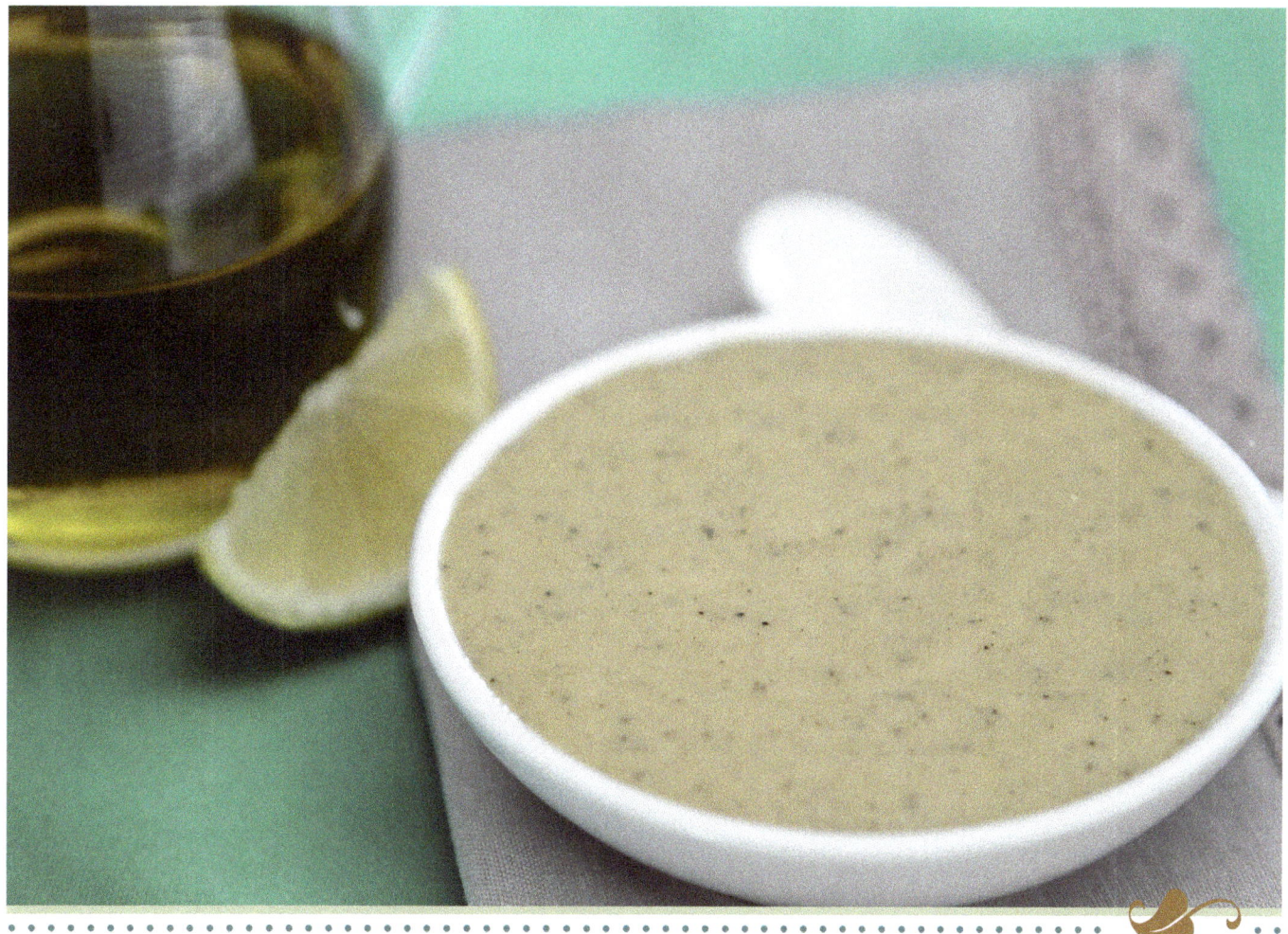

Tahini Vinaigrette

I made this dressing to go over my Rainbow Salad on page 91. It would complement any green salad. It is creamy but still very light.

Prep time: 10 minutes   Cooking time: none   Makes: ½ cup

Ingredients:

¼ cup olive oil
2½ Tbsp tahini (adjust to how creamy or light you prefer dressing)
3 tsp Nutritional Yeast Fakes
2 Tbsp lemon juice
1 Tbsp Apple Cider vinegar
1 tsp honey
½ tsp fine sea salt
¼ tsp ground pepper

Method:

Add all of the ingredients to a small bowl and whisk together. Check seasoning and consistency and adjust to your liking.

Serve over your favourite green salad.

Store in fridge for up to 7 days in an airtight container.

GRAVY, SAUCES AND DRESSINGS

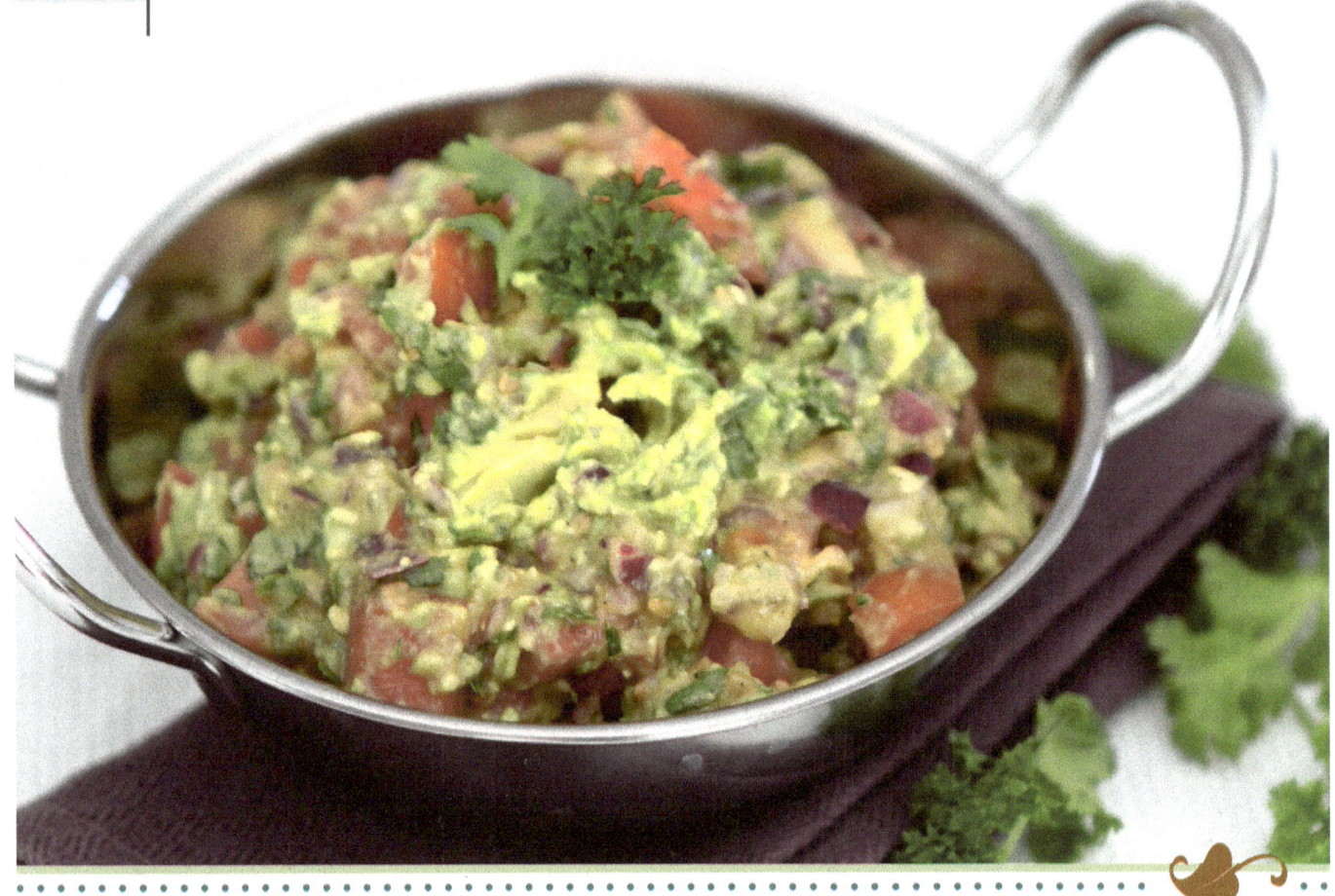

Spicy Guacamole Salsa

You can serve this tasty salsa with any type of meat, chicken or fish. Excellent with finger foods and as a dip.

Prep time: 15 minutes Cooking time: none Makes: 3 cups

Ingredients:

- 3 tomatoes, diced
- ½ small red onion, finely diced
- 1 Tbsp coconut vinegar
- 1 Tbsp avocado oil
- ⅛-¼ tsp chili powder, or to taste
- Juice of 2 limes
- Sea salt and pepper, to taste
- 2 avocados, mashed lightly
- ¼ cup coriander leaves, finely chopped
- ¼ cup fresh parsley, finely chopped

Method:

To a medium bowl add diced tomatoes and onion. Add vinegar, oil, chili powder and lime juice.

Season with sea salt and pepper to taste.

Add lightly mashed avocados, coriander and parsley and stir through.

White (Nut) Sauce

This is tastier than the usual dairy white sauce. Cashews are so versatile. Thanks to my daughter in law Natalie, who is a raw food chef, I get to discuss the many ways to use nuts in place of dairy. To turn it into a cheezy dairy free sauce, add 1-2 tablespoons of Nutritional Yeast Flakes.

Prep time: 8 minutes plus soaking time   Cooking time: 5 minutes   Makes: 2 cups

Ingredients:

- 1 cup raw cashews or macadamias
- Hot water and ⅓ tsp sea salt for soaking
- 2 tsp ghee or coconut oil
- ½ large leek, sliced thinly or ½ a small white onion
- 1 cup almond milk or water
- ¾ tsp mustard powder
- Pinch of nutmeg or to taste
- Pinch sea salt and white pepper

Method:

Add nuts and salt to a bowl, cover with hot water. Allow to soak for 30-60 minutes. Strain through a metal sieve and rinse.

While you wait. Heat a small frying pan on medium-low heat, add ghee. Gently cook leek or onion until soft but not brown (adding a pinch of sea salt to onions will prevent browning).

Add to a blender the drained nuts, almond milk/water, leek/onion, mustard, nutmeg, salt and pepper.

Blend until you have a smooth, creamy consistency.

Serve over vegetables or add to any recipe that requires a white sauce.

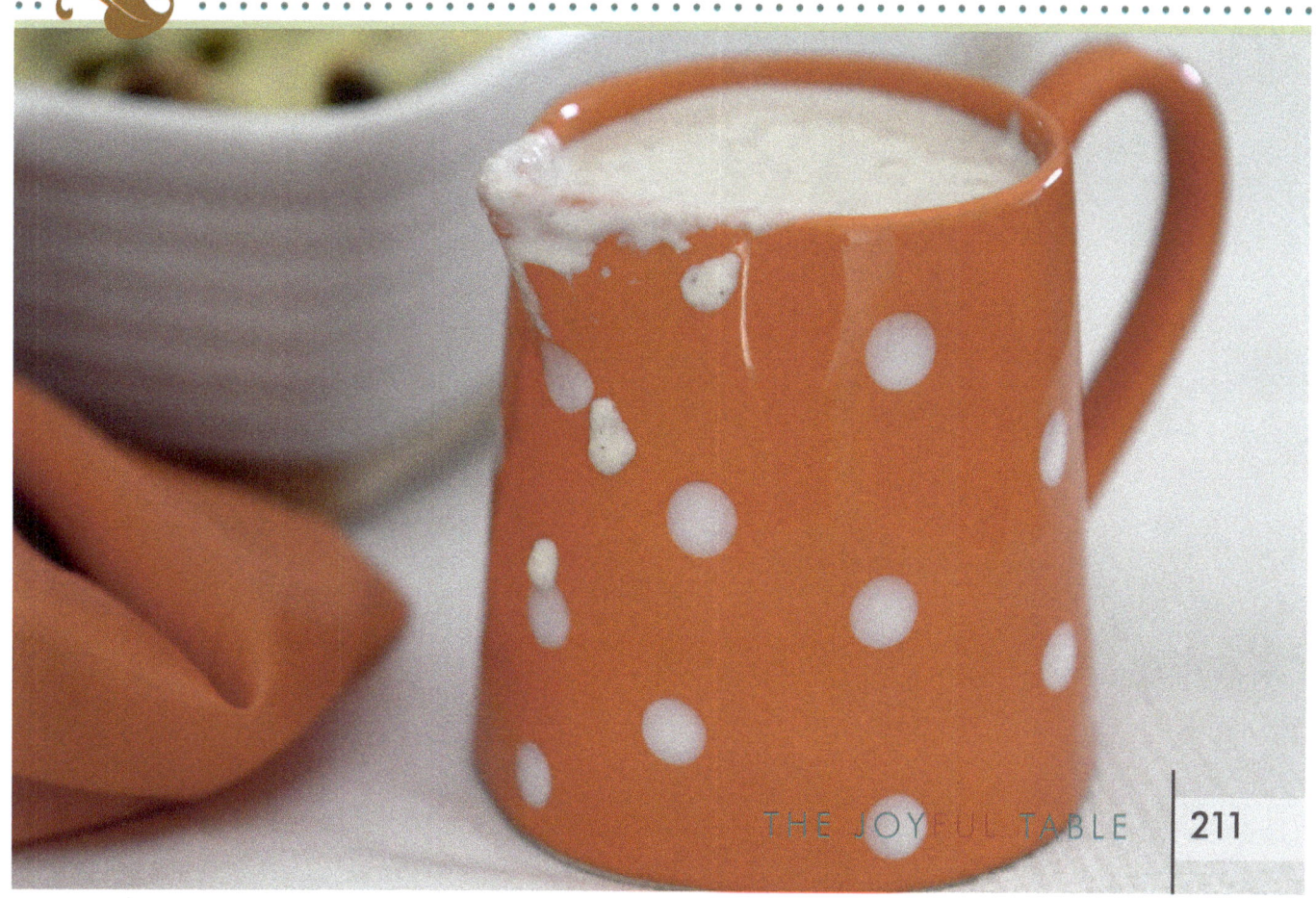

GRAVY, SAUCES AND DRESSINGS

White (Cauliflower) Sauce

Cauliflower produces a lovely silky white sauce, delicious over veggie noodles. Only milk can be used when making this sauce, almond or macadamia milk is best (water isn't suitable).

Prep time: 8 minutes Cooking time: 15 minutes Makes: 3½ cups approximately

Ingredients:

- 1 cauliflower, chopped into small pieces
- ½ tsp sea salt
- ¼ tsp pepper
- ½ cup almond milk, add gradually to reach required consistency

Method:

Steam cauliflower in a double saucepan for 10-15 minutes, or until tender, time may alter depending on size of cauliflower pieces.

Transfer to a blender, add salt and pepper. Blend on high (use tamper stick to push the cauliflower onto the blades) until you get a smooth and creamy consistency.

Add almond milk gradually. Use variable speed, then increase to high after each addition until you reach consistency required for your recipe.

When making a white sauce for veggie noodles, don't add milk. Vegetables release their own liquid, wait to adjust consistency.

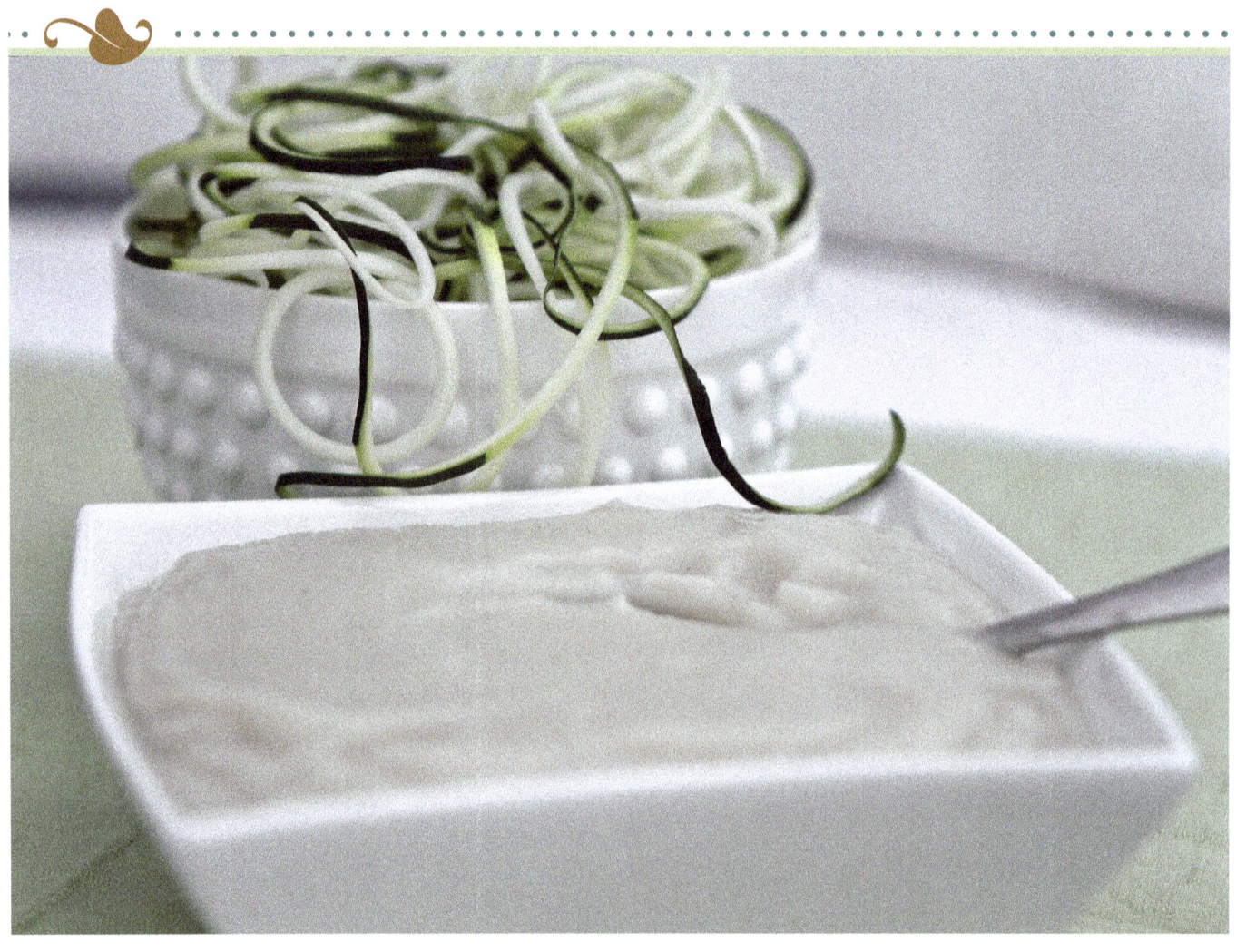

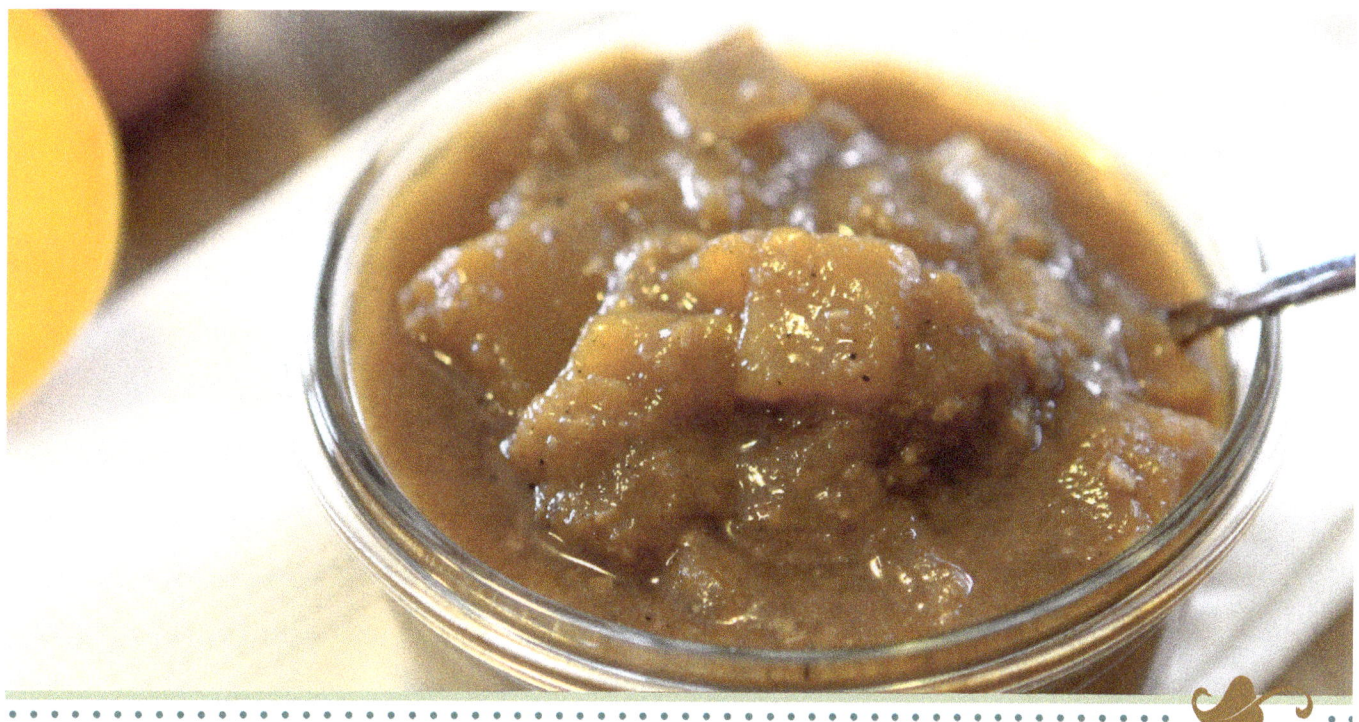

Apple and Mango Chutney

You can make this recipe as mild or spicy as you like. Apple and Mango chutney goes wonderfully with Crumbed chicken on page 192. It is also delicious with fish.

Prep time: 15 minutes   Cooking time: 30 minutes   Makes: 3 cups

Ingredients:

- 2 medium apples, chopped into 1cm(⅓in) pieces
- 3 mangoes, skin removed and chopped or 6 frozen cheeks
- ½ cup coconut sugar or to taste
- 1 cup water, plus extra ¼ cup during cooking if needed
- 3 tsp garlic, minced
- 2 tsp ginger, minced
- ½ cup white wine vinegar
- 1 tsp cinnamon
- ½ tsp ground cardamom
- ⅛-¼ teaspoon ground chili powder, adjust to taste
- 2 tsp sea salt
- ⅛ tsp pepper
- Juice of 2 limes

Method:

Peel the apples, remove the seeds and chop. Mango can be chopped into larger pieces, it will breakup as it cooks.

Add coconut sugar and water to a heavy based saucepan and bring to the boil.

Add apples, mangoes, garlic and ginger to the pot. Simmer uncovered for 10 minutes.

Then add the remaining ingredients and stir well. Bring back to boiling point. Reduce to a simmer.

Stir occasionally, cook until the mixture starts to thicken, approximately a further 15 minutes. Remove from heat and let the chutney cool to room temperature.

Spoon chutney into airtight glass jars and refrigerate. Chutney will have a fuller flavour after being in the fridge for 2-3 days but can be eaten right away. Store in the fridge, chutney will keep for 6-7 weeks. Serve with chicken or fish.

MUFFINS, CAKES AND SLICES

Banana and Blueberry Muffins 217

Lemon Poppy Seed Muffins 219

Brownies 221

Chocolate Chip Cookies 223

"Anzac" Biscuits 225

Gingerbread Cookies 227

Marzipan Cookies 229

Blueberry Thumbprint Biscuits 231

Banana Bread 233

Zucchini Bread 235

Scones 237

Fruity Nut Scones 239

Cinnamon Pecan Rolls 241

Carrot Cake with Lemon Cream Icing 243

Vanilla Cupcakes 245

Orange and Almond Cake 247

Lamington Cake 249

Macaroon and Chocolate Slice 251

Pistachio Macaroons 253

Coconut Rough Bites 255

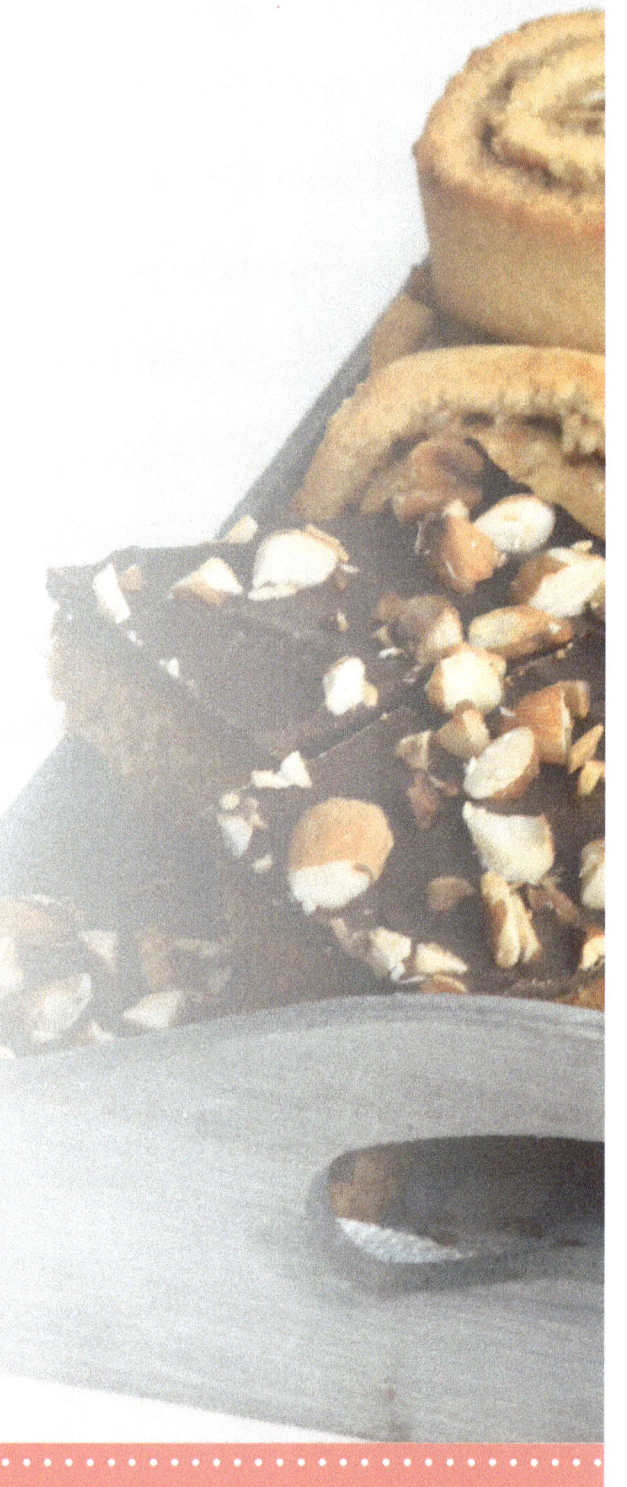

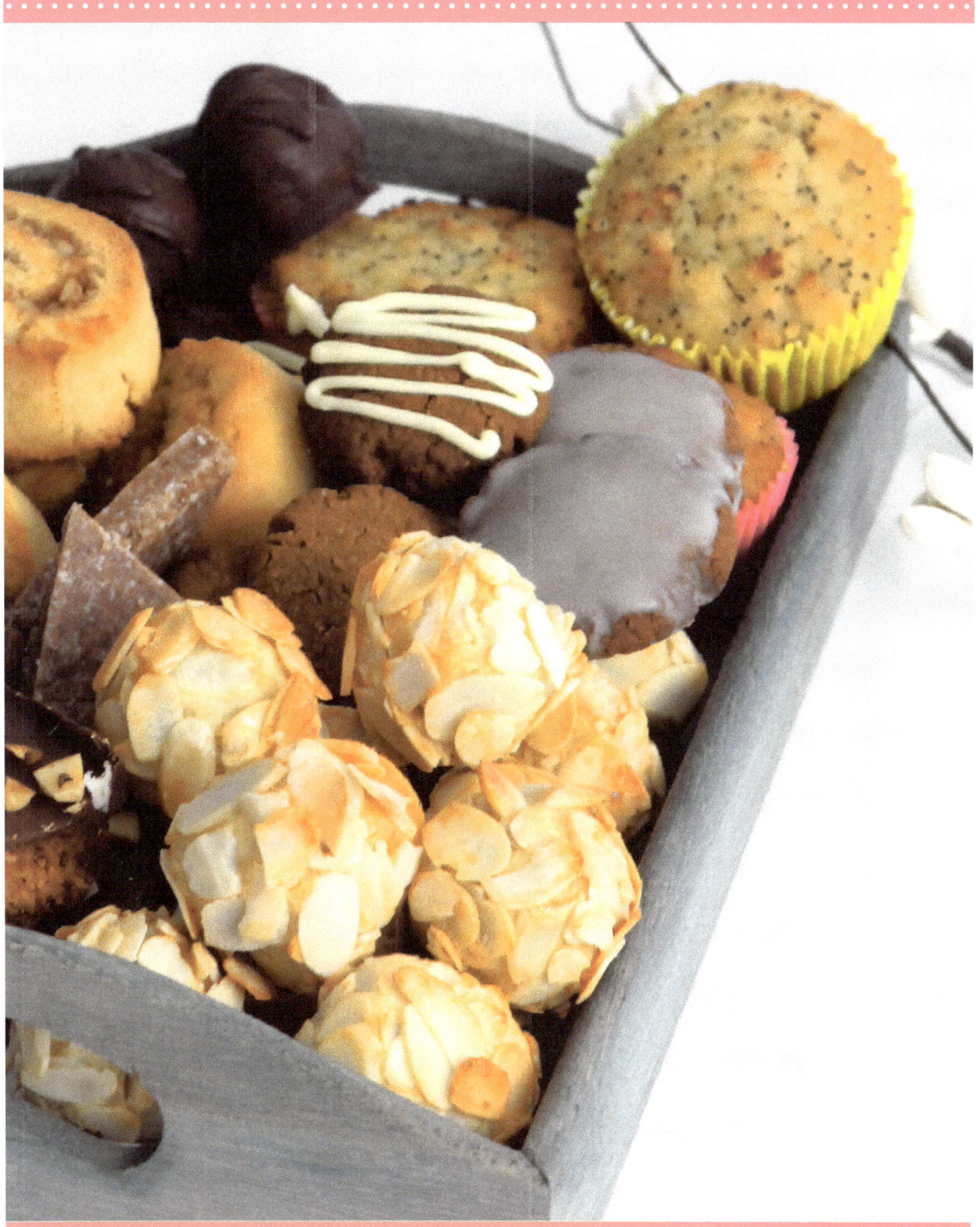

216 | MUFFINS, CAKES AND SLICES

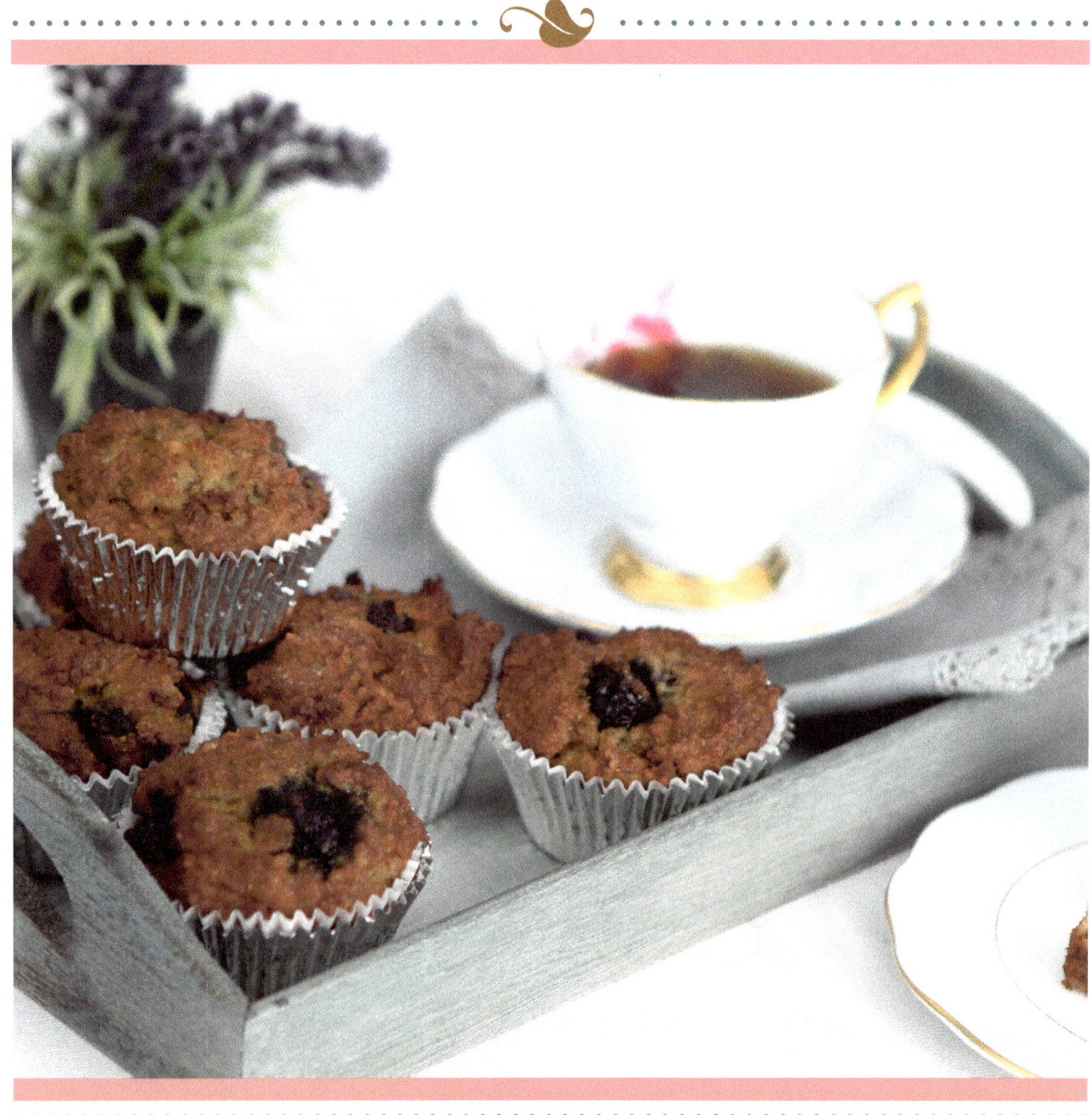

Banana and Blueberry Muffins

These muffins freeze well and are lovely and moist. I make them to take with us on family holidays. Muffins become a healthy breakfast at the airport.

Prep time: 20 minutes   Cooking time: 30 minutes   Makes: 12

Ingredients:

- 2½ cups almond meal/flour
- ¼ cup coconut flour, sifted
- 1½ tsp baking soda
- ¼ tsp fine sea salt
- ¼ cup macadamia oil
- 3 large eggs
- 1 Tbsp honey
- 2 cups (4-5) mashed ripe bananas
- 1 cup frozen blueberries

Method:

Preheat oven to 170c/340f. Place paper liners/patty pans in a muffin tin.

To a large bowl, add almond meal, coconut flour, baking soda and salt, stir to combine.

To a medium bowl, add macadamia oil, eggs and honey, whisk together well. Pour wet ingredients into the dry ingredients and mix until combined.

Add mashed banana to the batter and mix through. Add frozen blueberries, mix gently through the batter, trying not to burst the berries.

Spoon into muffin tin. Bake for 30 minutes or until golden brown. Let the muffins cool in the pan for 15 minutes then transfer to a wire rack to finish cooling.

Store in an airtight container in the fridge. Suitable to freeze.

MUFFINS, CAKES AND SLICES

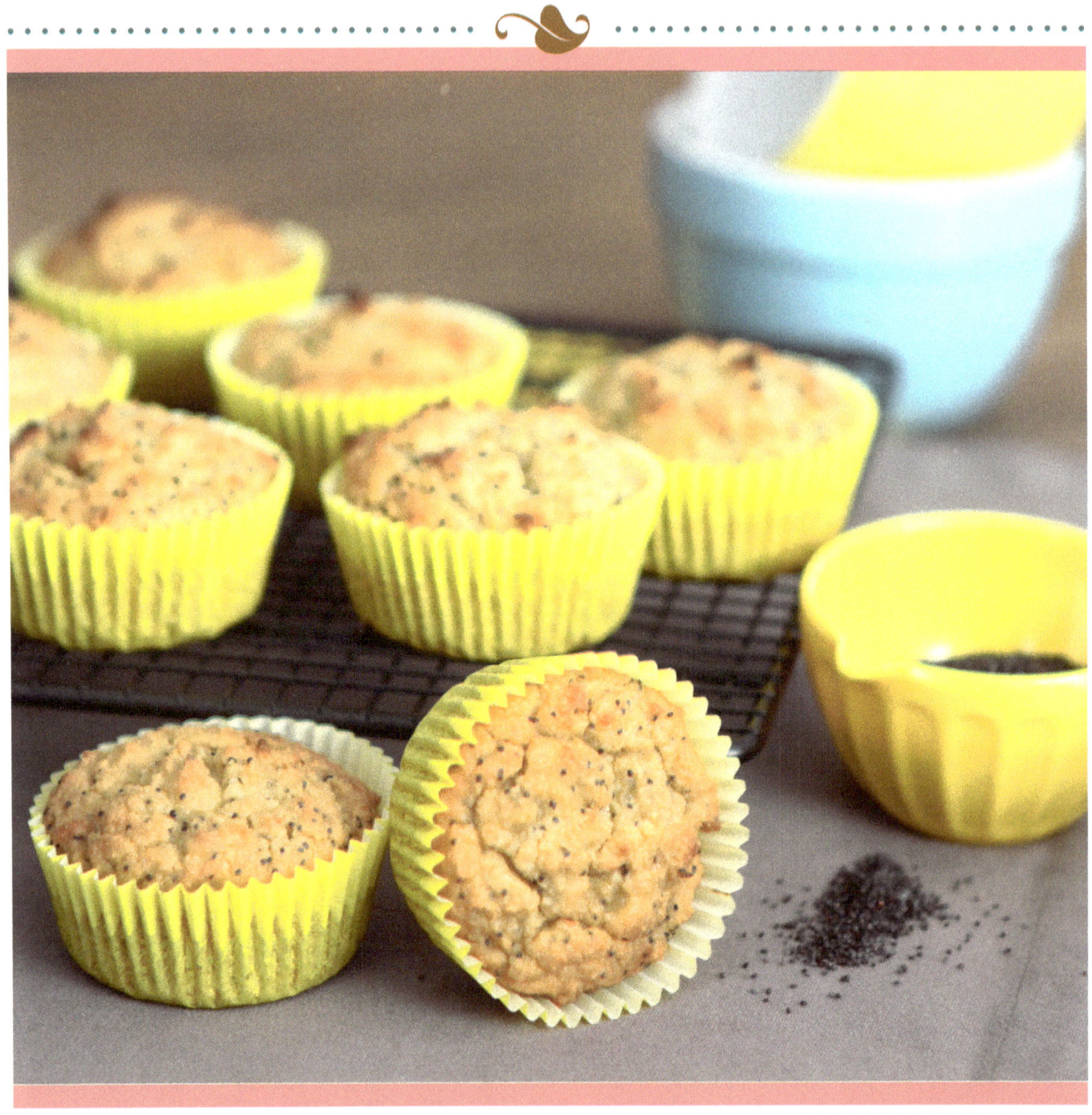

Lemon Poppy Seed Muffins

These lemon zesty muffins are light for a Paleo muffin. Citrus fruit is known for being high in vitamin C, but it is also high in vitamin B and E, calcium, iron, phosphorus, magnesium, potassium, copper and zinc. That's a good reason to add a squeeze of lemon juice into as many recipes as possible.

Prep time: 20 minutes Cooking time: 25 minutes Makes: 8 large

Ingredients:

- 3 large eggs
- ½ cup coconut milk
- ¼ cup ghee or coconut oil
- ¼ cup honey
- ¼ cup lemon juice
- 2 Tbsp lemon zest
- ½ tsp vanilla extract
- 1½ cups almond meal/flour
- ¼ cup coconut flour
- 2 Tbsp arrowroot flour
- ½ tsp baking soda
- ¼ tsp fine sea salt
- 1-1½ Tbsp poppy seeds

Method:

Preheat oven to 160c/320f. Add paper liners/patty pans to a muffin tin.

To a food processor add, eggs, coconut milk, ghee, honey, lemon juice, zest and vanilla. Process to combined well.

Add almond meal, coconut flour, arrowroot flour, baking soda and salt. Process until you have a smooth and creamy mixture with all ingredients well incorporated. Remove blade and stir in poppy seeds.

Spoon batter evenly throughout the muffin tin. The batter will be thick, use a spoon to press and spread the batter to all sides of the muffin liners.

Bake for 25 minutes or until just starting to brown and middle is just firm, don't over cook. Allow to cool for 10 minutes in muffin tin, remove to a wire rack to finish cooling.

Store in an airtight container. Suitable to freeze.

MUFFINS, CAKES AND SLICES

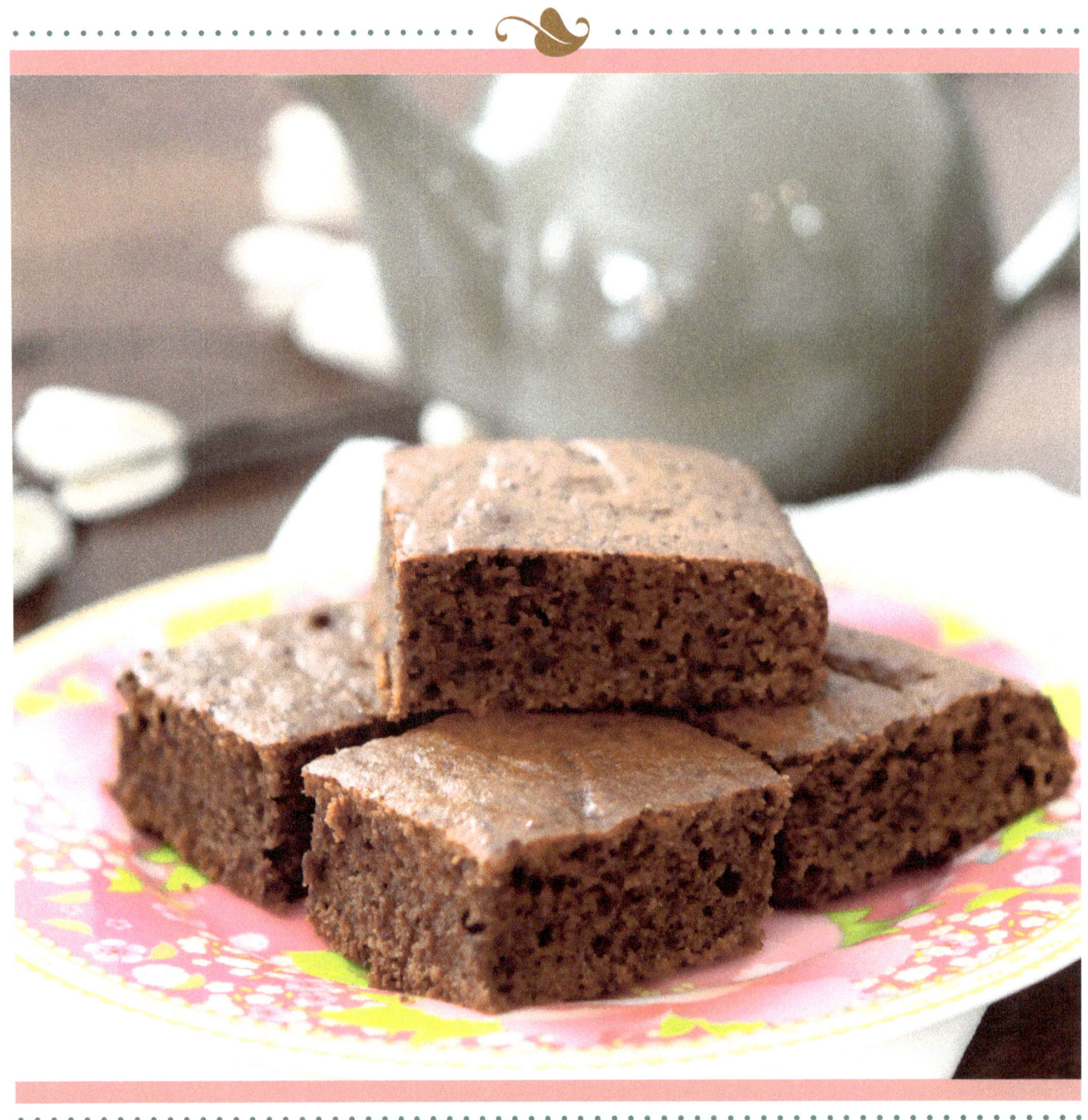

Brownies

This is a fudgy brownie, which can also be used for a dessert (warmed and topped with dairy free cream). Also delicious frosted with Chocolate Ganache, page 283. I enjoy them plain as a treat with a cup of dandelion tea. The batter is so yummy you may be licking the spatula just like I do.

Prep time: 15 minutes Cooking time: 20 minutes Makes: 12

Ingredients:

- 1¼ cups almond meal/flour
- ¼ tsp baking soda
- ¼ tsp fine sea salt
- 100g/3.5oz block 85% organic dark chocolate (soy free, paleo friendly)
- 10 Medjool dates, pitted
- 3 large eggs
- ½ cup coconut oil, softened
- 3 Tbsp cashew butter/spread
- 1 Tbsp honey or to taste
- 2 tsp vanilla extract
- Optional ½ cup chopped nuts of choice

Method:

Preheat oven to 160c/320f. Line or grease a 27x17cm (10.5x6.5in) slice tin with baking paper or coconut oil.

To a food processor add, almond meal, baking soda, salt and roughly broken up chocolate. Process until chocolate resembles the almond meal.

Add dates and process until they are broken up.

Add eggs, coconut oil, cashew butter, honey and vanilla. Process until mixture is smooth. Remove blade (if you are adding nuts, stir through batter).

Transfer batter to the prepared tin. Spread batter out evenly and smooth the top with a spatula.

Bake for 20 minutes, do not over cook, you want a moist fudge texture. Brownies should have slightly risen and just browning on the edges. Cool completely before cutting into squares.

Once cooled the top will change to a darker brown. The longer brownies are left after baking, the more fudge-like they become (best baked one day ahead). Store in an airtight container.

222 | MUFFINS, CAKES AND SLICES

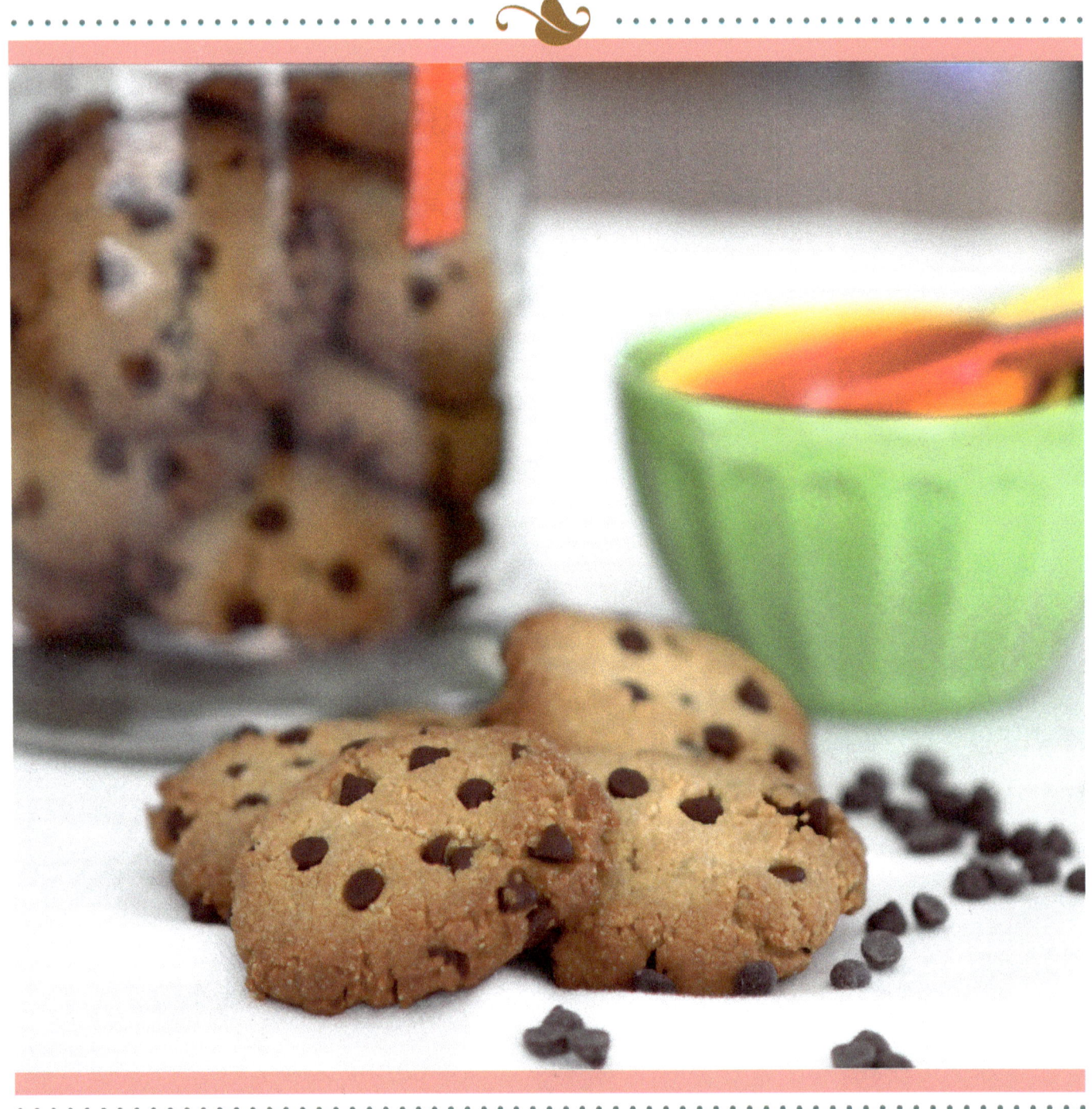

Chocolate Chip Cookies

This is the most baked recipe in our house. Usually almond meal makes for a softer texture, due to its moisture content. If you watch them carefully, turning often to get them to dry out nicely without burning, you will be rewarded with a lovely crisp cookie.

Prep time: 15 minutes Cooking time: 15 minutes Makes: 20

Ingredients:

- 2½ cups almond meal/flour
- ½ tsp baking soda
- ¼ tsp fine sea salt
- ¼ cup coconut oil
- 2 Tbsp honey, or adjust to your taste
- 1 Tbsp vanilla extract
- ½ cup dark chocolate chips, soy-free paleo friendly
- Variation: swap choc chips for ½ cup chopped macadamia nuts

Method:

Preheat oven to 150c/300f. Line 2 baking trays with baking paper.

To a food processor add, almond meal, baking soda and salt. Pulse a couple of times to combine.

Add coconut oil, honey and vanilla, process until well combined. If coconut oil is solid, check it has been well incorporated into the mixture.

Remove blade from food processor and stir through the chocolate chips or macadamia nuts by hand.

Scoop a tablespoonful of dough into your hand, press mixture together and form a cookie shape, place on prepared baking tray. Press dough down gently to flatten.

Bake for 15-18 minutes or until golden, keeping an eye on them while baking. The secret to giving them a crunch, is using the low temperature to slowly dry out the almond meal, turn frequently to produce an even colour. (This recipe with macadamia nuts is just as delicious). Cool for 15 minutes before removing from trays.

Store in an airtight container to prevent cookies softening. They freeze well.

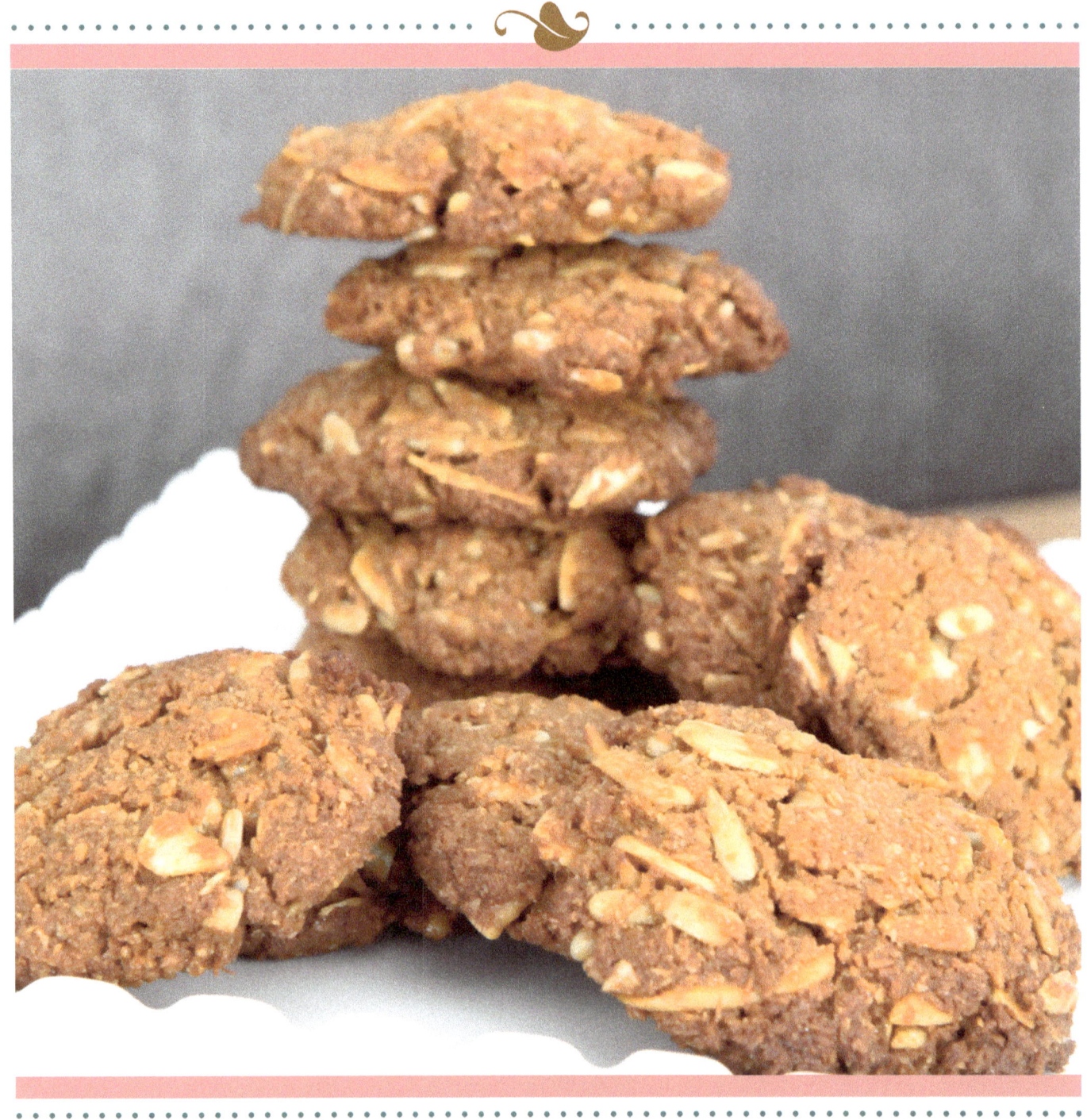

"Anzac" Biscuits

"Anzac" biscuits have long been associated with the "Australian and New Zealand Army Corps". They go back to World War 1, when our troops where stationed on the shores of Gallipoli. My grandfather was one of them. Anzac tiles, as they were called then, where part of a soldiers rations with beef bully. They were used as bread because the ingredients didn't spoil easily but were very hard to eat. The mothers, wives and girlfriends of Australian troops back home got wind of the terrible Anzac tiles and were reportedly concerned that their boys were not getting enough nutrients. These women used the recipe for Scottish oatcakes as a base and developed what we know of today as the Anzac biscuit. I have altered the ingredients to make them Paleo friendly.

Prep time: 15 minutes Cooking time: 20 minutes Makes: 28

Ingredients:

- 1½ cups almond meal/flour
- 1 cup flaked almonds
- 1 cup desiccated coconut
- ½ cup sunflower seeds
- ⅓ tsp fine sea salt
- ⅓ cup honey
- 1 Tbsp organic molasses, unsulphured
- ¼ cup ghee or organic butter
- 1 tsp baking soda
- 2 Tbsp filtered water

Method:

Preheat oven to 140c/285f. Line 2 baking trays with baking paper.

Add to a large bowl, almond meal, flaked almonds, coconut, sunflower seeds and salt. Mix to combine.

To a small saucepan, add honey, molasses and ghee. Heat gently, don't allow to boil. Add baking soda and water together in a small cup and add to heated honey mixture. Mix through and when it froths remove from heat.

Make a well in dry ingredients and pour in frothing honey mixture. Mix well to combine.

Scoop out rounded tablespoons of mixture and press together in your hands to make the mixture come together. Form a round patty shape 5cm(2ins) in diameter and place on prepared tray, gently flattening.

Bake for 20 minutes or until golden brown and firm to the touch.

Let cool on the trays for 10 minutes while they crispen up further, then transfer to a wire rack to completely cool.

Store in an airtight container to keep the biscuits crunchy.

226 | MUFFINS, CAKES AND SLICES

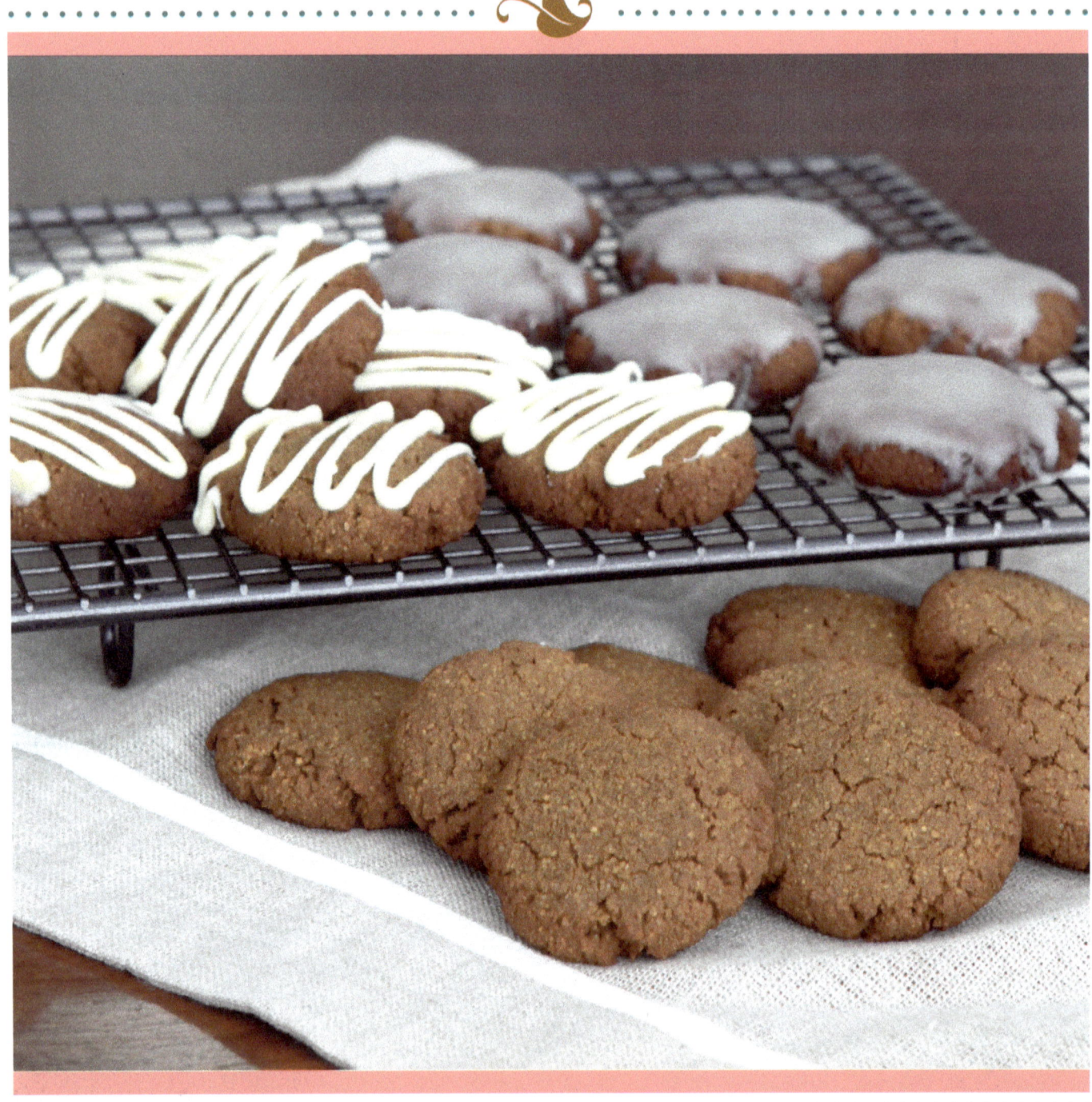

Gingerbread Cookies

These cookies are one of my grandchildren's favourites. Gingerbread is traditionally for Christmas time but who wants to wait for once a year to eat them, definitely not my family.

Prep time: 15 minutes Cooking time: 13-15 minutes Makes: 24

Ingredients:

- ½ cup almond meal/flour
- ½ cup coconut flour
- ¼ cup coconut sugar
- 4 Medjool dates, pitted
- 1 tsp cinnamon
- ¾ tsp ground ginger
- ½ tsp baking soda
- ⅛ tsp fine sea salt
- 2 Tbsp organic molasses, unsulphured
- 2 large eggs
- ¼ cup ghee
- White organic chocolate or use any choice of glaze on page 284 to decorate

Method:

Preheat oven to 160c/320f. Line 2 baking trays with baking paper.

To a food processor add, almond meal, coconut flour, coconut sugar, dates, spices, baking soda and salt. Pulse to combine.

Add molasses, eggs and ghee, process until mixture comes together and gathers at the sides of the bowl. Scrape mixture down and pulse a few times. Mixture will firm up a little as the coconut flour soaks up the moisture. Remove blade and stir through the dough left on bottom of bowl.

Roll cookie dough into 24 small balls and place on prepared baking trays, leaving 5cms(2ins) between them. To make a nice round cookie shape, place a small square of baking paper over a ball of dough and use the flat bottom of a glass to press down gently through the paper. Repeat for each ball of dough.

Bake for 13-15 minutes, or until the bottoms of the cookies are brown. Let cookies completely cool before handling.

For Christmas I melt white chocolate over a double saucepan, pour melted chocolate into a snap lock bag and snip a very small piece from the corner. Drizzle chocolate across the cookies making a pattern. Or make a glaze and spread over the top of the cookies.

Store completed cookies in an airtight container in the fridge. I have kept these cookies for up to 3 weeks and they freeze well.

MUFFINS, CAKES AND SLICES

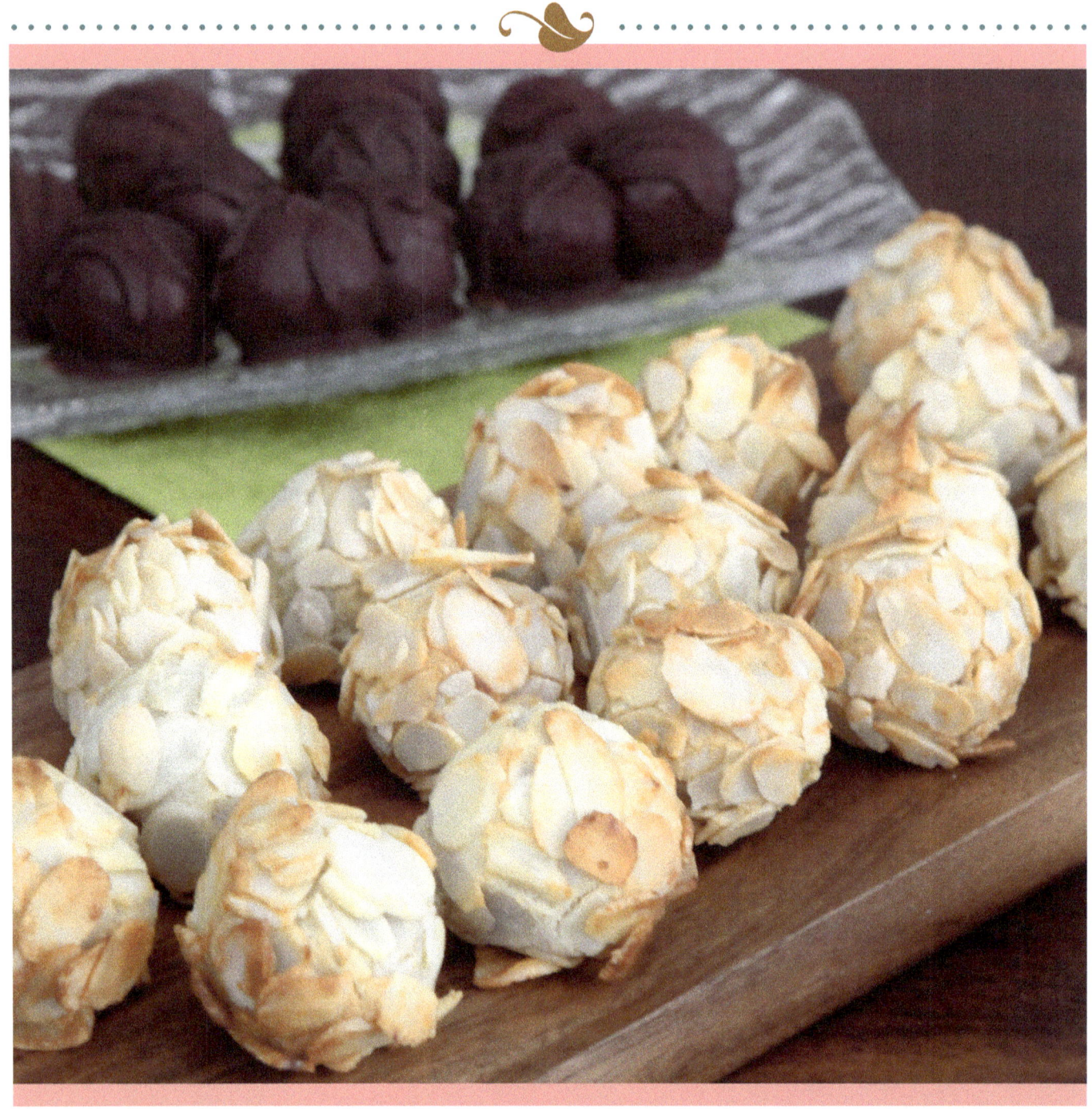

Marzipan Cookies

These were created with all three of my marzipan loving daughters in law in mind. Then I realized you can't have marzipan without chocolate! See the chocolate option at the bottom of the page.

Prep time: 20 minutes, plus refrigeration time Cooking time: 15 minutes Makes: 20

Ingredients:

- 3 cups almond meal/flour
- ⅓ cup honey
- 1 large egg white
- 2½ tsp organic almond extract
- Pinch of fine sea salt
- 1 large egg white, for coating
- 1 ½ - 2 cups almond flakes, for coating

Method:

To a food processor add, almond meal, honey, egg white, almond extract and salt. Process until all ingredients have combined and formed together. Remove and wrap dough to seal and prevent drying out, refrigerate for 1 hour.

Just before removing dough from fridge, preheat oven to 160c/320f. Line a baking tray with baking paper.

Shape chilled dough into 20 small balls. Add egg white to a small bowl and whisk with a fork to break it up. Add almond flakes to a plate. Dip 2 or 3 balls into egg white at a time and roll to coat.

Transfer to plate with almond flakes. Press as much almond flakes into the dough as possible. I like to place almond flakes into my palms and press the flakes into the marzipan ball, I find more stick that way. If you find missing spots just poke extra fakes in sideways.

Place on prepared baking tray. Repeat until tray is full. Bake for 15 minutes or until almond flakes have started browning. Cool before serving.

Store at room temperature in an airtight container for up to 1 week.

Chocolate Marzipan Balls: Omit egg whites from recipe. Prepare dough as above. After shaping balls, skip almond flakes and baking. Place balls on a tray and then into the freezer to firm up.

Make your own or melt paleo friendly chocolate in a double saucepan, let it cool slightly. Dip each marzipan ball into chocolate. Use 2 forks to cradle each ball, let excess chocolate drip off and place on a lined tray to set.

After they have started to set, drizzle a little extra chocolate across the tops to decorate. Store in fridge in an airtight container for up to 10 days.

230 | MUFFINS, CAKES AND SLICES

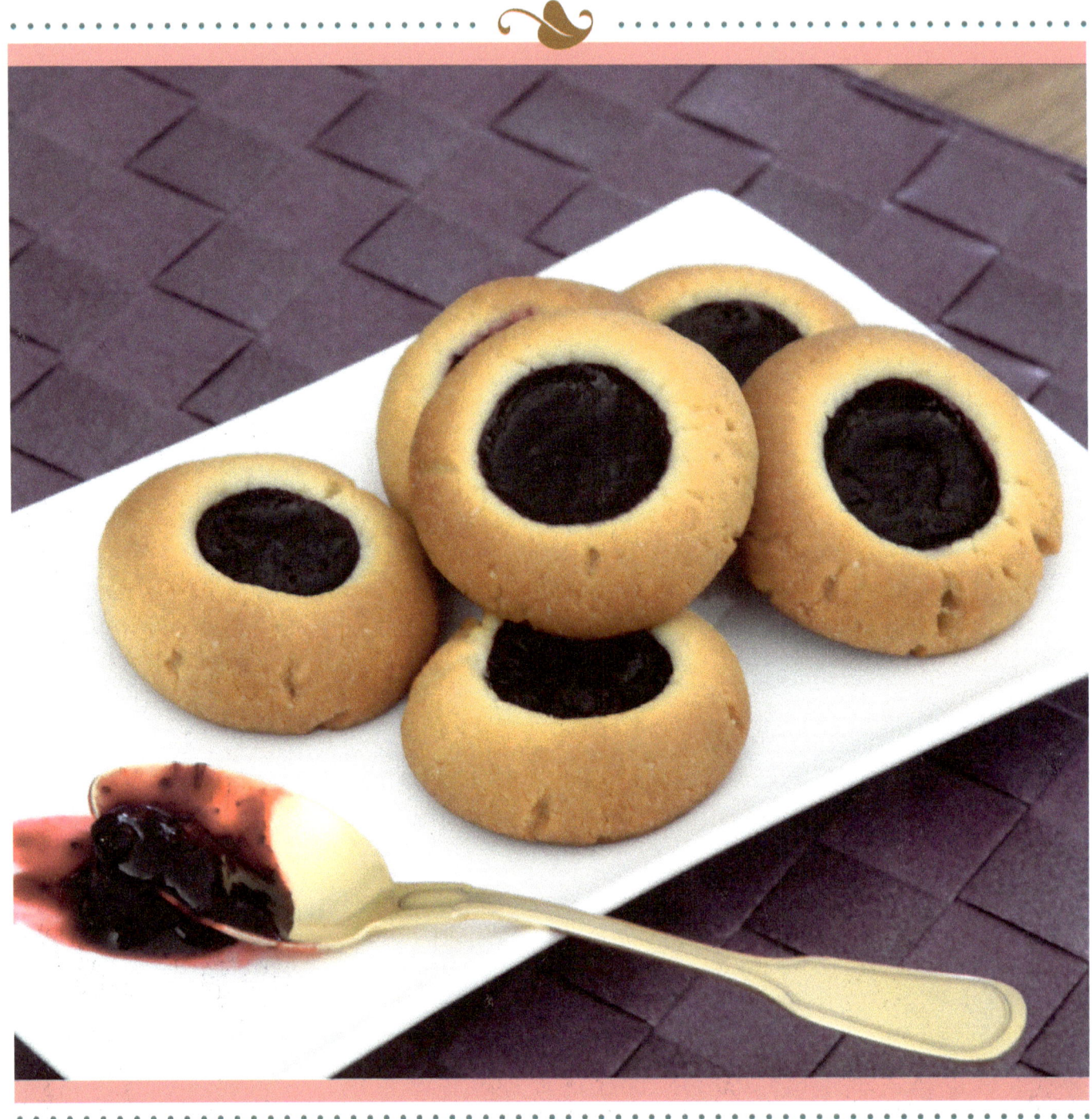

Blueberry Thumbprint Biscuits

This biscuit recipe was made as a surprise for my daughter in law, Ashleigh. A few years back, when she was dating my son Mark, she lived 4 hours away in a country town and often mailed him a box of thumbprint biscuits. (She is still spoiling him).

Prep time: 15 minutes   Cooking time: 12 minutes   Makes: 20

Ingredients:

- 2½ cups almond meal/flour
- 3 Tbsp desiccated coconut
- ⅓ tsp fine sea salt
- ¼ tsp baking soda
- ⅓ cup ghee, room temperature
- 2 Tbsp honey
- ¼ cup blueberry spread page 290 or organic jam of choice

Method:

Preheat oven to 150c/300f. Line a baking tray with baking paper.

To a food processor add, almond meal, coconut, sea salt and baking soda. Pulse to combine. Add ghee and honey, process until a smooth, light dough forms and comes together. Scoop out scant tablespoons of dough and roll into balls. Place on prepared baking tray.

Use your thumb to press an indent into the centre of each ball of dough, being careful not to split the biscuit. Place ½ a teaspoon of blueberry spread or organic jam into the centre of each biscuit.

Bake for 12-14 minutes or until light brown, the biscuits will be slightly soft to touch but will firm up as they cool. Turn tray while cooking to help brown evenly. Leave on tray to completely cool before serving.

THE JOYFUL TABLE

232 | MUFFINS, CAKES AND SLICES

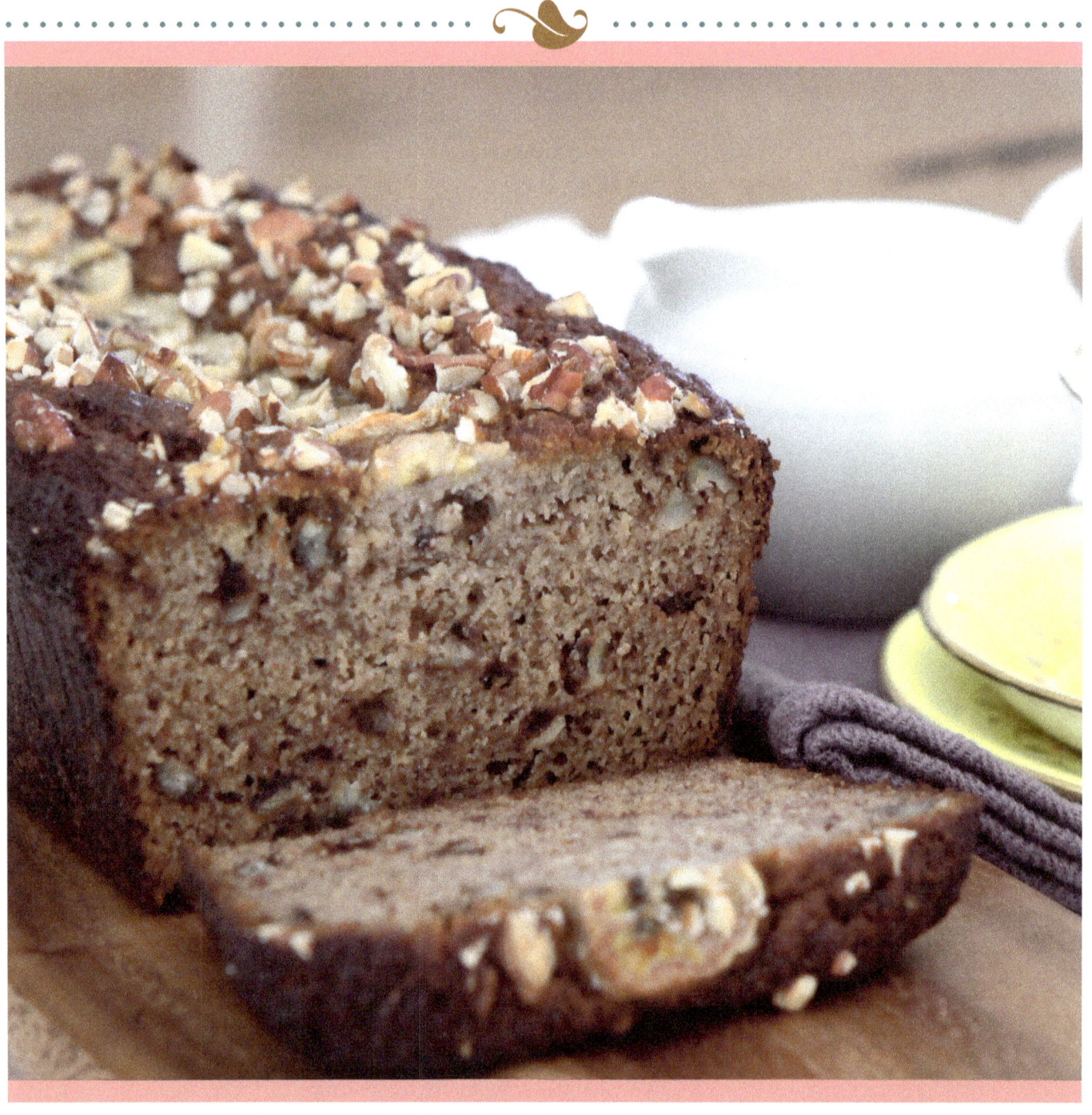

Banana Bread

My grandchildren love my Banana Bread and ask me to bake it for them all the time. It's so easy to make and friends can't believe that something that tastes this good can be healthy too! For a change, bake in muffin tins.

Prep time: 10 minutes Cooking time: 1 hour Makes: 1 loaf

Ingredients:

- 3 ripe bananas (1½ cups mashed)
- 3 large eggs
- ¼ cup coconut oil, melted
- 3 medjool dates, pitted
- 1 Tbsp honey
- 1 Tbsp vanilla extract
- 2 ¼ cups almond meal/flour
- 1 tsp baking soda
- ½ tsp fine sea salt
- ½ cup chopped pecans plus extra to sprinkle on top

Method:

Preheat oven to 160c/320f. Grease and line the base of a loaf tin.

To a food processor, add the bananas, eggs, coconut oil, dates, honey and vanilla. Process until smooth.

Add almond meal, baking soda and salt, process just until combined.

Remove blade and mix in nuts by hand. Pour batter into the prepared loaf tin. Sprinkle top with extra chopped pecans.

Bake for approximately 1 hour, or until a skewer or toothpick inserted comes out clean. (Turn during cooking as almond meal browns easily.)

Let cool in tin for 20 minutes before removing to finish cooling on a wire rack.

Store in a sealed container in the fridge for up to 1 week. Freezes well, slice before freezing and place baking paper between slices.

234 | MUFFINS, CAKES AND SLICES

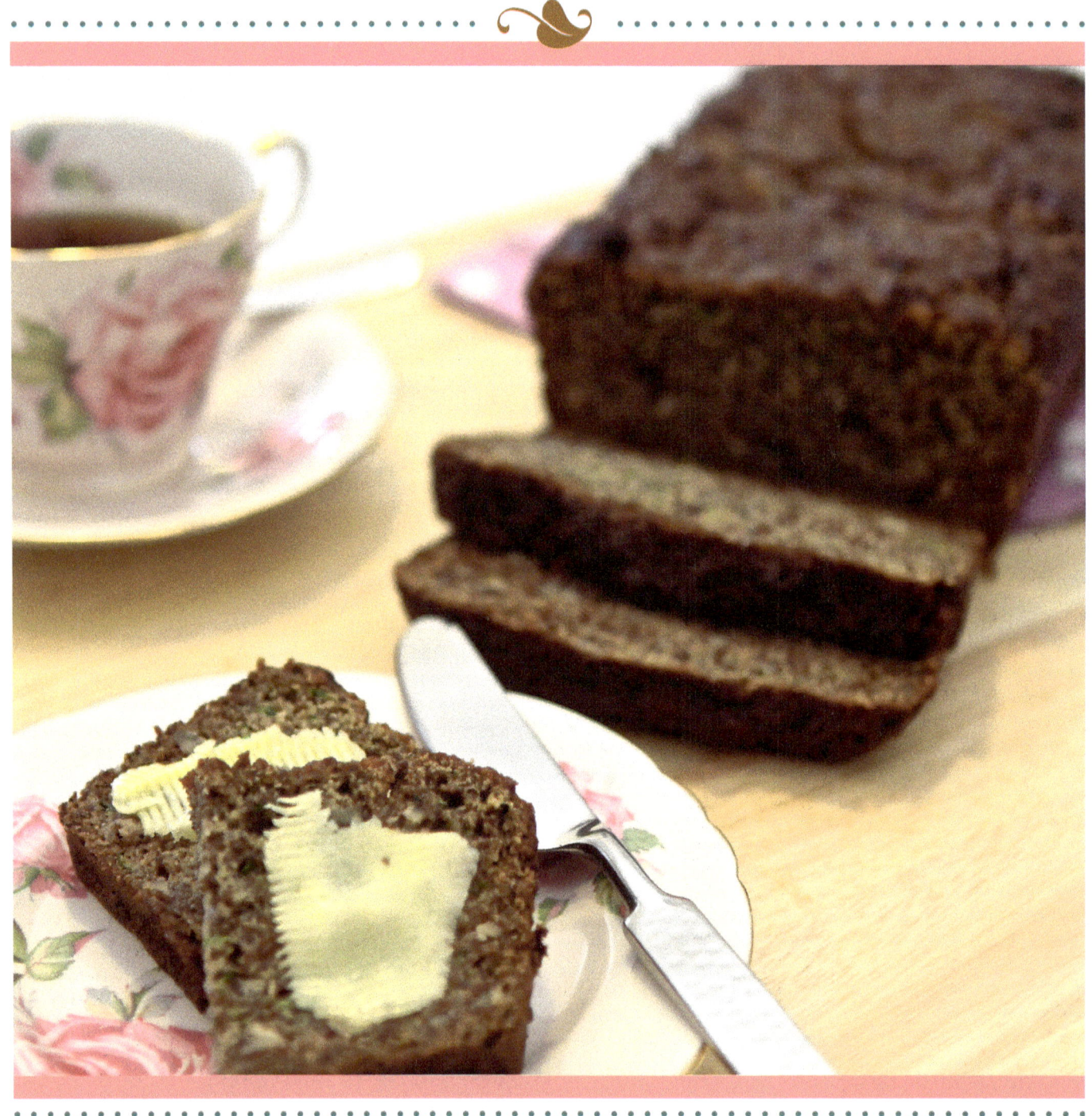

Zucchini Bread

An excellent way to get vegetables into kids. I have also included a Nut Free option.

Prep time: 20 minutes   Cooking time: 1 hour   Makes: 1 loaf

Ingredients:

- 1½ cups grated zucchini (skin left on)
- ¾ cup flaxseed meal
- ⅓ cup coconut flour, sifted
- ½ cup almond meal, for nut free substitute with sunflower meal 1:1 ratio
- ¾ cup chopped pecans or walnuts (omit for nut free)
- 1 tsp baking soda (if using sunflowers sub with 3 tsp baking powder)
- ⅓ tsp fine sea salt
- 3 large eggs
- ½ cup honey
- ⅓ cup coconut cream or yoghurt
- 1 Tbsp vanilla extract

Method:

Preheat oven to 160c/320f. Grease and line the base of a loaf tin with baking paper. Grate zucchini and set aside.

In a large bowl, combine flaxseed, coconut flour, almond meal, nuts, baking soda and salt. Stir to thoroughly mix.

Add the eggs, honey, coconut cream and vanilla to a medium bowl and beat to combine. Pour into dry ingredients and stir until moistened. Mix in zucchini making sure it is distributed evenly.

Spoon batter into prepared loaf tin, smooth over top. Bake approximately 1 hour or until a skewer or toothpick inserted comes out clean. This is a very moist cake. Turn during cooking for even colour. Let cool in tin for 20 minutes before you finish cooling on a wire rack.

Best kept in an airtight container. If stored in the fridge, it will keep for up to 10 days. Also freezes well.

MUFFINS, CAKES AND SLICES

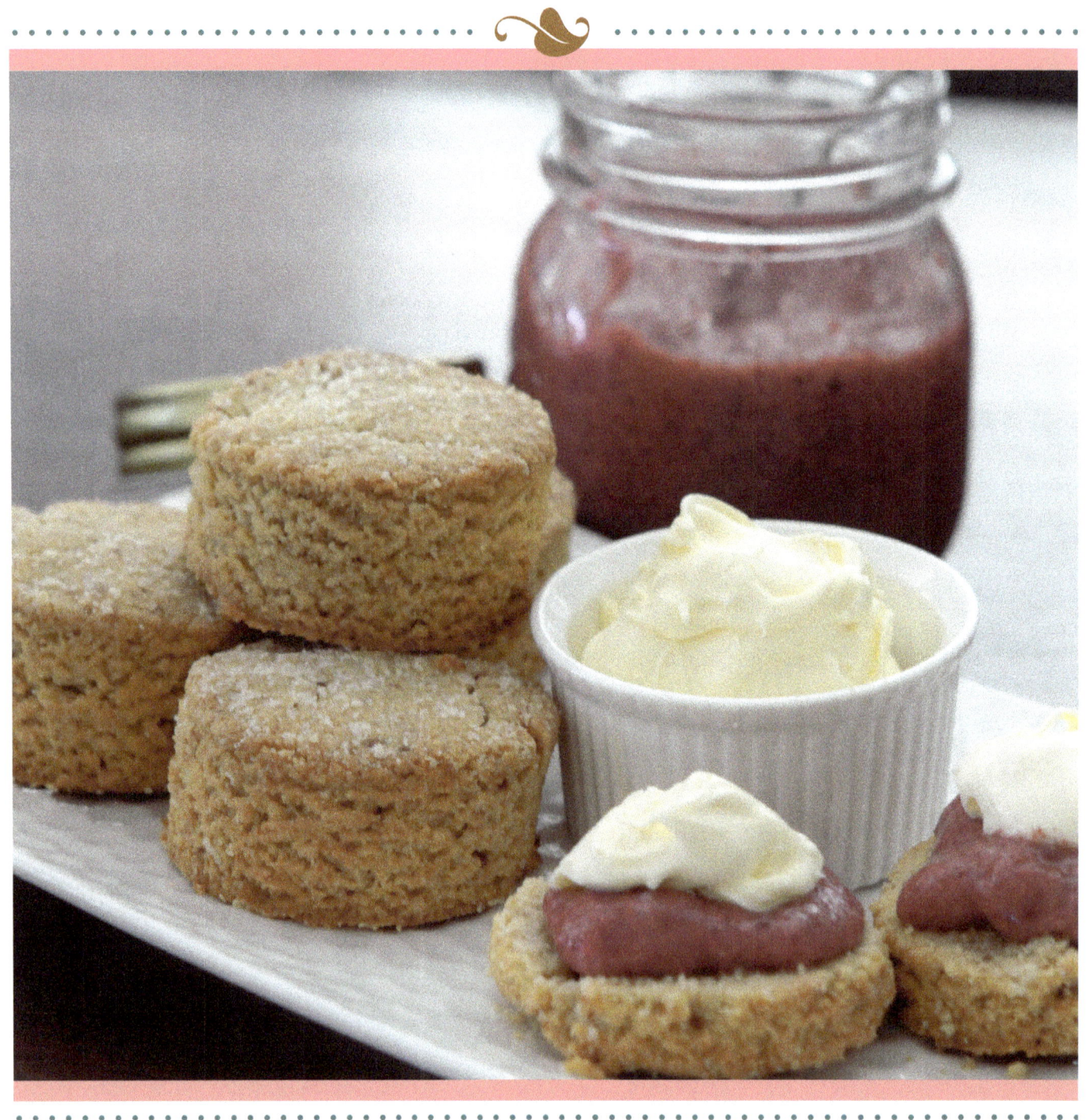

Scones

I love this recipe, I don't miss wheat scones at all and even family and friends that aren't gluten free love them. They are so quick and easy to bake. Serve warm with homemade fruit jam and dairy free cream of choice or spread with ghee or organic butter. Also great to serve with a hearty stew.

Prep time: 15 Cooking time: 15 Makes: 8-9

Ingredients:

- 3 cups almond meal/flour
- 1 Tbsp coconut sugar
- ¾ tsp baking soda
- ½ tsp fine sea salt
- 2 large eggs, room temperature
- 60gm/¼ cup ghee, melted and cooled slightly

Method:

Preheat oven to 160c/320f. Line a baking tray with baking paper.

To a large bowl, add almond meal, coconut sugar, baking soda and sea salt. Mix well to combine.

Whisk eggs in a small bowl, pour in melted ghee that has been slightly cooled. Whisk to combine.

Stir the wet ingredients into the dry. Use your hands to knead and make the dough come together.

Place the dough onto a sheet of baking paper. Use hands to shape and flatten the dough. Flatten to 2.5cms(1in) thick. If a little sticky use extra almond meal.

Use a 5.5cm(2.5in) scone cutter to cut scones out. Place on prepared tray and very lightly sprinkle a little almond meal on top of each scone, optional. (I find this gives a more traditional scone look after being baked.)

Bake for 15 minutes until scones have brown bottoms and golden on top.

MUFFINS, CAKES AND SLICES

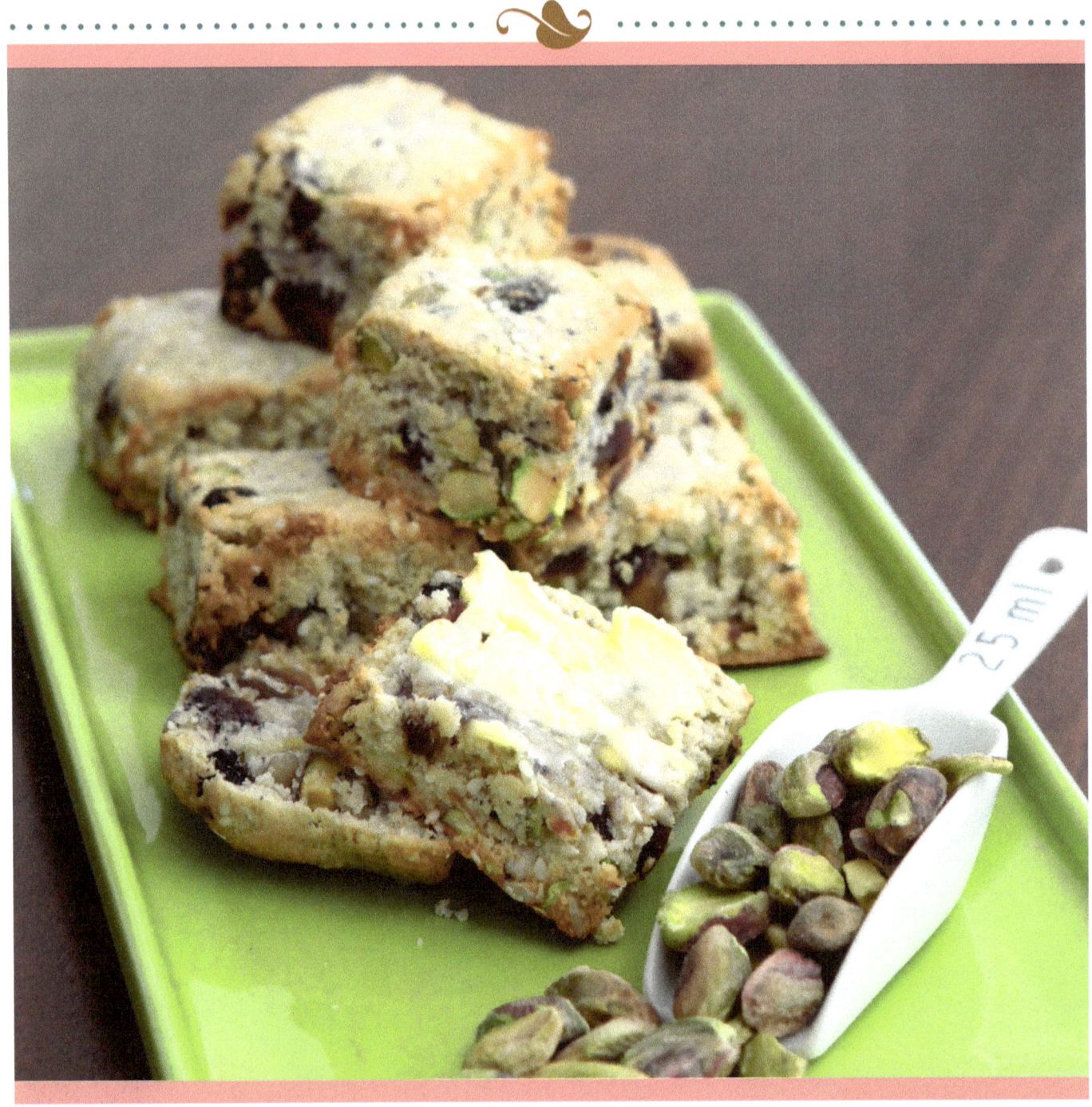

Fruity Nut Scones

Use these scones for your next High Tea, they will impress. I love the combination of these flavours, add your favourite fruits and nuts and see what you come up with.

Prep time: 20 minutes Cooking time: 15 minutes Makes: 12

Ingredients:

- 2½ cups almond meal/flour
- ¼ cup sesame seeds
- ¼ cup sunflower seeds
- 1 tsp baking soda
- ⅓ tsp fine sea salt
- ⅓ cup freeze dried blueberries or your favourite dried fruit (preservative free)
- 5 medjool dates, chopped into pieces
- ⅓ cup pistachios, coarsely chopped
- 2 Tbsp 100% maple syrup
- 1 large egg

Method:

Preheat oven to 160c/320f. Line a baking tray with baking paper.

Add to a large bowl, almond meal, sesame and sunflower seeds, baking soda and sea salt. Mix to combined. Add blueberries, dates and pistachios. Combined well.

To a small bowl add, maple syrup and egg, whisk together with a fork. Make a well in the centre of the dry ingredients and pour egg mixture in. Stir to combine; you may like to use your hands to knead mixture together.

Place dough on a sheet of baking paper that has a little almond meal sprinkled over it. Form into a 16x14cm(6.5x5.5in) rectangle with a thickness of 2.5cm(1in). Cut dough into 4x3 rows, making 12 scones.

Bake for 15 minutes or until just lightly browning, the bottoms will be a lot darker.

Serve warm with organic butter or ghee or just as they are.

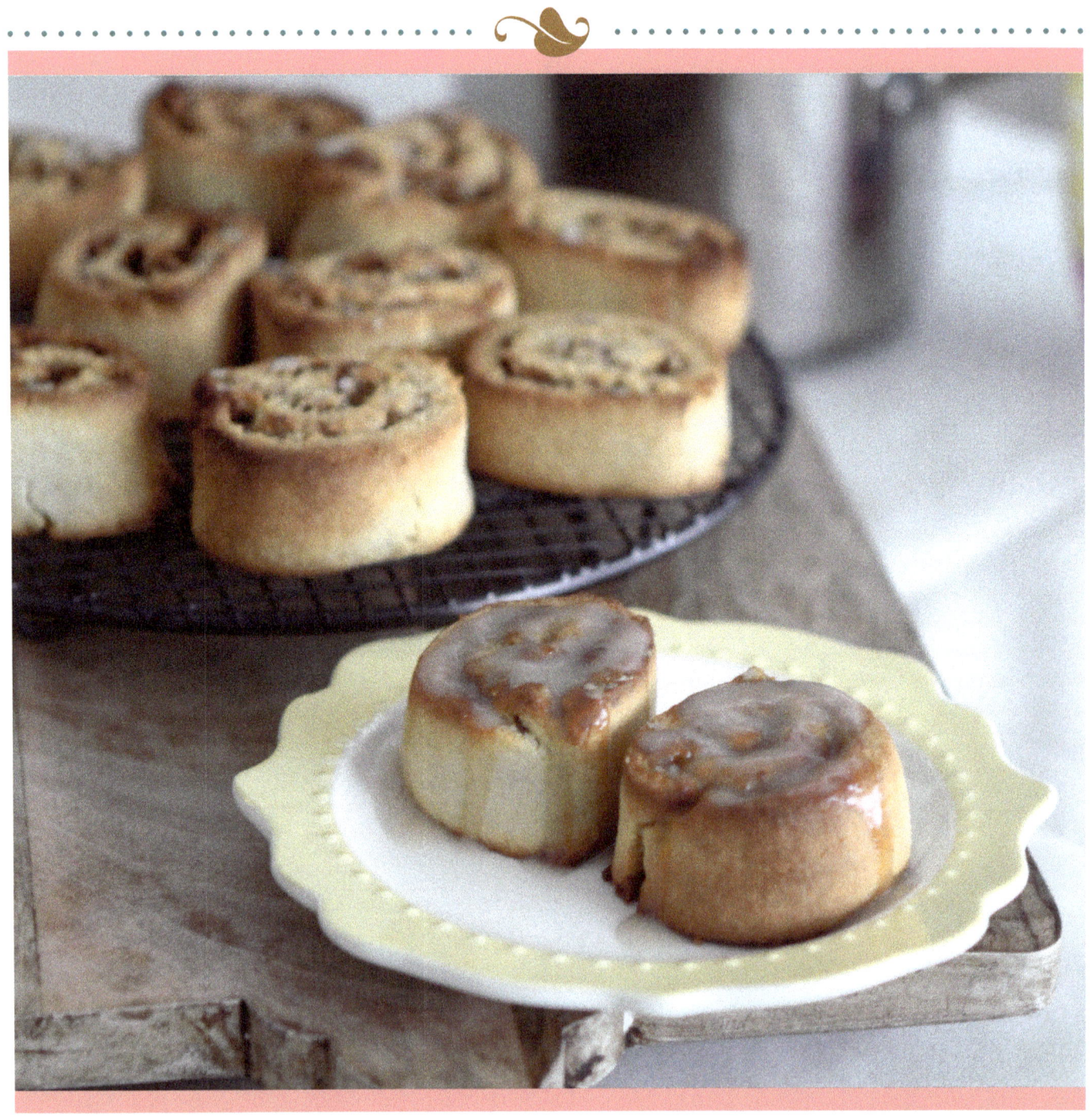

Cinnamon Pecan Rolls

I enjoy these Cinnamon and Pecan rolls served warm straight from the oven. You may like to drizzle vanilla or cinnamon glaze over your rolls, recipes on page 284.

Prep time: 20 minutes   Cooking time: 12 minutes   Makes: 12

Ingredients:

3⅓ cups almond meal/flour
¾ tsp gluten free baking powder
¼ tsp baking soda
¼ tsp sea salt
2 large eggs, room temperature

2 Tbsp coconut oil, melt and allowed to cool slightly
2 Tbsp honey
½ tsp organic almond extract

FILLING
¼-⅓ cup honey
1 Tbsp ground cinnamon
¾ cup pecans, finely chopped

Method:

Preheat oven to 160c/320f. Line a baking tray with baking paper.

To a large bowl add, almond meal, baking powder, baking soda and salt. Mix well to combine. To a medium bowl add, eggs and whisk. Continue whisking while you pour in coconut oil. Add honey and almond extract, blend well making sure coconut oil doesn't firm up. Add egg mixture to the almond meal. Mix well.

Knead until a smooth dough is formed. If you dampen your hands with water the dough shouldn't stick while kneading. Place dough on a large piece of baking paper. Shape dough into a rectangle and flatten. Cover with another sheet of paper. Using a rolling pin, roll out into a rectangle, approximately 27x40cm(10.5x15.75ins).

Remove top sheet of baking paper to add filling. Drizzle honey evenly over the dough. Use a flat knife to carefully spread honey. Sprinkle cinnamon over honey, then evenly cover with chopped pecans.

Start with long edge closest to you and begin to roll the edge of the dough away from you. Begin rolling tightly, using the baking paper to help you roll and keep the dough together. Press down on the paper as you roll but don't allow it to get caught up in the rolled dough. Continue rolling until you have a nice even log, mending any splits as you go. Keep the paper around the outside and roll the whole log gently, lengthening it out a bit as you roll.

With a sharp knife, cut the roll into approximately 3.5cm(1.5in) thick slices. (Wipe the knife to keep the cuts neat). Place slices on their side on the prepared baking tray, leaving space between them.

Bake for 12-15 minutes. The Cinnamon Pecan rolls should be golden in colour, with the dough towards the centre being soft but not too doughy. Their bottoms will be lovely and brown due to the honey dripping out. After removing from oven let cool for 10 minutes on the tray.

Serve warm or cold, either plain or glazed. Store in an airtight container. Can be kept for up to 5 days, if they last that long. Also suitable to freeze.

MUFFINS, CAKES AND SLICES

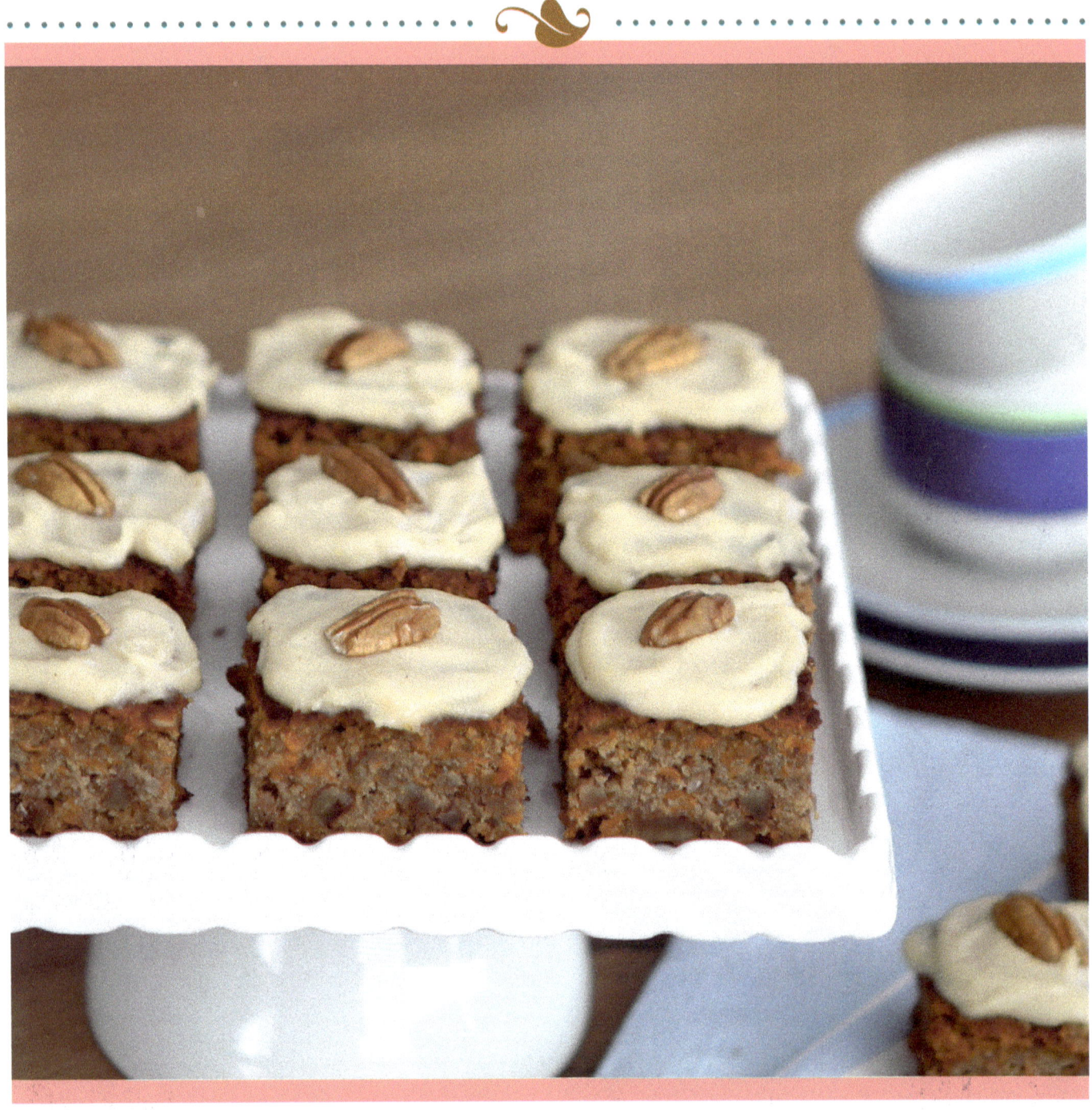

Carrot Cake
with Lemon Cream Icing

You cannot have carrot cake without icing. I have included my dairy free Lemon Cream icing recipe below.

Prep time: 20 minutes Cooking time: 45 minutes Serves: 16 pieces

Ingredients:

- 2 Tbsp chia seeds
- 100ml filtered water to soak chia seeds
- 1/3 cup coconut flour, sifted
- 1 1/2 baking soda
- 1 1/2 tsp cinnamon
- 1 tsp mixed spice
- 3/4 cup almond meal
- 1/4 cup golden flaxseed meal
- 1/4 tsp fine sea salt
- 2 cups grated carrot
- 1 cup pecans, chopped
- 3 large eggs
- 1/2 cup honey
- 2/3 cup macadamia nut oil or coconut oil
- 2 tsp vanilla extract
- Extra whole pecans to decorate

LEMON CREAM ICING

- Make Whipped Cashew Cream, recipe page 282 (use 1/2 the quantity)
- 1 Tbsp lemon juice
- 1 Tbsp lemon zest

Method:
Follow method for Whipped Cashew Cream, blending until whipped and smooth. To half the quantity add lemon juice and zest. Blender a further 30 seconds to combine well.

Method:

Preheat oven to 160c/320f. Grease and line a 22cm(8.5in) square cake tin. Soak chia seeds in water for approximately 10 minutes to form a gel, stir often so it doesn't form into lumps.

To a large bowl, sift in coconut flour, baking soda and spices. Add almond meal, flaxseed and salt, mix well to incorporate all ingredients. Add grated carrot and nuts to the dry mixture and stir through.

To a medium bowl add, eggs, honey, chia mixture, oil and vanilla. Whisk together well, making sure chia is well blended. Add the wet ingredients to the bowl of dry ingredients and combine well.

Spread batter into prepared cake tin and smooth top, the batter will start to thicken as the coconut flour soaks up the moisture.

Bake for 40-45 minutes, or until golden, test with a skewer to see if it comes out clean. Let cake cool in tin before removing.

Make your icing and spread over cooled cake and decorate with whole pecans. I find it easier to cut cake first, spread each square with icing and place a whole pecan on top.

Store in the fridge, but best served at room temperature.

MUFFINS, CAKES AND SLICES

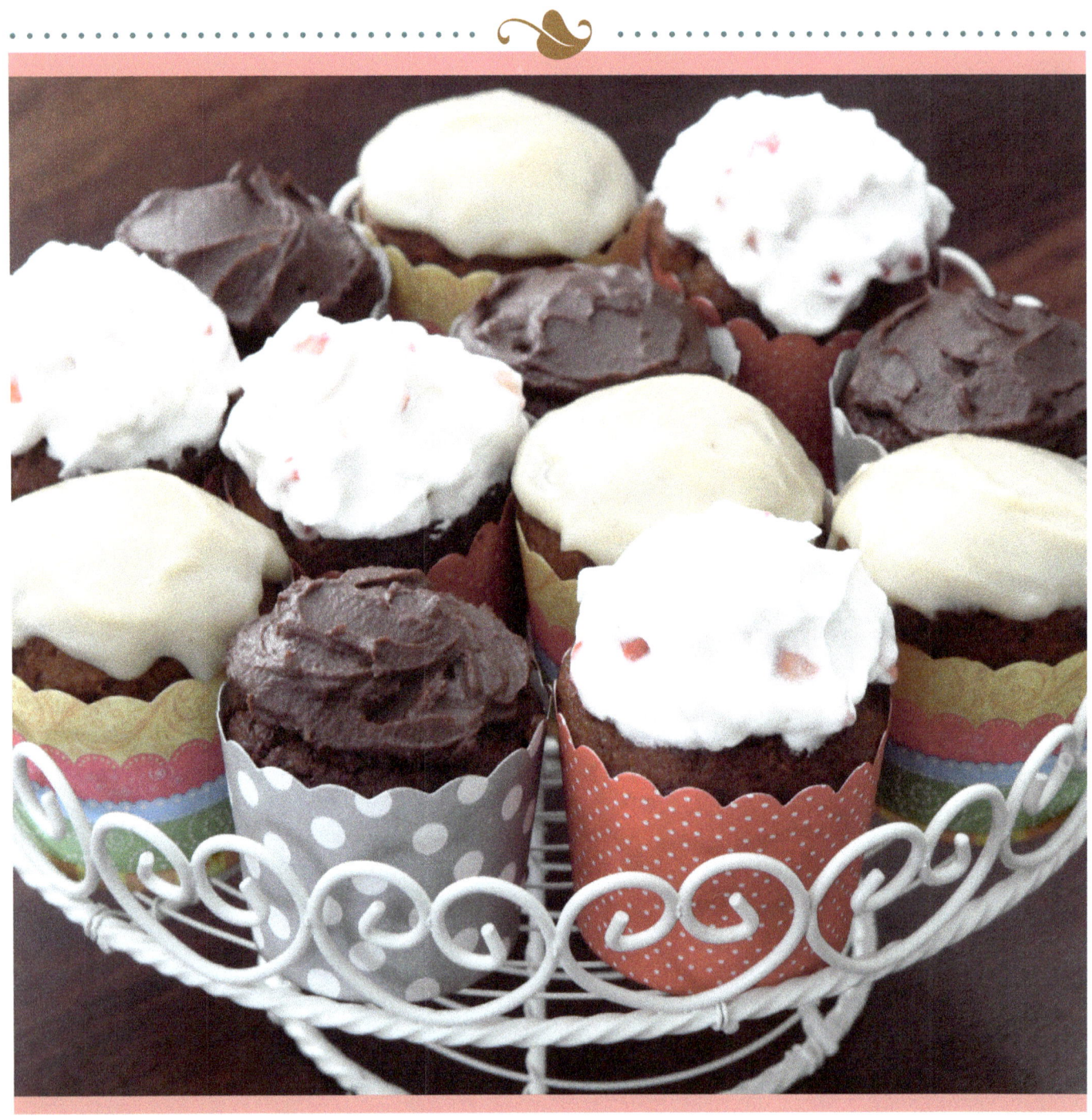

Vanilla Cupcakes

This is a simple and tasty recipe. Add cacao, fruit or nuts to this basic recipe for different flavours. I have included a couple of my favourites below.

Prep time: 15 minutes Cooking time: 23 minutes Makes: 10

Ingredients:

- 4 large eggs
- ½ cup honey
- ¼ cup macadamia oil
- ¼ cup coconut milk or almond milk
- 1 Tbsp vanilla extract
- ¾ tsp baking soda
- ½ tsp fine sea salt
- 2 cups almond meal/flour
- 2 Tbsp coconut flour, sifted

Method:

Preheat oven to 160c/320f. Place paper baking cups in a muffin tin.

To a large bowl add, eggs, honey, macadamia oil, coconut milk and vanilla. Beat with a handheld electric beater until well combined. Add baking soda and salt to bowl and beat to mix through.

Add almond meal and coconut flour. Beat until well combined and aerated.

Spoon ¼ cup of batter into each paper cup. Bake for 23-25 minutes or until light brown. Let cool on a wire rack for 1 hour before icing.

Cupcakes that are not iced can be stored in an airtight container at room temperature but iced cakes need to be store in fridge.

Top with Vanilla Macadamia or Chocolate frosting or your choice from Topping and Spreads section.

CHOCOLATE CUPCAKES

Use the ingredients and method for Vanilla Cupcakes with the addition of; ¼ cup cacao powder. Add cacao with the flours. Bake and store the same as Vanilla cupcakes.

Serve topped with frosting of choice and garnish with grated chocolate or coconut flakes.

STRAWBERRY CUPCAKES

Use the ingredients and method for Vanilla Cupcakes with the addition of; 1 cup of finely chopped fresh strawberries.

Add strawberries after the flours have been well beaten into the wet ingredients. Gently stir strawberries through the batter. Bake and store the same as Vanilla cupcakes.

246 | MUFFINS, CAKES AND SLICES

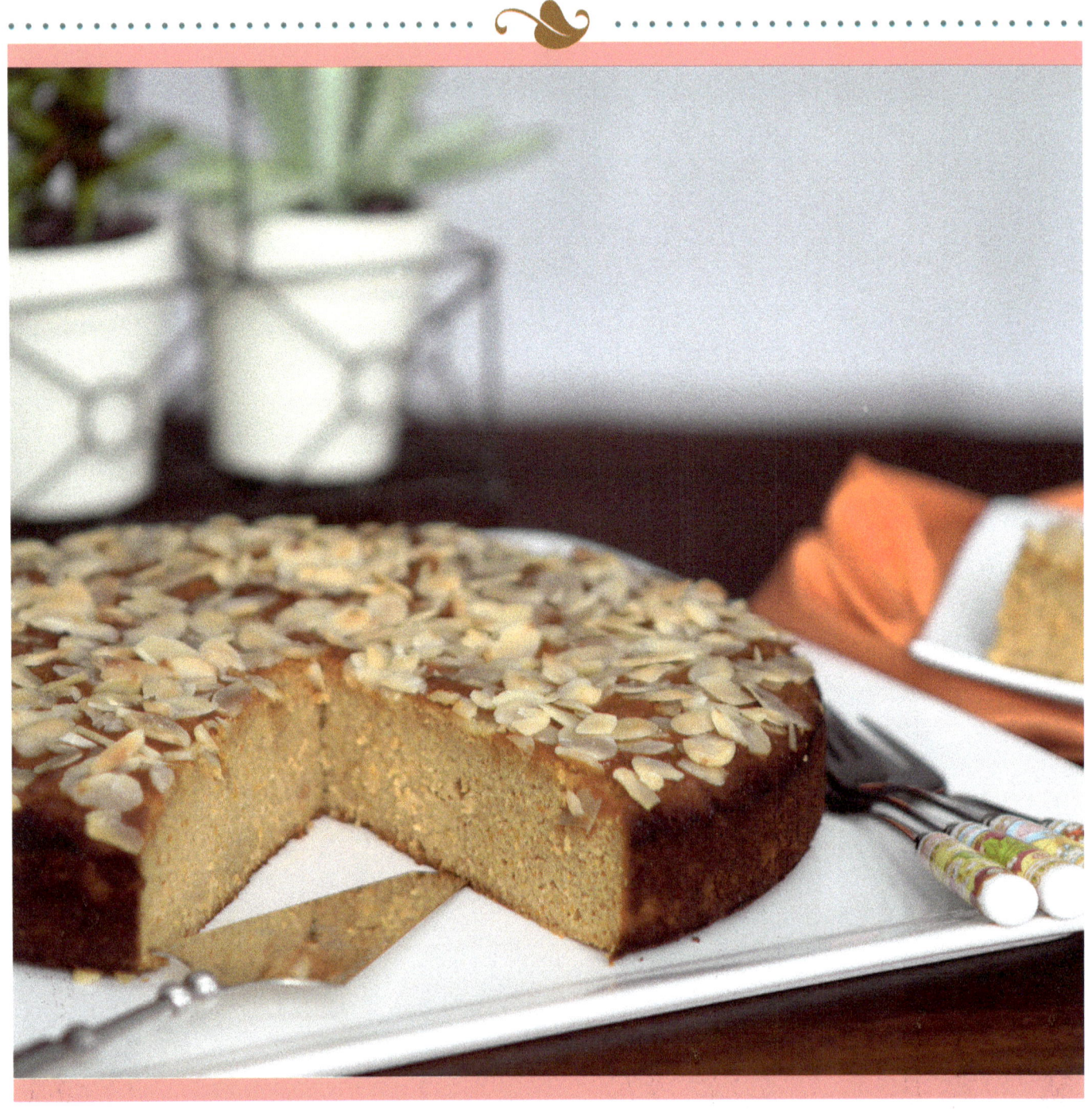

Orange and Almond Cake

This was one of the first gluten free cakes I made. I find if you change the water during the cooking of the oranges, you get a better flavoured cake (reduces any bitterness from the skins). It is delicious on it's own or served with dairy free cream. A good size to take to a party, not just gluten/grain free eaters will enjoy it.

Prep time: 20 minutes Cooking time: 55 minutes plus oranges Serves: 12-14

Ingredients:

- 2 navel oranges
- 6 large eggs, at room temperature
- ¾ cup coconut sugar
- 2 Tbsp honey
- 2 tsp vanilla extract
- 3½ cups almond meal/flour
- 2 tsp gluten free baking powder
- 1½ tsp ground cinnamon
- ½ tsp fine sea salt
- ¾ cup almond flakes, for topping

Method:

Wash oranges well and place unpeeled into a full saucepan of hot water, bring to the boil and reduce heat. Make sure the oranges are covered well, simmer for 30 minutes. Drain off the cooking water and replace with fresh hot water and continue to simmer the oranges for a further 20 minutes or until soft. Drain and leave to cool.

Preheat oven to 160c/320f. Grease the sides and line the base of a 25cm(9.75in) spring form cake tin with baking paper. Place your sheet of baking paper over the base and clip closed the sides, have 2-3cm(1in) hanging out, this will make it easier to remove when placing cake on a serving plate (I also find it easier to remove if you grease the baking paper).

To a food processor add, eggs, coconut sugar, honey and vanilla. Blend well. Add cooled oranges cut into quarters, leaving the skins on. Blend until oranges have been incorporated into mixture and you have a smooth consistency. Scrape down sides and lid of food processor.

Add almond meal, baking powder, cinnamon and salt. Blend well to combined.

Pour batter into prepared cake tin. Spread evenly and top with almond flakes. Press very lightly over the nuts to prevent falling off once cooked.

Bake for 55 minutes or until the top is golden brown, you may want to turn the cake around during cooking as almond meal can brown very easily.

Let cool in tin for at least 30 minutes, then run a flexible spatula around the sides of the cake and remove the spring form sides. Let sit to completely cool before sliding cake off the base. Gently loosen paper and slide onto a large serving plate.

Store covered at room temperature, cake becomes moister the longer it sits. A great cake to make ahead of time.

MUFFINS, CAKES AND SLICES

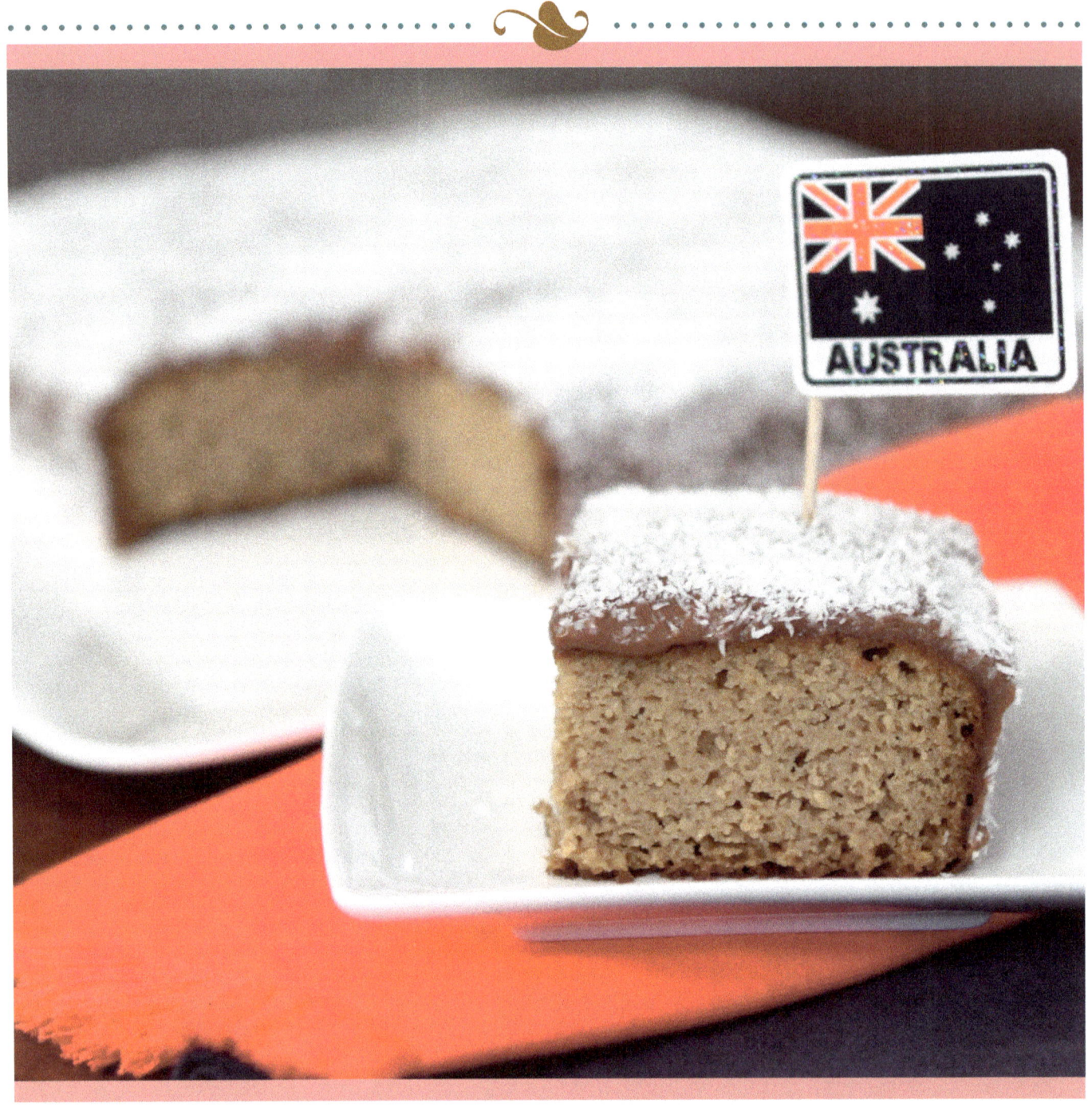

Lamington Cake

My mother made Lamingtons when I was a kid, it was a sign guests were coming. It is such an Australian icon. So for Australia Day I decided to create my own version. Traditionally a vanilla sponge cake was cut into 4cm cubes, dipped into chocolate icing and rolled in coconut. The Lamington was invented in early 1900 and named after Lord Lamington, who served as Governor of Queensland.

Prep time: 15 minutes Cooking time: 30 minutes Serves: 8-12

Ingredients:

- 6 large eggs
- ¾ cup cashew milk or nut milk of choice
- 1 cup coconut sugar
- ½ cup ghee or coconut oil
- 2 tsp vanilla extract
- 1½ cups almond meal/flour
- ⅔ cup coconut flour, sifted
- 1½ teaspoons baking soda
- 1 tsp gluten free baking powder
- ¼ teaspoon sea salt
- Chocolate frosting from page 280
- Coconut to sprinkle over frosted cake

Method:

Preheat oven to 170c/340f. Line the bottom and sides of a 22cm(8.5in) square cake tin with baking paper.

To a blender add, eggs, milk, coconut sugar, ghee and vanilla. Blend using variable speed for 10 seconds. Turn to high speed for a further few seconds, until creamy and sugar has dissolved.

To a large bowl add, almond meal, sift in coconut flour, baking soda, baking powder and salt. Stir to combine. Pour the wet mixture from the blender into the bowl. Mix well to thoroughly combine.

Pour batter into prepared cake tin and smooth over with a spatula.

Bake for 30 minutes, or until the cake is coming away from sides and springs back when you touch the centre. Remove from oven, let cool in the tin for 20 minutes.

Place a wire cooling rack upside down on top of the cake tin, holding both together, turn cake tin upside down so the cake slides out onto the rack. Let the cake finish cooling upside down.

Make your chocolate frosting while the cake is cooling. Place the frosting in the fridge to firm up, but must remain spreadable. When cake is completely cooled place your serving plate upside down on the cake and turn over ready for coating.

Coat the top and sides of your cake with chocolate frosting. Use a spoon to sprinkle coconut evenly over top and sides. You will need to turn your plate on a few angles to get the coconut on the sides, use a pastry brush to dust off excess coconut from the plate. Place in fridge to set the frosting.

Option: To make traditional lamingtons, place the cooled cake in the fridge for 1 hour to firm up, cut into squares. Using a knife or spatula, spread the chocolate frosting thinly over all four sides. Roll cake squares into coconut to coat all sides, then refrigerate to set.

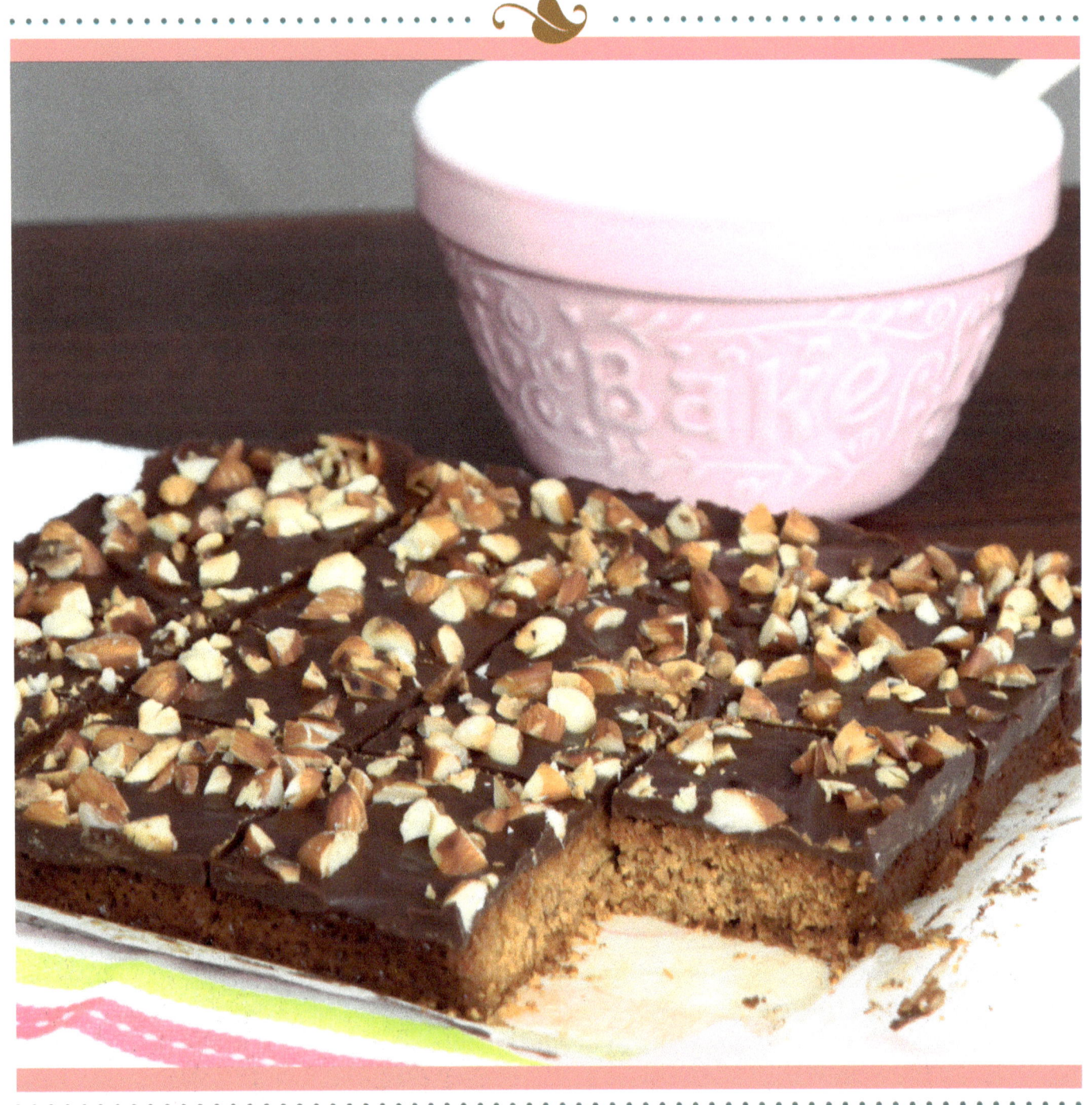

Macaroon and Chocolate Slice

This slice has a lovely crunch to it and by adding almond butter, it not only adds flavour but the creamy nut butter helps reduce the amount of sweetener needed.

Prep time: 18 minutes Cooking time: 15 minutes Makes: 16

Ingredients:

- 250gms/1 cup almond butter/spread or sunflower butter for nut free
- ¼ cup coconut oil, melted
- 3 Tbsp honey
- 2 tsp vanilla extract
- 1½ cups desiccated coconut
- 3 Tbsp golden flaxseed meal
- ¼ tsp fine sea salt
- ¾ cup dark chocolate chips, for topping (no soy, paleo friendly)
- ⅓ cup toasted chopped almonds or toasted coconut to decorate top

Method:

Preheat oven to 170c/340f. Line a 20cm(8in) square cake tin with baking paper, leaving a small overhang for lifting out.

To a large bowl add, almond butter, melted coconut oil, honey and vanilla. Using a hand held electric beater, beat well until you have a creamy texture.

Add coconut, flaxseed and salt to the wet ingredients. Mix well to combine.

Transfer mixture to prepared baking tin. Use the back of a metal spoon to spread mixture evenly across the base, pressing firmly down.

Bake for approximately 15 minutes or until the edges start to brown, it will still be a little soft on top but not gooey, it firms up when cooled. Cool in tin. Don't refrigerate before pouring the melted chocolate over the slice (it will spread more evenly).

Meanwhile, toast chopped almonds in a small frying pan with ½ teaspoon of coconut oil until lightly brown.

Melt the dark chocolate chips in a double saucepan and spread over the baked macaroon slice. Immediately sprinkle over toasted almonds or coconut before it hardens.

Refrigerate until the chocolate sets. Remove from tin by lifting out with the baking paper. Allow to sit at room temperature before cutting into squares.

Store in an airtight container in the fridge.

THE JOYFUL TABLE

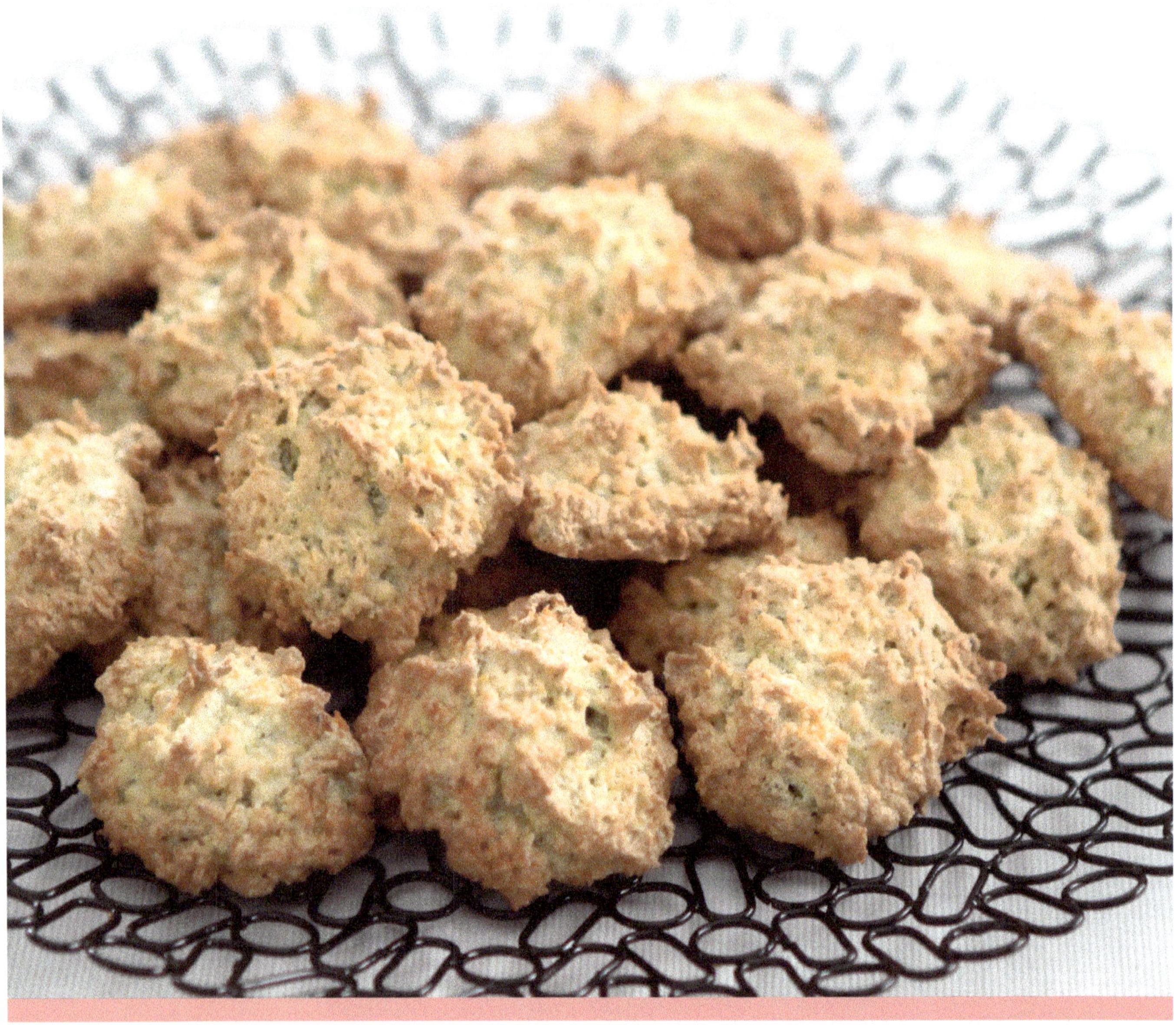

MUFFINS, CAKES AND SLICES

Pistachio Macaroons

These little macaroon treats have a light meringue texture. Normally almond meal is used but for a little difference I have ground pistachio nuts. Cook them in a slow oven so they can dry out without getting too brown, treat them like you would a pavlova and you will be rewarded with a delicious crispy, light treat.

Prep time: 18 minutes
Cooking time: 40 minutes plus 30 minutes with oven off Makes: 28

Ingredients:

- ¾ cup/100g pistachios
- 4 large egg whites, room temperature
- ¼ tsp fine sea salt
- ½ cup organic maple syrup, heated
- Zest of 1 lemon, finely grated
- 1¾ cups desiccated coconut

Method:

Preheat oven to 130c/270f. Line 2 baking trays with baking paper.

Add pistachios to a blender. Blend on a low speed to breakup nuts to the texture of almond meal. Set aside.

Heat maple syrup but don't let it boil. Set aside.

To a large stainless steel or glass bowl, add egg whites. Using an electric hand-held beater whisk egg whites until you have soft peaks. Add salt. Continue to beat, slowly drizzle hot maple syrup into the beaten egg whites. Beat for a further 1-2 minutes or until you have a thick and glossy mixture. Add lemon zest and beat to combine.

Use a spatula and gently fold in ground pistachios and coconut, don't over mix. Mixture should resemble a thick and fluffy meringue or pavlova texture. Drop heaped tablespoons of mixture onto prepared trays. (While baking you may need to turn trays around to prevent uneven browning).

Bake for 40 minutes, then turn off oven and leave to continue drying out for a further 30 minutes. If the macaroons look like over browning open oven door slightly. Transfer to a wire rack to cool.

Store in a glass airtight container. If you find they start to go soft the next day, just pop back into a low oven and dry out.

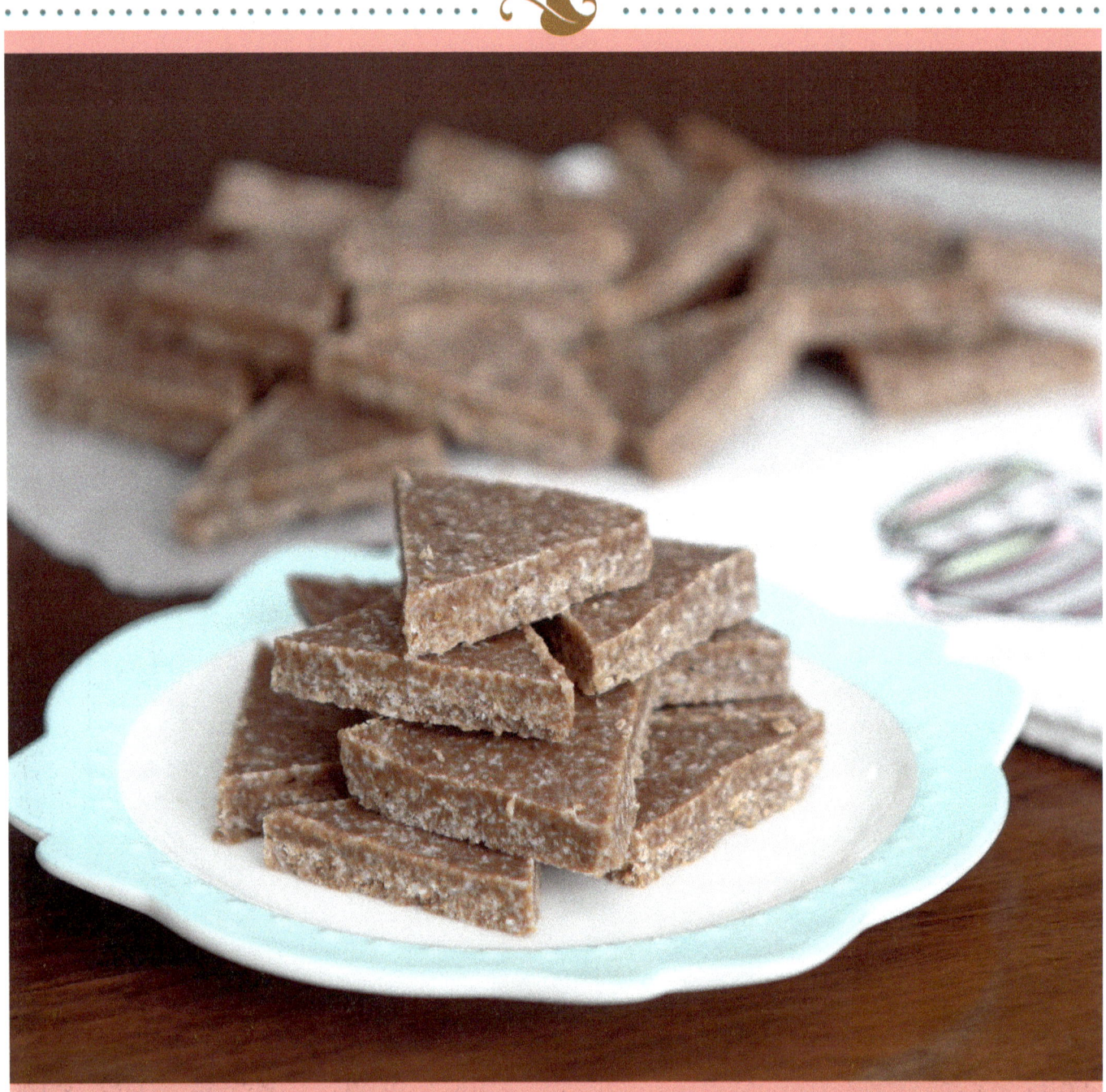

Coconut Rough Bites

These yummy little bites are so easy to make. You can also make them into individual chocolates by pressing mixture into mini silicon cups or molds.

Prep time: 10 minutes Cooking time: none Makes: 36 bites

Ingredients:

- 15 medjool dates, pitted
- 2½ Tbsp cacao powder
- 50gms/1.8ozs cacao butter, melted or 3 Tbsp coconut oil, melted
- 1½ tsp vanilla extract
- ⅛ tsp fine sea salt
- 3 cups desiccated coconut, divided

Method:

Line a 22cm (8.5in) square baking tin with baking paper, leaving an overhang to make it easy to remove the set coconut rough from tin.

To a food processor add, dates and process until broken into pieces. Add cacao powder, cacao butter, vanilla, salt and 2 cups of coconut. Process until all ingredients are well incorporated and mixture is moist, approximately 1 minute (you still need to see the coconut in the mixture).

Add the remaining 1 cup of coconut and pulse several times to incorporate into the mixture. If you like a finer texture add all the coconut at once or a rougher texture, leave 2 cups to add at the end.

Press mixture firmly into prepared baking tin, making sure all corners are packed down. Place in fridge to set or if you can't wait, place in the freezer.

Remove by lifting the overhang of baking paper, place on a chopping board and cut into bite size shapes (triangles, squares or fingers).

Store in an airtight container in the fridge. (I use cacao butter as it stays firmer, if using coconut oil make sure to serve straight from the fridge).

DESSERTS

Apple Pie 258

Lemon Meringue Pies 261

Strawberry Crumble 262

Chocolate Mousse Cake
with Strawberry Sauce 265

Hazelnut Sticky Date Pudding
with Caramel Sauce 266

Apple and Pear Crumble 269

Blueberry Chocolate Chia Puddings 270

Chocolate Dessert Cake 273

Individual Strawberry Cheesecakes 274

Raw Raspberry Cheesecake 276

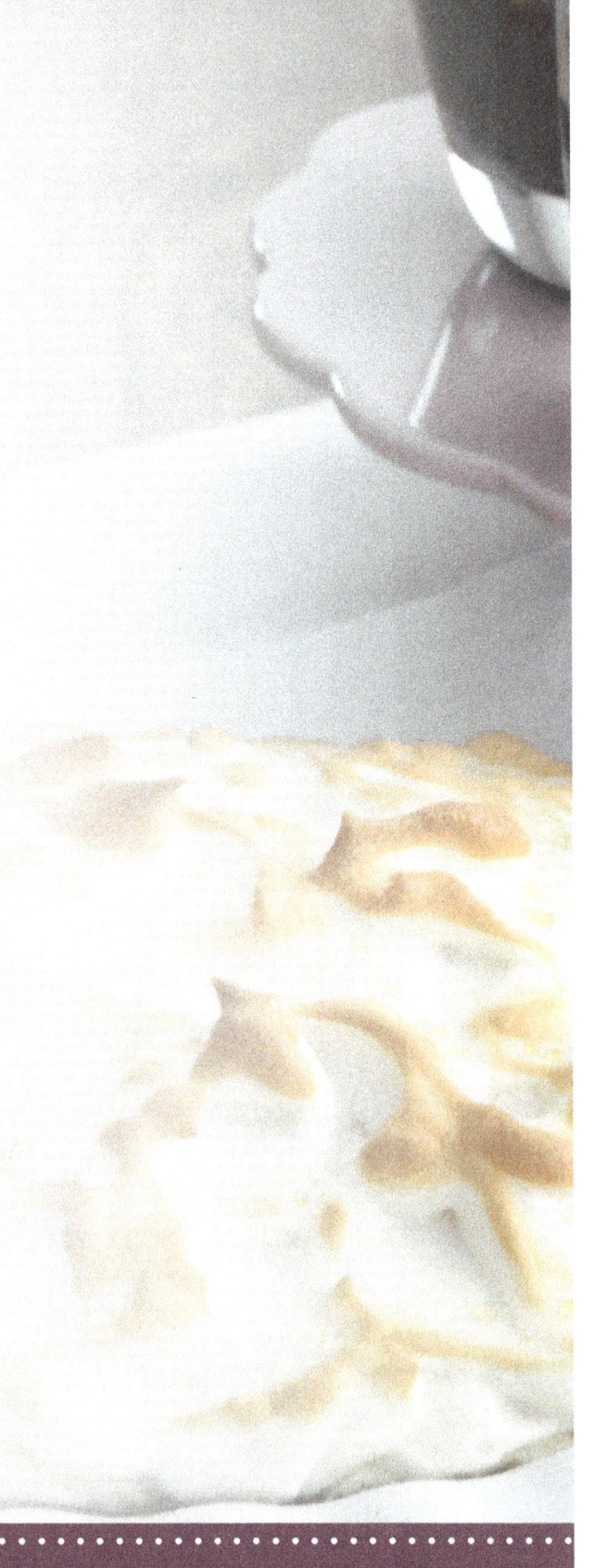

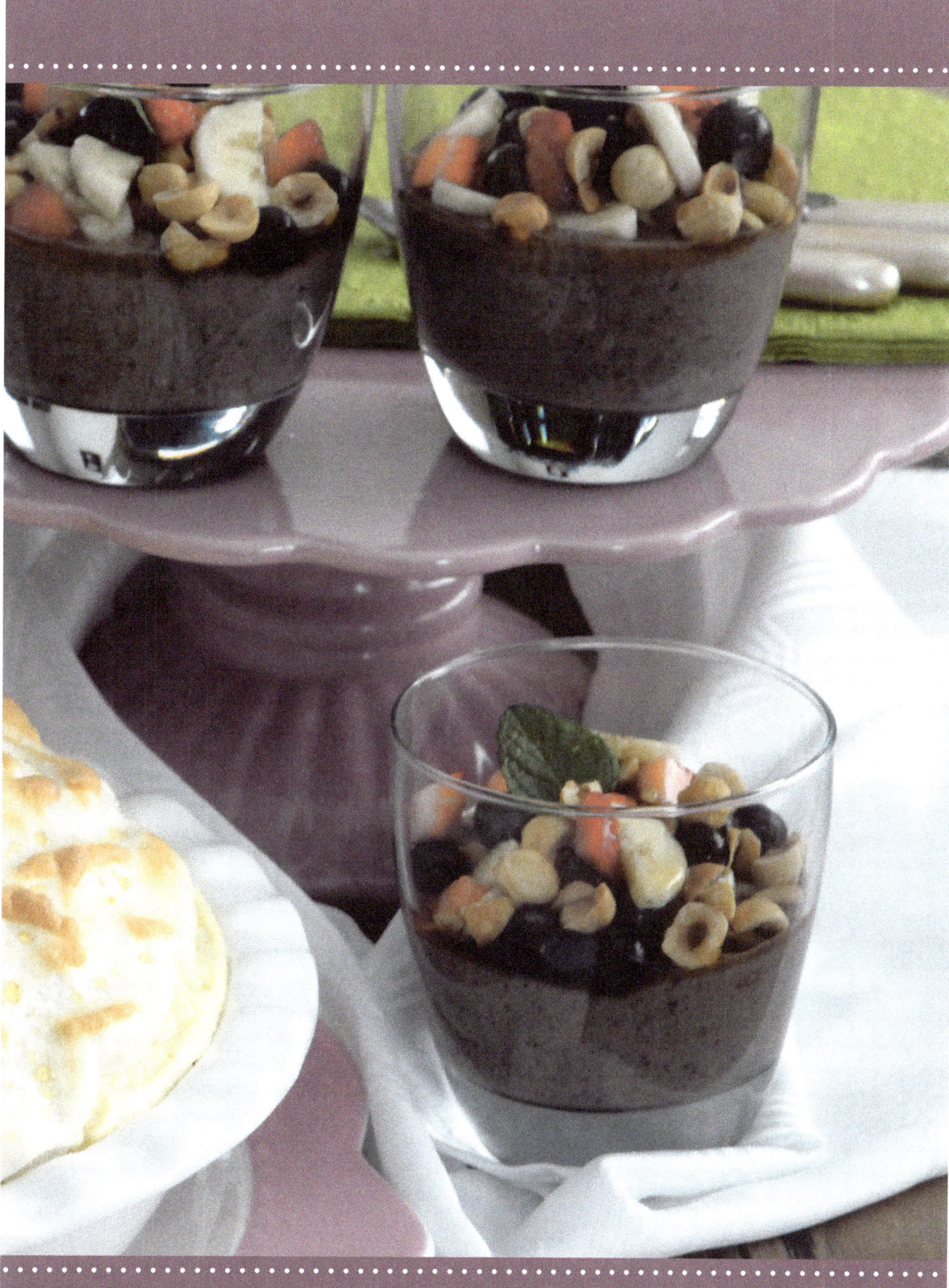

Apple Pie

Apple Pie is always a favourite. I have used my Sweet Coconut Piecrust for this recipe. It stays crisp even with all the moist apple filling. Double the piecrust recipe so you have enough to make the base and top. You can choose to make a crisscross pattern or to totally cover your pie. Serve warm with your choice of dairy free cream or custard.

Prep time: 25 minutes Cooking time: 25 minutes Serves: 6

Ingredients:

- 2 x recipe for Sweet Coconut Piecrust page 85
- 1.1kg/7 apples, peeled, cored and sliced thinly
- 3 Tbsp 100% maple syrup
- 2 Tbsp ghee or coconut oil
- Juice of 1 small lemon
- 1 tsp vanilla extract
- 1½ tsp ground cinnamon
- 1 tsp mixed spice
- ¼ tsp fine sea salt

Method:

Prepare piecrust as per recipe on page 85. Bake base and set aside to cool. Wrap and seal the other half of the pastry to prevent drying out while preparing the filling.

To a large saucepan, add thinly sliced apple and the remaining ingredients.

Cook over low-medium heat, uncovered for 10 minutes stirring occasionally while juice is released from apples. Reduce heat and cover for 3-4 minutes to finish cooking apples (they should still be in slices, not mushy). Remove lid and stir through the juices on the bottom of pan. The juice will have thickened and clinging to the apples. Remove from heat.

Place remaining half of pastry dough between 2 sheets of baking paper and roll out to a rectangle ready to cut into strips. Preheat oven to 160c/320f.

Spoon apples and juice into the prebaked piecrust.

Use a pizza cutter to cut strips approximately 2.5cm(1in) wide. Cut 8 in total, 4 for each layer. The longest strips going across the centre will need to be 24cm(9.5ins) long, the others a little shorter. Take a long metal spatula or similar, dusted in arrowroot flour and slide under strips. Place one at a time on top of the filled pie, spaced evenly. Repeat crossing over with second layer of strips. Press ends of strips neatly onto the rim of the piecrust.

Bake for 25-30 minutes or until strips have started to brown and are firm. Let sit for 10 minutes before serving.

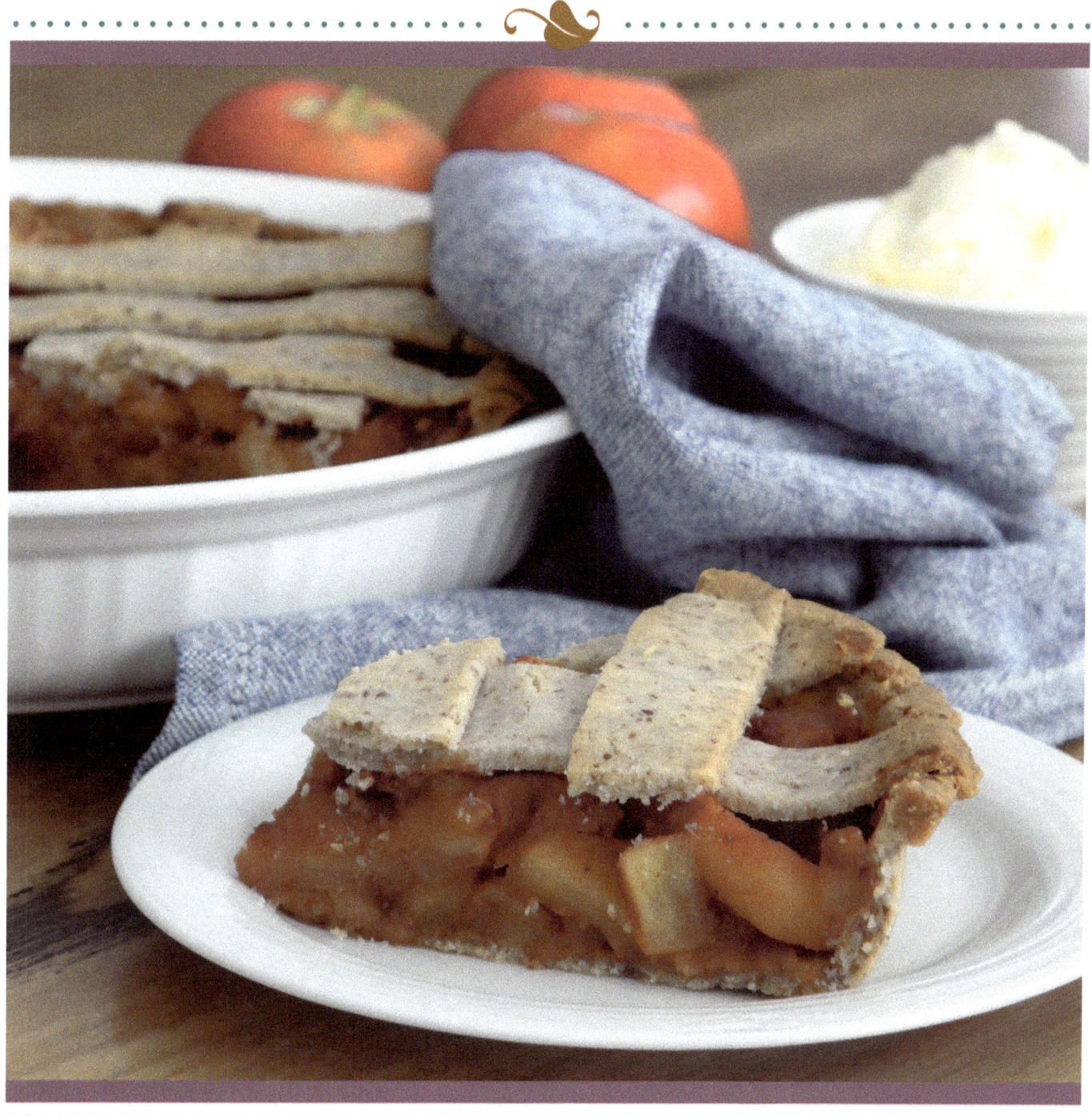

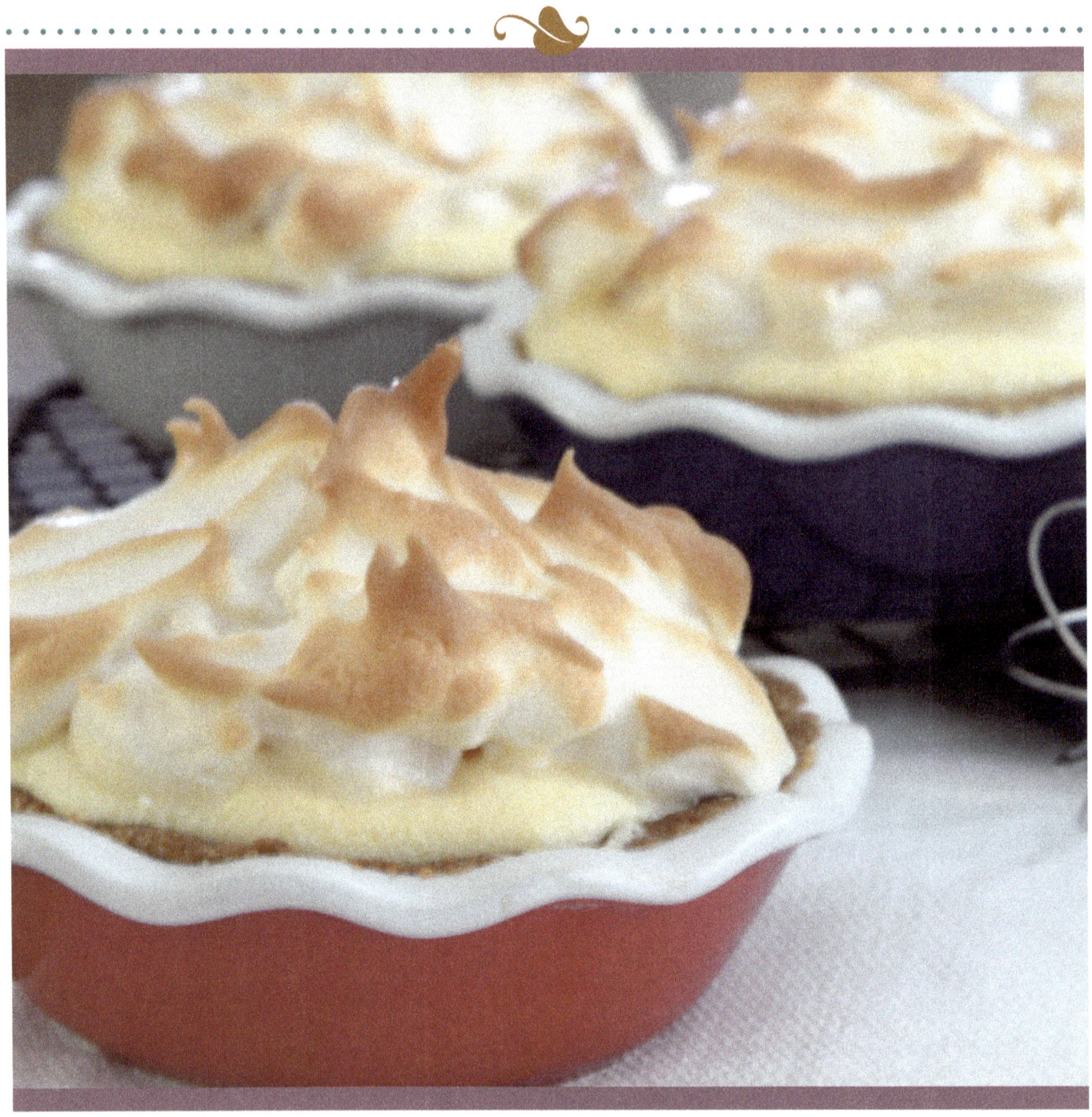

Lemon Meringue Pies

I received rave reports from the family over these little yummy pies. They loved the light texture of the lemon filling. The piecrust and lemon filling can be made earlier in the day or even the day before. You will need to make your meringue only 1-2 hours before serving. These quantities will also make one large pie.

Prep time: 30 minutes Cooking time: 10 minutes plus pie crust
Makes: 4 small pies

Ingredients:

2 x Sweet Piecrust recipe page 86

LEMON FILLING
- 6 egg yolks
- ½ cup 100% maple syrup
- 125ml/½ cup lemon juice
- 30ml/2 Tbsp filtered water
- 1 Tbsp unflavoured gelatin powder, for setting
- 1½ Tbsp lemon zest, finely grated
- 3 egg whites
- ¾ tsp cream of tartar

MERINGUE TOPPING
- ⅓ cup 100% maple syrup, heated
- 5 egg whites
- 1 tsp cream of tartar
- 1 Tbsp arrowroot flour

Method:

Prepare double quantity of Sweet Piecrust as per recipe on page 86, for the 4 pie dishes. Place pastry lined pie dishes on a baking tray. Bake for 10 minutes. Follow instructions to prevent base rising. Set aside to cool after baking.

Prepare Lemon filling: Use a medium stainless steal or glass bowl that will fit onto a saucepan or use a double boiler. Add 2.5cm(1in) of water to saucepan, bring to a gently boil.

Add to the bowl, egg yolks and maple syrup. Use an electric hand-held beater and whip the egg yolks and maple syrup until light and fluffy. Add lemon juice. Place bowl over saucepan or pour mixture into the top of a double boiler. Use a large whisk, to whisk egg yolk/lemon mixture until it becomes thick and foamy, the colour will lighten.

Add the water to a cup and sprinkle the gelatin over the water to soften. Add the gelatin mixture and lemon zest into the heated yolk/lemon mixture and whisk through. This whole process takes approximately 4 minutes. Remove from heat.

Beat the egg whites with cream of tartar until you have stiff peaks. Fold into the lemon mixture and pour into baked pie shells. Allow too set before topping with meringue.

Prepare Meringue Topping: Preheat oven to 170c/340f. Heat maple syrup in a saucepan but don't allow to boil.

Beat egg whites with cream of tartar until stiff peaks form. Slowly drizzle hot maple syrup into beaten egg whites while you continue beating on medium-high. Stop and sprinkle over arrowroot flour. Continue beating for a further 1-2 minutes until you have a lovely stiff glossy mixture.

Spoon onto the filled pies and spread all the way to the edges. Scoop the mixture so it stand ups. Place pie dishes on a baking tray, place in the oven and bake for approximately 6-8 minutes, until lightly golden. Or place under the grill for 1 minute, watch very carefully. You are just lightly toasting the top of the meringue. Set aside to cool, serve at room temperature.

THE JOYFUL TABLE

Strawberry Crumble

This is a very quick and easy dessert to make, prepared and baked all in a total of 30 minutes. Serve with cream of your choice or dairy free vanilla custard, or with both!

Prep time: 15 minutes Cooking time: 15 minutes Serves: 6

Ingredients:

Ghee for greasing
3 punnets/750g fresh strawberries
¼ cup almond meal/flour
2 Tbsp coconut sugar
¾ tsp organic almond extract

TOPPING
1 ¼ cups almond meal/flour
½ cup desiccated coconut
2 Tbsp coconut sugar
1 tsp organic vanilla powder or 1 ½ tsp vanilla extract
Pinch fine sea salt
⅓ cup ghee, melted
½ cup flaked almonds

Method:

Preheat oven to 170c/340f. Grease a deep pie dish with ghee.

Cut off green stalks from strawberries. Place strawberries upside down on their flat tops where you cut the stalks from, to cover the base of the dish. Place a second layer pointing down to fit between the spaces left from the first layer of strawberries (you may have to cut some strawberries in half to squeeze them in).

Sprinkle a ¼ cup of almond meal and 1 tablespoon of coconut sugar over the strawberries. With your thumb over the opening of the almond extract bottle, allow even drops to sprinkle over the strawberries. Approximately ¾ teaspoon in total (it's far too tricky to sprinkle from a teaspoon, so just give a guess from the bottle).

To prepare topping: to a medium bowl add, almond meal, coconut, coconut sugar, vanilla powder, and salt. Mix to combine. Melt ghee and pour over the dry ingredients. Mix well until everything is moist. Add flaked almonds and gently mix. (If you don't have vanilla powder, add extract to ghee and mix through together).

Spoon the crumble topping over the strawberries.

Bake for 15-20 minutes or until lightly brown on top and strawberries are heated through. (If left too long in oven strawberries will become mushy.)

DESSERTS | 263

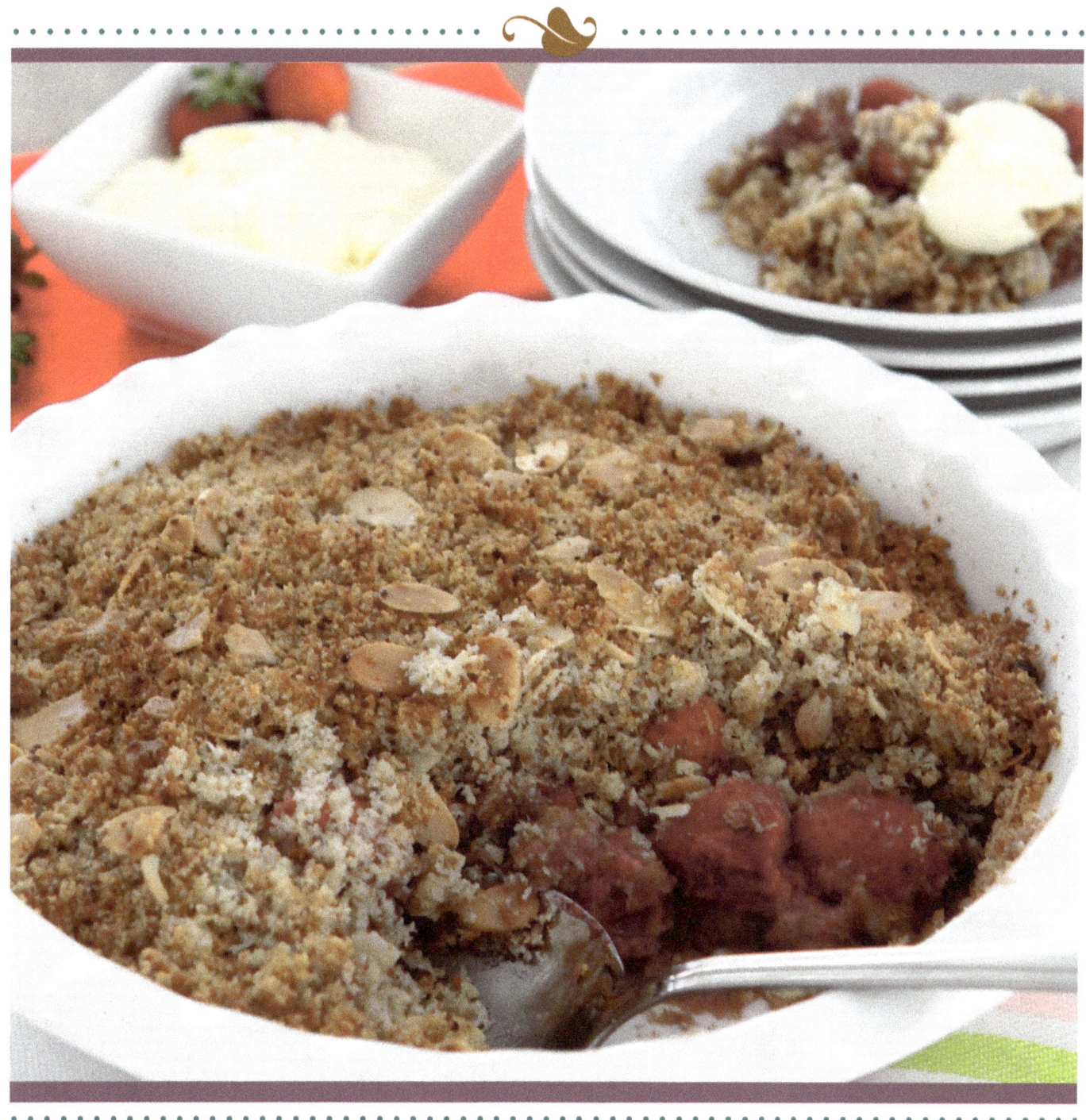

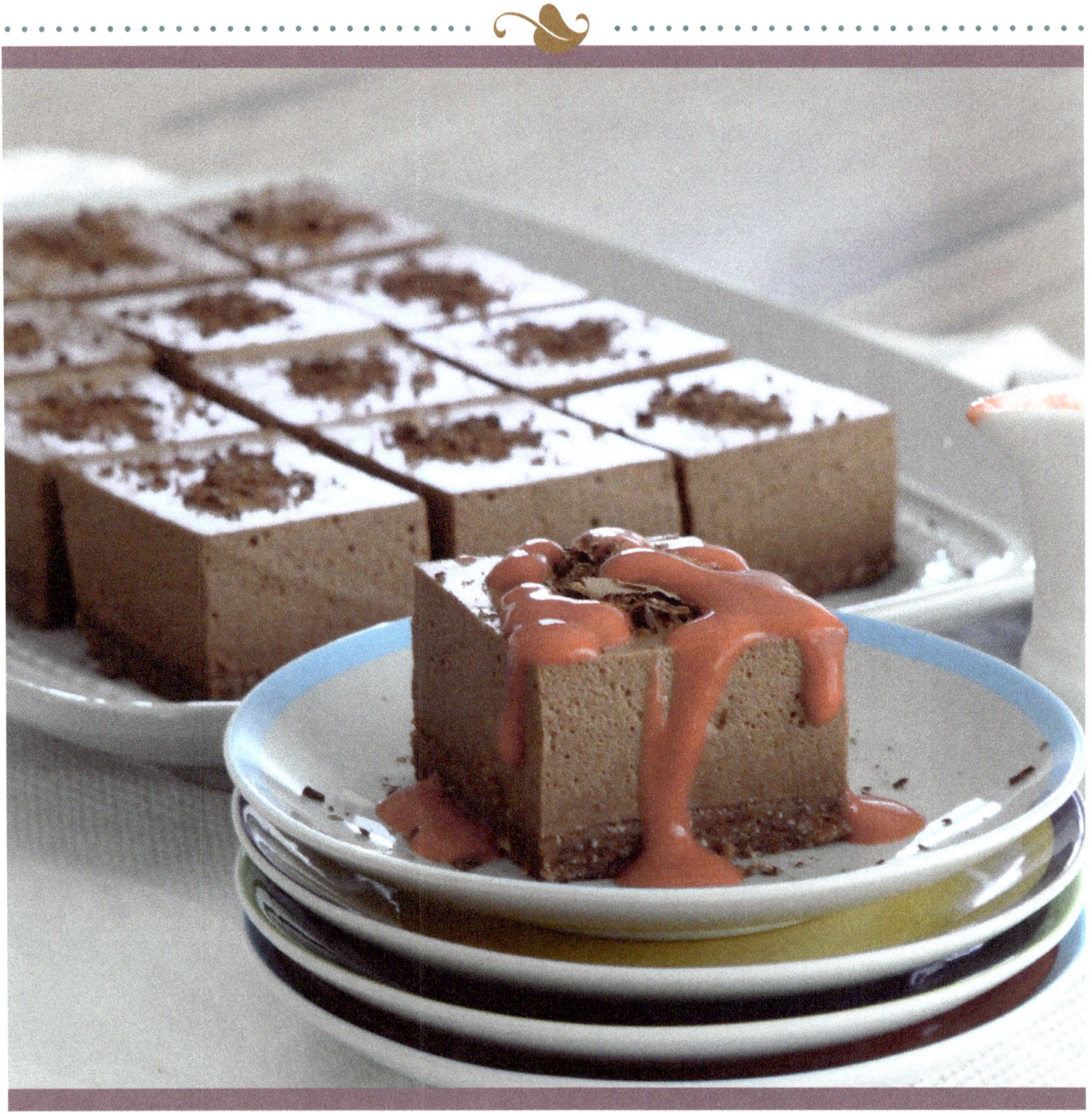

Chocolate Mousse Cake with Strawberry Sauce

A lovely light chocolaty mousse, sits on top of a brazil nut crust, drizzled with strawberry sauce. I hope I've enticed you to make this yummy dessert that doesn't just taste good but is good for you. Make a day ahead.

Prep time: 25 minutes plus chilling time 2-3 hours
Cooking time: none   Serves: 8-12

Ingredients:

BASE
- 10 medjool dates, pitted
- 1 cup raw brazil nuts
- 1 cup coconut
- 2 Tbsp cacao powder

CHOCOLATE MOUSSE
- 4 eggs separated, room temperature
- 700ml/2.8 cups coconut milk
- ½ cup 100% maple syrup
- 2 Tbsp unflavoured gelatin, for setting
- ½ cup raw cacao powder

STRAWBERRY SAUCE
- 1½ cups strawberries (fresh or frozen ½ thawed)
- 2 tsp honey or to taste

Garnish:
Shaved 85% dark chocolate

Method:

To a food processor add all the ingredients for the base. Process until mixture is well combined. Takes approximately 2½-3 minutes to come together. Press mixture between your fingers, if mixture sticks together it's ready.

Line a 22cm(8.5in) square cake tin with baking paper, leaving an overhang for easy removal. Press mixture firmly and evenly into cake tin. Place in fridge.

Separate egg yolks from whites. Cover egg whites and set aside at room temperature.

To a medium saucepan add, egg yolks, coconut milk and maple syrup, whisk well to combine. Sprinkle over gelatin, let sit for 30 seconds to soften, then whisk into mixture. Add cacao powder and whisk through. Heat mixture on low-medium heat. Continue whisking until mixture just comes to a light simmer. Turn off heat.

Pour into a large bowl and set aside to cool. Cover to prevent a skin forming and place in the fridge. (If a skin forms don't mix it in, scrape off.) Check from time to time to see if cool, it will start to slightly thicken but you don't want it to set before the egg whites are added.

Beat egg whites until you have stiff peaks. Fold half the beaten egg whites into chocolate mixture. Repeat with the other half until you have a smooth texture. Pour into cake tin over base, being careful to not let the mousse go behind the baking paper. Place back into the fridge to set firm.

To remove from tin run a knife carefully around the mousse so it's not sticking to the paper. Lift out using overhang and place on a chopping board. Use a large sharp knife to cut into portions.

Use a potato peeler to shave a piece of 85% dark chocolate to decorate the Mousse Cake.

Serve with chocolate shavings over each serving portion and drizzle with strawberry sauce.

To make Strawberry Sauce: Add strawberries and honey to a blender. Blend for a few seconds to create a smooth sauce. Pour into a small jug and serve over your Chocolate Mousse Cake portions.

Hazelnut Sticky Date Pudding with Caramel Sauce

This rich flavourful but light textured pudding dripping in caramel sauce, is the perfect winter dessert treat. Hazelnuts are a great source of vitamins and minerals but are best know for their high antioxidant content.

Prep time: 20 minutes Cooking time: 45 minutes Serves: 6-8

Ingredients:

- 1½ cups/15 Medjool dates, pitted
- 1 cup boiling water
- 1 tsp baking soda
- 3 large eggs
- ½ cup canned coconut cream
- ¼ cup ghee or coconut oil

- 2 Tbsp coconut sugar
- 2 tsp cinnamon
- 1 tsp vanilla extract
- 1½ cups hazelnut meal
- ¼ cup coconut flour

CARAMEL SAUCE

- 400ml/14oz canned coconut cream
- ⅓ cup 100% maple syrup

- 2 Tbsp ghee or organic butter
- 1 tsp vanilla extract

Method:

Preheat oven to 170c/340f. Grease the sides and line the base of a 20cm(8in) round spring form cake tin. To a small bowl add, dates, baking soda and boiling water. Set aside and allow to cool.

To a food processor add all the remaining ingredients except for the date mixture. Process until well combined.

Add date mixture and blend for 10 seconds to incorporate into batter (I like to see some bits of dates in the mixture).

Pour batter into prepared cake tin. Smooth over top with a spatula.

Bake for 45-50 minutes or until golden. The top will be firm but still a little soft underneath, this is ready. It will finish cooking while it sits. Let sit for 15 minutes before loosening sides of cake tin and remove. To serve, place individual servings in dessert bowls and pour over Caramel sauce.

Caramel Sauce: While the pudding is cooking prepare the sauce. In a saucepan combine all the sauce ingredients and heat on medium. Stir frequently until it starts to slowly simmer. Reduce to low.

Gently simmer for 20-25 minutes or until the caramel reduces a little and thickens slightly, the colour turns a shade darker. Watch it doesn't burn. Allow too cool slightly before serving warm over the pudding.

DESSERTS | 267

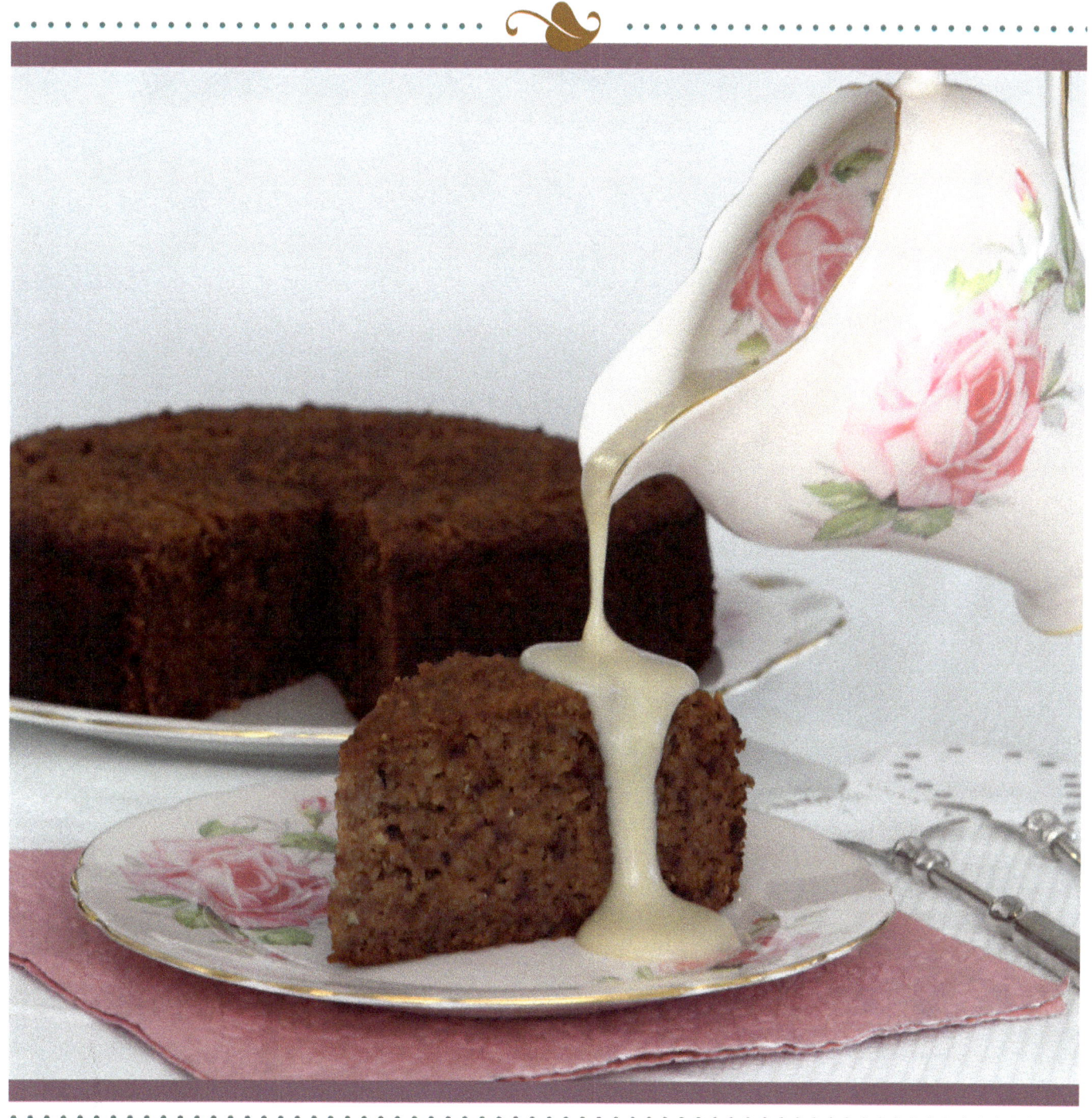

268 DESSERTS

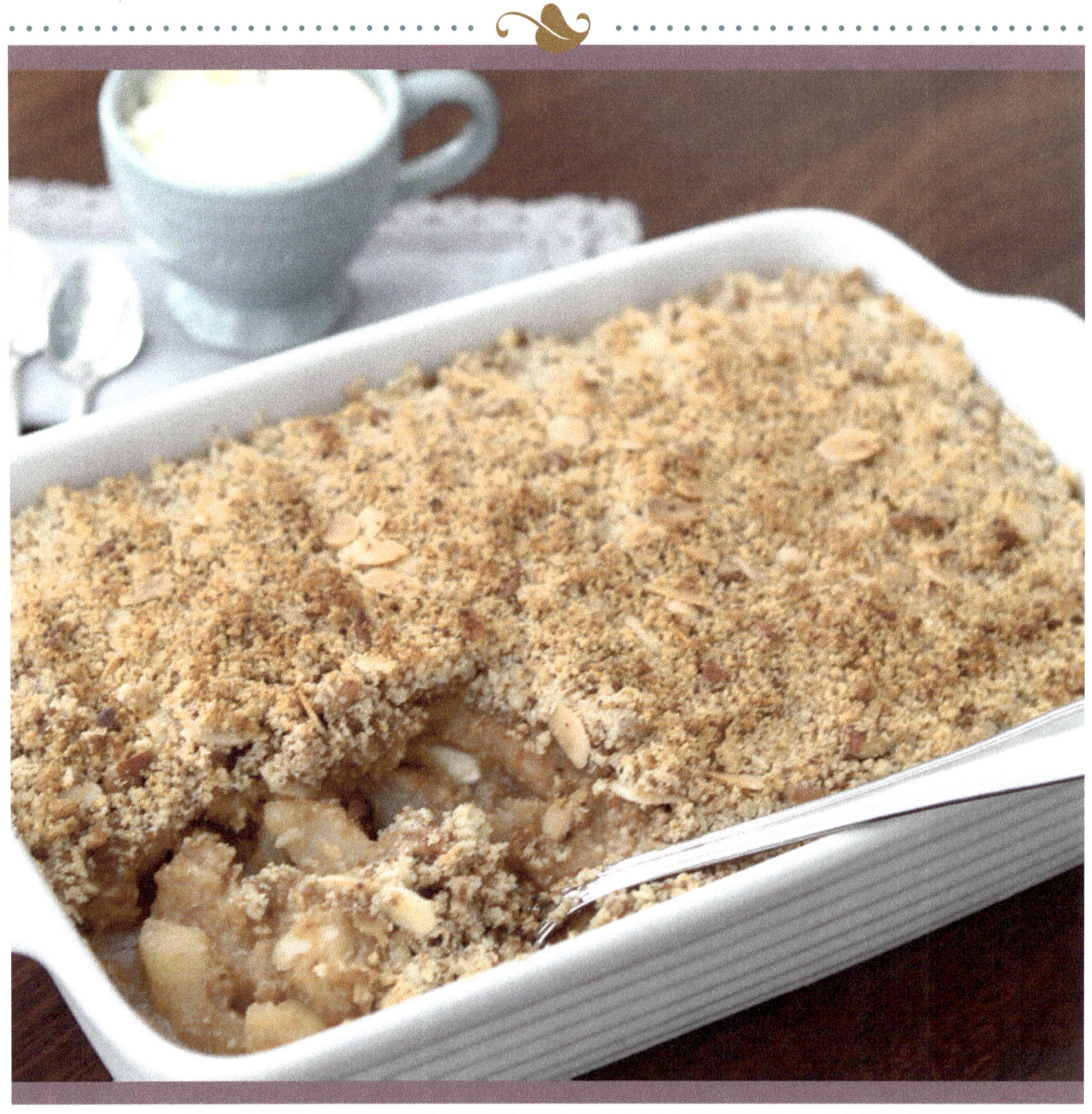

Apple and Pear Crumble

Such an easy to prepare and inexpensive dessert when fruit is in season. This dessert is often on our families Sunday lunch table. I prepare the fruit the night before. Just as we sit down for lunch, I spread the topping over the fruit and pop into the oven. Perfect size for our family but you may want to adjust the quantities to suit yours.

Prep time: 20 minutes Cooking time: 35 minutes Serves: 8–10

Ingredients:

- 1kg/2.2lb red apples, peeled
- 1kg/2.2lb pears, peeled
- ½ cup filtered water
- 3 Tbsp 100% maple syrup
- 2 tsp ground cinnamon
- 1½ tsp mixed spice
- ¾ tsp ground ginger
- Pinch fine sea salt

TOPPING MIXTURE

- 2 cups almond meal/flour
- ½ cup desiccated coconut
- ½ cup pecans, chopped
- 2 Tbsp organic coconut sugar
- ½ tsp ground cinnamon
- ½ tsp mixed spice
- ⅓ cup ghee
- ½ cup flaked almonds

Method:

Cut fruit into quarters and remove core, then slice thinly.

Add fruit, water, maple syrup, spices and salt to a large saucepan over medium heat. Mix gently to combine and bring to a simmer. Cook covered for 15 minutes or until fruit is tender.

Meanwhile prepare topping mixture and preheat oven to 160c/320f.

To a large bowl add all the topping ingredients except for ghee and flaked almonds. Mix to combined.

Rub the ghee through topping mixture with your hands until you have a mixture resembling breadcrumbs. Gently stir through flaked almonds.

Spoon apple and pear mixture including juice into a greased 30x20cm(12x8in) ceramic or glass baking dish. Top with crumble mixture and press lightly down with your hand.

Bake for 20-25 minutes or until the top is golden brown. Allow to sit a few minutes before serving. Serve with dairy free cream or custard (see Whipped Cashew cream page 282).

Blueberry Chocolate Chia Puddings

This is a quick and easy dessert that is so good for you. You can dress it up with fruit and nuts and serve to guests or make a single serve for yourself, when a chocolate fix is needed.

Prep time: 10 minutes Cooking time: none Serves: 4

Ingredients:

- 1½ cups canned coconut milk
- ⅓ cup chia seeds
- 2 Tbsp cacao powder
- 2 Tbsp honey
- ½ cup frozen blueberries
- ½ small banana
- ¼ cup hazelnuts, roughly chopped and toasted
- Extra fruit and honey to top puddings

Method:

Roughly chop hazelnuts and toast in a preheated oven until lightly brown. Set aside.

To a blender add coconut milk, chia, cacao powder, honey, blueberries and banana. Blend on high until fruit is smooth.

Spoon mixture evenly between 4 dessert glasses or you can use fancy jars. Place in the fridge for 20–30 minutes.

Just before serving, chop up fresh fruit and place on each pudding. (I like to use strawberries, blueberries and the remaining half of the banana).

Sprinkle the chopped hazelnuts over the fruit and drizzle with a little honey. For a bit more colour I like to add a mint leaf.

DESSERTS 271

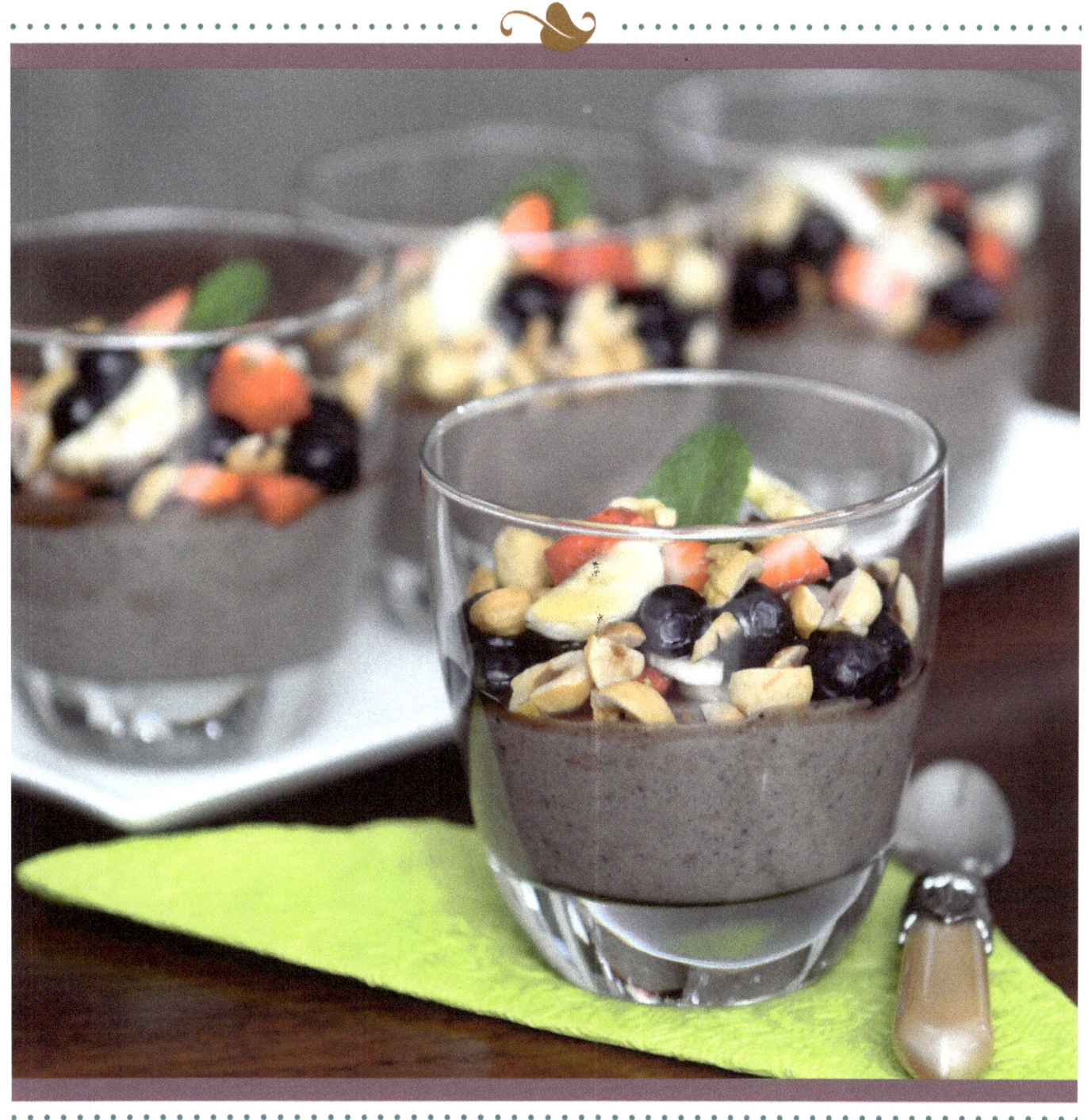

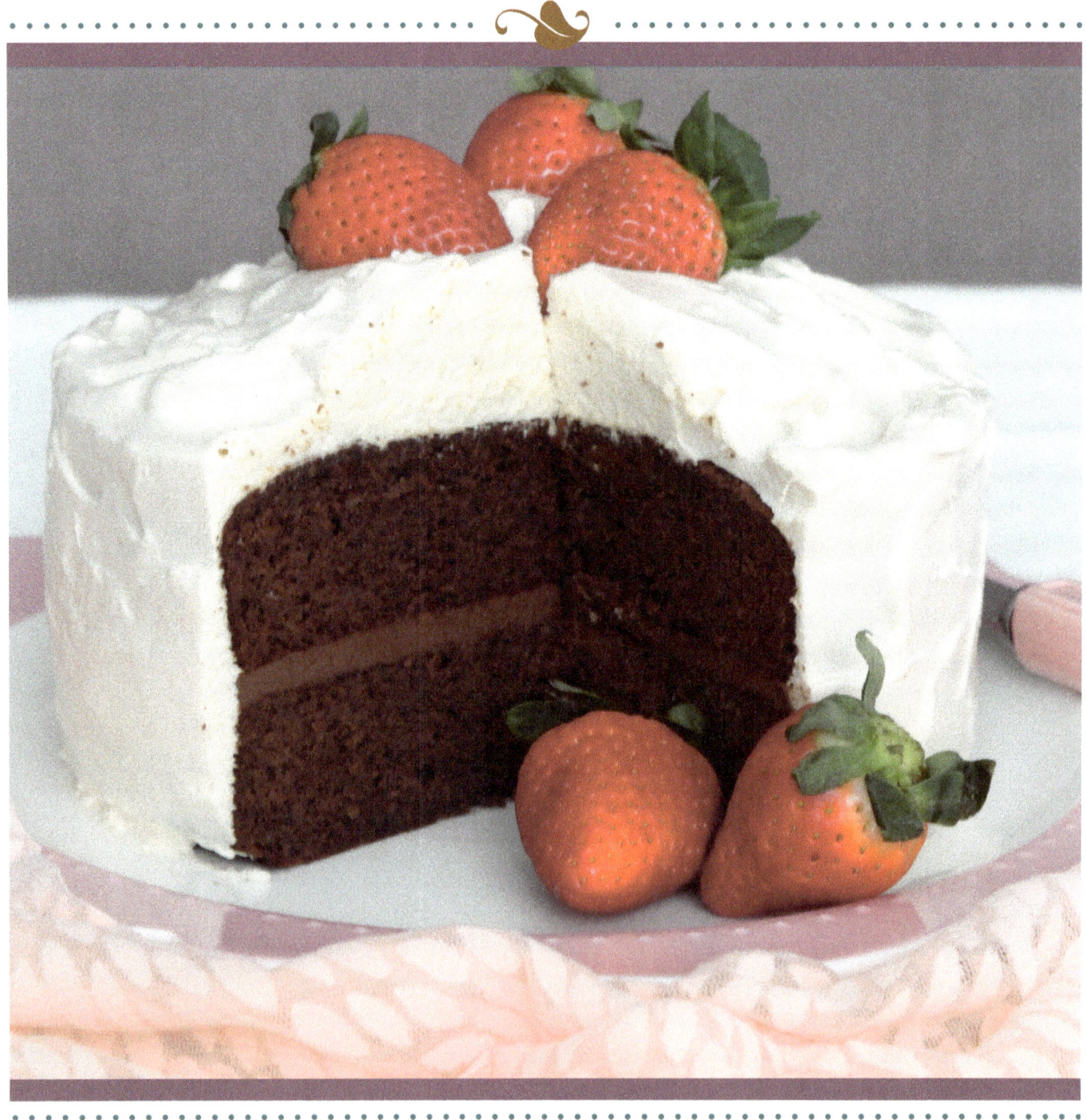

Chocolate Dessert Cake

This dessert cake is moist and fudgy. It is perfect to use for a Birthday Cake. I have included quantities for both a single and 2 layered cake. This cake becomes more moist the second day.

Prep time: 20 minutes
Cooking time: 40 minutes 1 cake / 30 minutes 2 layered cake Serves: 8-10

Ingredients:

- 3 cup almond meal/flour
- 6 Medjool dates, pitted
- ⅓ cup cacao powder
- 1 tsp baking soda
- ½ tsp fine sea salt
- 4 large eggs
- ⅓ cup honey
- 3 Tbsp coconut oil, softened
- ½ cup almond milk or milk of choice
- 1 Tbsp vanilla extract

2 LAYERED CAKE

- 4 cups almond meal/flour
- 8 Medjool dates, pitted
- ½ cup cacao powder
- 1⅓ tsp baking soda
- ¾ tsp fine sea salt
- 5 large eggs
- ½ cup honey
- ¼ cup coconut oil, softened
- ¾ cup almond milk
- 1½ Tbsp vanilla extract

Method:

Preheat oven to 160c/320f. Grease and line the base of a 20cm(8in) round spring form cake tin. If you are making a 2 layered cake use two 20x4cm(8x1.5in) round sandwich cake tins.

To a food processor add, almond meal, dates, cacao powder, baking soda and salt.

Process together until dates have broken up. Add eggs, honey, coconut oil, milk and vanilla. Process until well blended into a smooth batter.

Pour the batter into prepared cake tin or tins. Use a spatula to smooth the top. Bake for 40 minutes or 30 minutes for the two smaller sandwich cakes.

The cake should be ready when it comes away from the sides of tin and centre springs back when lightly pressed. Don't over cook, it should be a moist cake. Let cool in the tin before removing.

Serve topped with Marshmallow Frosting on page 286 or Vanilla Macadamia Frosting on page 281. If you are making the 2 layered cake, place one upside down so the two flat bottoms sit together. Spread your choice of frosting in the middle to sandwich them together. Frost or ice the top and sides to complete your Chocolate Dessert Cake. (I like to use Chocolate Ganache as the filling, page 283 and Marshmallow Frosting, always looks impressive.)

Individual Strawberry Cheesecakes

These little cheesecakes will impress your guests and can be made a day ahead, just bring them out of the freezer 30 minutes before serving. You can also make one large cheesecake with this recipe.

Prep time: 35 minutes Cooking time: none Serves: 6

Ingredients:

BASE
1½ cups almond meal/flour
6 medjool dates, pitted
2 Tbsp cacao powder
2 Tbsp desiccated coconut
2 tsp vanilla extract
¼ tsp fine sea salt

FILLING
50gm/1.8ozs cacao butter, chopped finely or shaved
3½ cups cashews, soaked
¼ cup honey or coconut nectar
1 tsp vanilla extract
½ cup freshly squeezed lemon juice

TOPPING
2 cup frozen strawberries
1-2 Tbsp honey or to taste
1 cup of the filling

Method:

Place cashews in a bowl with ⅓ teaspoon of sea salt and hot water, let them soak while you prepare base.

Place all the base ingredients into a food processor and blend until well combined. Takes approximately 4 minutes, check by pressing some mixture between your fingers. If it sticks together it's ready.

Divide the mixture between 6 dessert glasses, approximately 3 tablespoons per glass. Press firmly into the base of the glass (I find it's best to use your fingers for this job). Set aside in the fridge while you make the cheesecake filling.

Drain cashews and rinse well. Transfer cashews to a high-speed blender. Add all the remaining ingredients for the cheesecake filling. Start with variable speed, use the tamper to push the mixture onto the blades. Turn to high speed and blend until you get a lovely creamy, smooth texture. Scrape down the sides often.

Set aside one cup of the filling mixture. Divide the remainder between the dessert glasses. Spread evenly over the base mixture and place in the freezer.

For the topping, reuse the blender. Add the cup of filling you set aside and all the topping ingredients.

Blend until creamy and smooth. Use the tamper to push the frozen fruit onto the blades. Divide the strawberry topping between the dessert glasses, spread evenly.

Place in the freezer for an hour to set, then transfer to the fridge until ready to serve. Decorate with fresh strawberries.

DESSERTS | 275

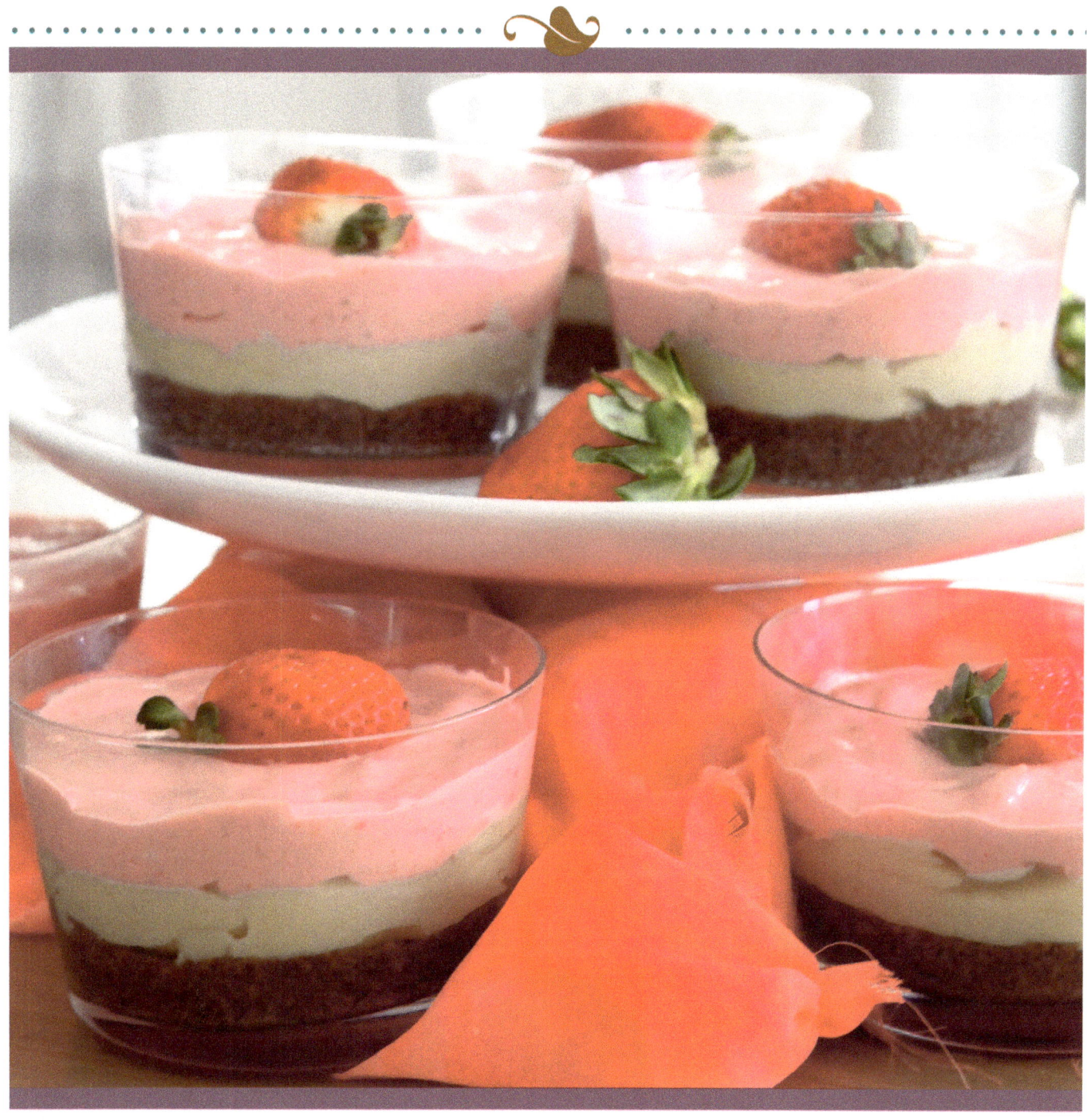

Raw Raspberry Cheesecake

I've used brazil nuts in the base of this raw cheesecake. You get some extra nutrients eating this dessert. Vitamin E, manganese, magnesium, oleic acid, and brazil nuts also contain the highest source of selenium, which is essential for immune support and thyroid function. The tartness of the raspberries make it a very refreshing dessert.

Prep time: 30 minutes Cooking time: none Serves: 8

Ingredients:

BASE
- 10 medjool dates, pitted
- 1 cup raw brazil nuts or almonds
- 1 cup desiccated coconut
- 2 Tbsp cacao powder

CHEESECAKE FILLING
- 2½ cups raw cashews, soaked
- 10 medjool dates, pitted
- 2 cups frozen raspberries
- 2 tsp vanilla extract
- ½ cup coconut water
- ¼ cup coconut oil
- Juice of 1 large lemon

Method:

Soak cashews in hot water with ⅓ teaspoon of sea salt for 30-60 minutes. Grease a 20 or 22cm(8.5in) spring form cake tin with coconut oil. To a food processor add all the ingredients for the base. Process until mixture is well combined. Takes about 2½-3 minutes to come together. Press mixture between fingers, if mixture sticks together it's ready.

Press mixture firmly into base of tin. Place in fridge to firm up while you start on the cheesecake filling.

Wipe out your food processor for this next step. Add dates, raspberries and vanilla. Process until all ingredients are well combined, approximately 2 minutes. Spoon into a bowl and set aside.

There's no need to wipe out food processor.

Add rinsed and drained cashews and the remaining cheesecake filling ingredients. Blend until very smooth and well combined, with no grainy bits. This will take approximately 5 minutes. Stop from time to time to scrape down sides of bowl. When you have a lovely smooth and creamy consistency, add the set aside raspberry mixture. Blend until well combined.

Spread the cheesecake mixture over your base and cover. Place in the freezer for several hours or overnight. Allow too sit out at room temperature for 40 minutes before serving. Top with raspberries.

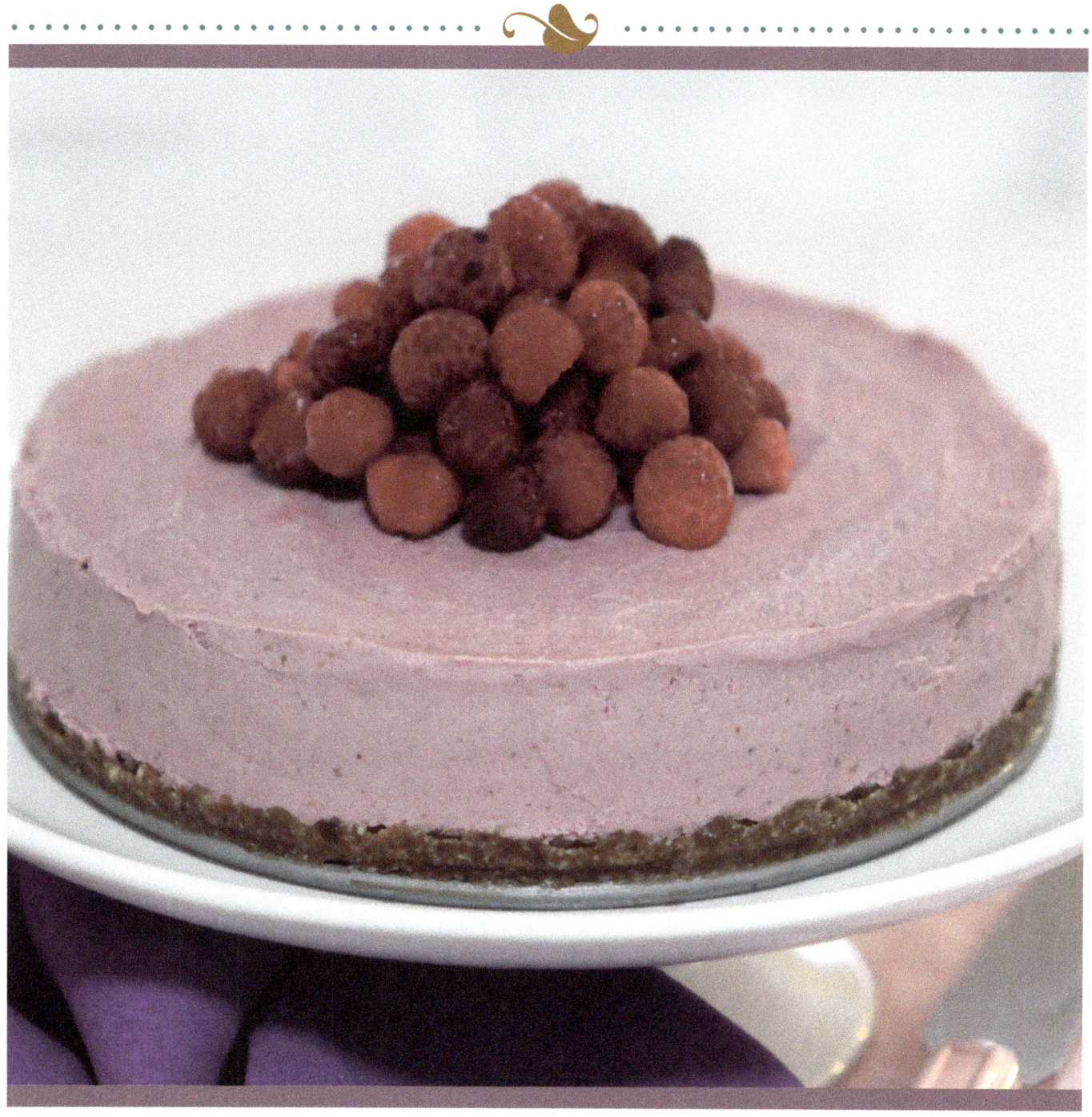

TOPPINGS & SPREADS

Chocolate Frosting 280

Vanilla Macadamia Frosting 281

Whipped Cashew Cream........................... 282

Chocolate Ganache 283

Cookie and Cake Glazes 284

Marshmallow Frosting 286

Strawberry Preserve 288

Fruity Chia Jam 289

Blueberry Spread....................................... 290

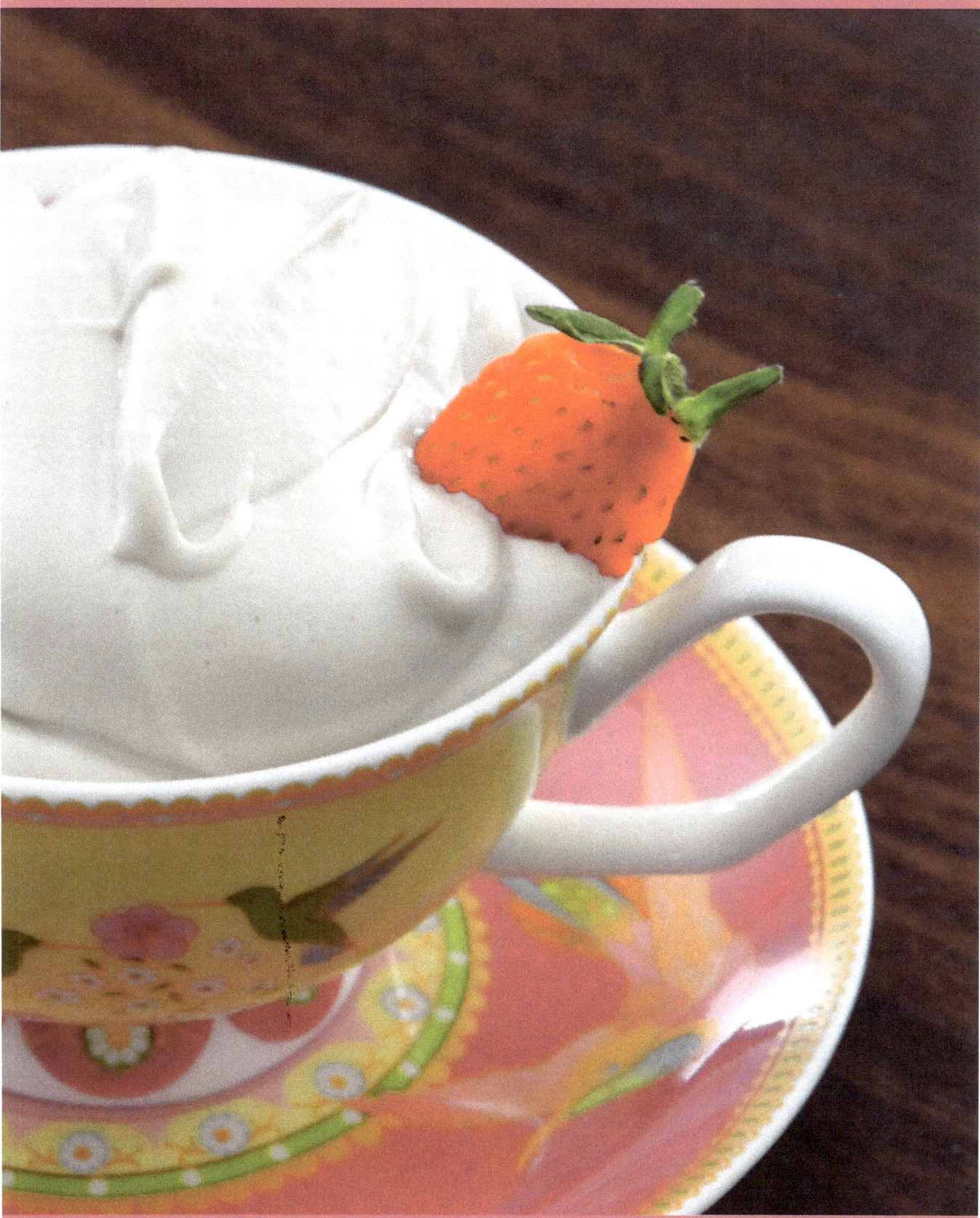

Chocolate Frosting

This is a lovely rich chocolate frosting to use on cupcakes, brownies or a large cake.

Prep time: 10 minutes, plus soaking time Cooking time: none Makes: 1½ cups

Ingredients:

- ¾ cup raw cashews, soaked
- 2-3 Tbsp cacao powder, adjust to your taste
- ½ cup canned coconut cream
- ¼ cup coconut oil
- 1-2 Tbsp honey, or to taste
- 2 tsp vanilla extract

Method:

Soak cashews in filtered water with a pinch of sea salt for 30–60 minutes, drain and rinse well.

Add cashews and cacao powder to a high-speed blender and blend until finely ground. Add coconut cream, coconut oil, honey and vanilla, to the nut mixture and blend on high until smooth and creamy.

Place in the fridge for a while to firm up, but still spreadable.

After coating your cake or cupcakes, store them in the fridge until ready to serve.

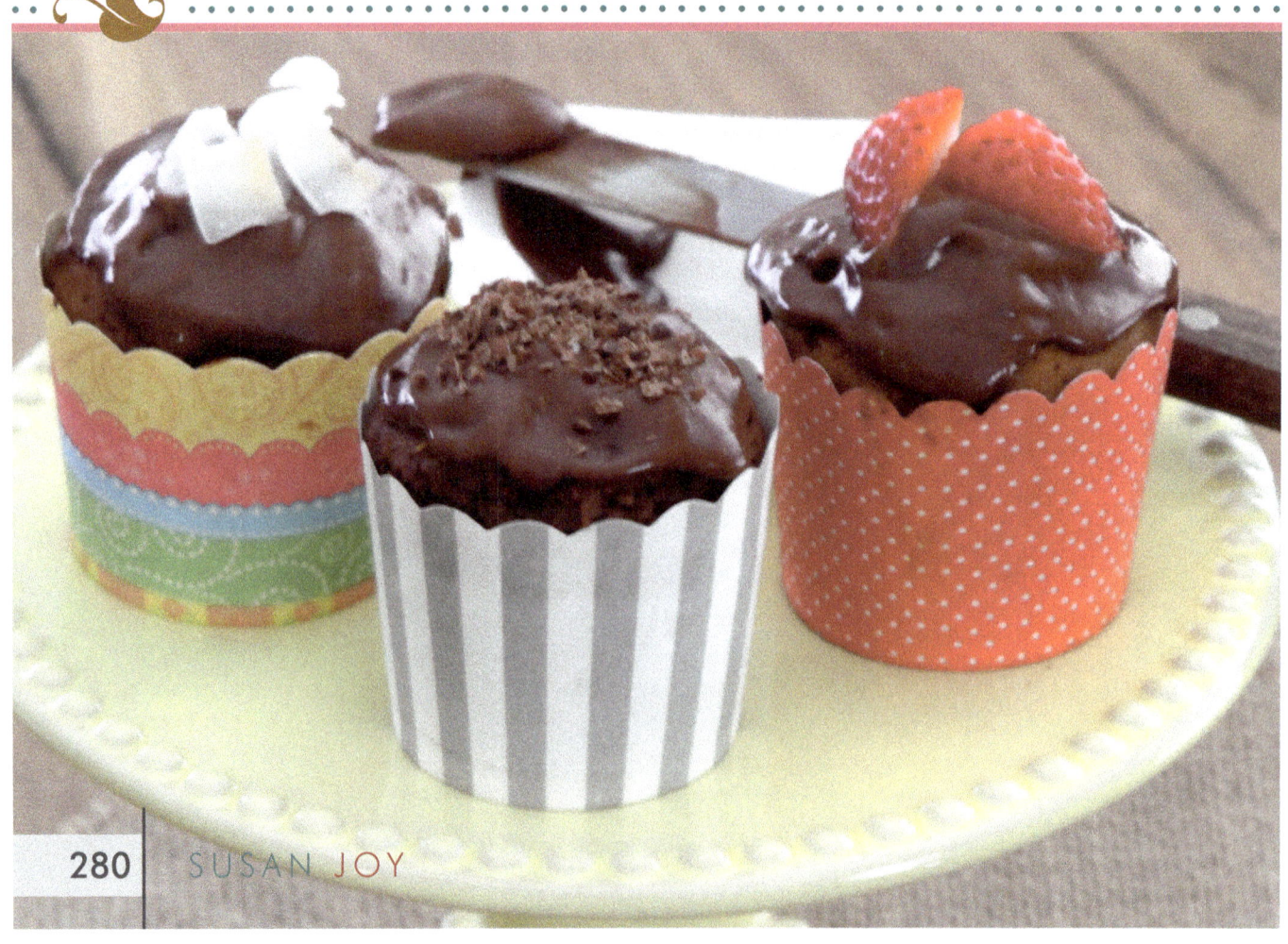

TOPPINGS & SPREADS | 281

Vanilla Macadamia Frosting

Blended macadamia nuts create a very smooth and sweet texture, this is ideal for making a healthy frosting. Delicious on vanilla and chocolate cupcakes.

Prep time: 8 minutes   Cooking time: none   Makes: 1½ cups

Ingredients:

- 1 cup macadamia nuts
- ¼ cup almond meal/flour
- ¼ cup coconut milk
- 2 Tbsp coconut oil
- 1-2 Tbsp honey or to your taste
- 2 tsp vanilla extract
- 1 tsp lemon juice

Method:

Add all the ingredients to a high-speed blender and blend until smooth and creamy. Use the tamper stick to help push nuts onto the blades, this will help to make the process faster. If you are making a double-layered cake, double this recipe, so you have enough for the filling.

If a firmer frosting is required, place in the fridge. After frosting your cake or cupcakes, store them in the fridge until ready to serve. Keeps in the fridge for up to 4 days.

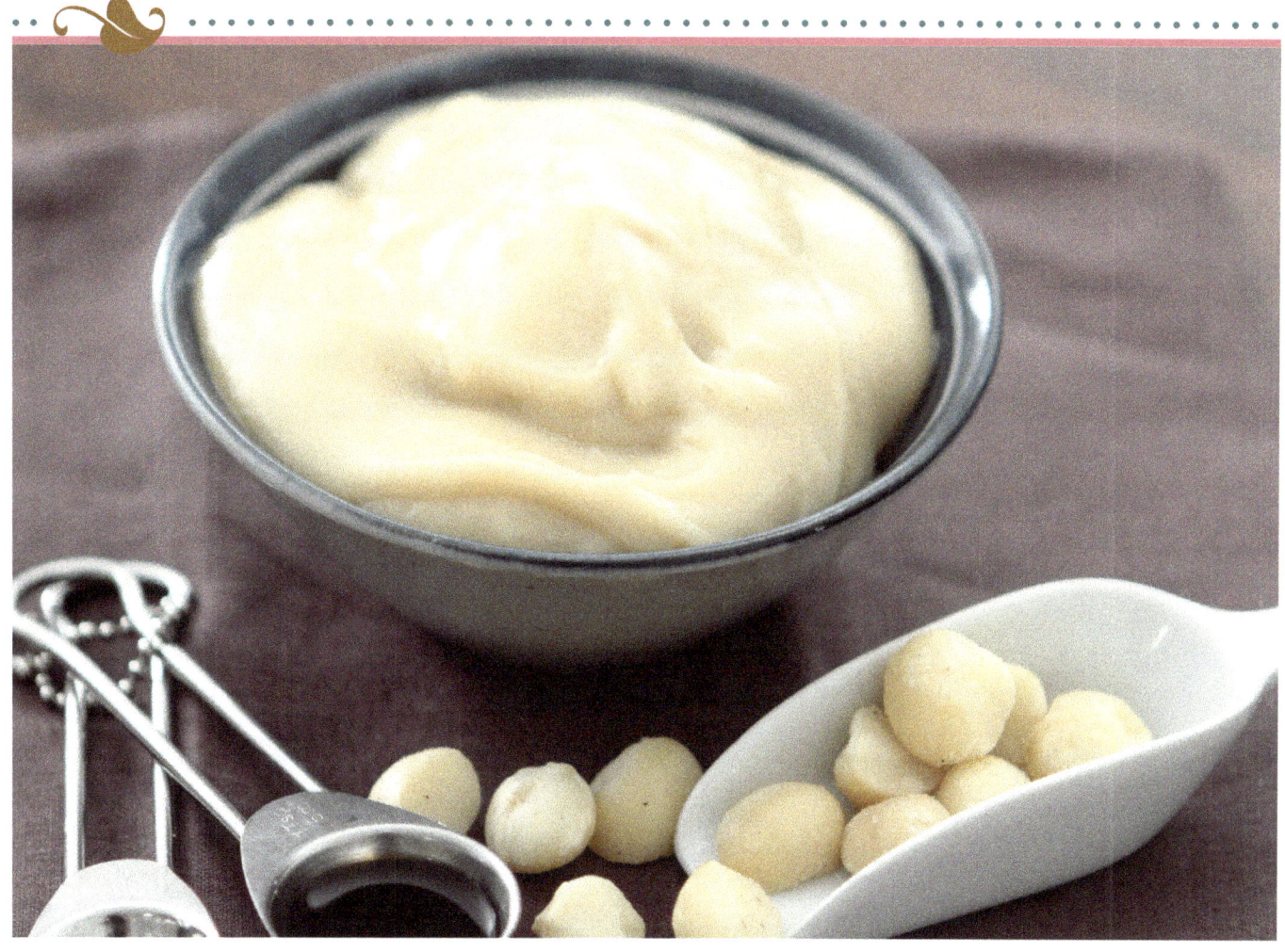

TOPPINGS & SPREADS

Whipped Cashew Cream

This is a great alterative to coconut cream for dolloping on your healthy desserts. Blended cashews become lovely and creamy, this makes them so versatile. By using water when whipping, you get a much lighter cream.

Prep time: 10 minutes plus soaking time Cooking time: none Makes: 2 cups

Ingredients:

- 2 cups raw cashews, soaked
- ½ tsp sea salt
- 1-2 Tbsp honey or to taste
- 1 Tbsp vanilla extract
- ¾ cup filtered water

Method:

Add cashews and salt to a bowl and cover with plenty of hot water.

Soak for 30-60 minutes, drain through a metal sieve and rinse well with clean filtered water and drain.

To a blender, add cashews, honey, vanilla and water. Blend until you have a light and smooth consistency, scrapping down the sides a few times to incorporate well. (When placed in the fridge, cream firms up slightly).

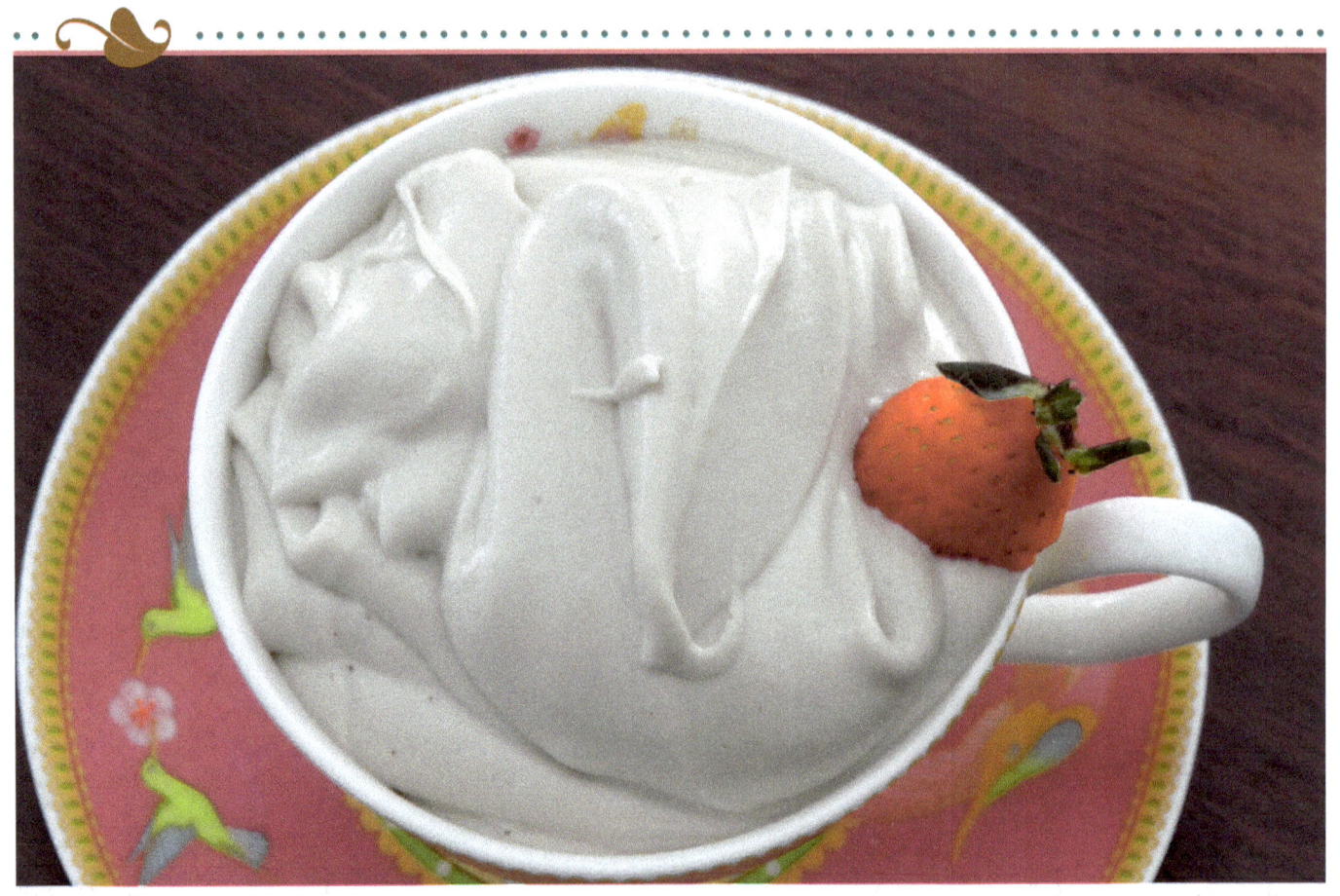

Chocolate Ganache

This is for a treat only. Use on a birthday cake or to drizzle warm over a dessert pudding or just about anything that needs yummy chocolate sauce dripping all over it. Only use dark chocolate, preferably 70 - 85%, with no soy or additives.

Prep time: 5 minutes Cooking time: 6 minutes Makes: 1½ cup

Ingredients:

- 1 cup canned full fat coconut cream
- 100g/3.5ozs 85% dark chocolate, chopped
- 2 tsp honey
- 2 tsp vanilla extract
- ⅛ tsp fine sea salt

Method:

Add coconut cream to a small saucepan over medium-low heat. Remove from heat just before cream starts to boil.

Add chocolate a little at a time, whisking as it melts in the cream. When melted add honey, vanilla extract and sea salt. Whisk to combine.

Pour into a bowl and set aside. Let cool for 15 minutes before placing in fridge to continue cooling. Watch carefully as you don't want the ganache to become too firm and not spreadable.

If you are pouring over a pudding, skip refrigeration.

Keeps for up to 4 days stored in an airtight glass container in the fridge.

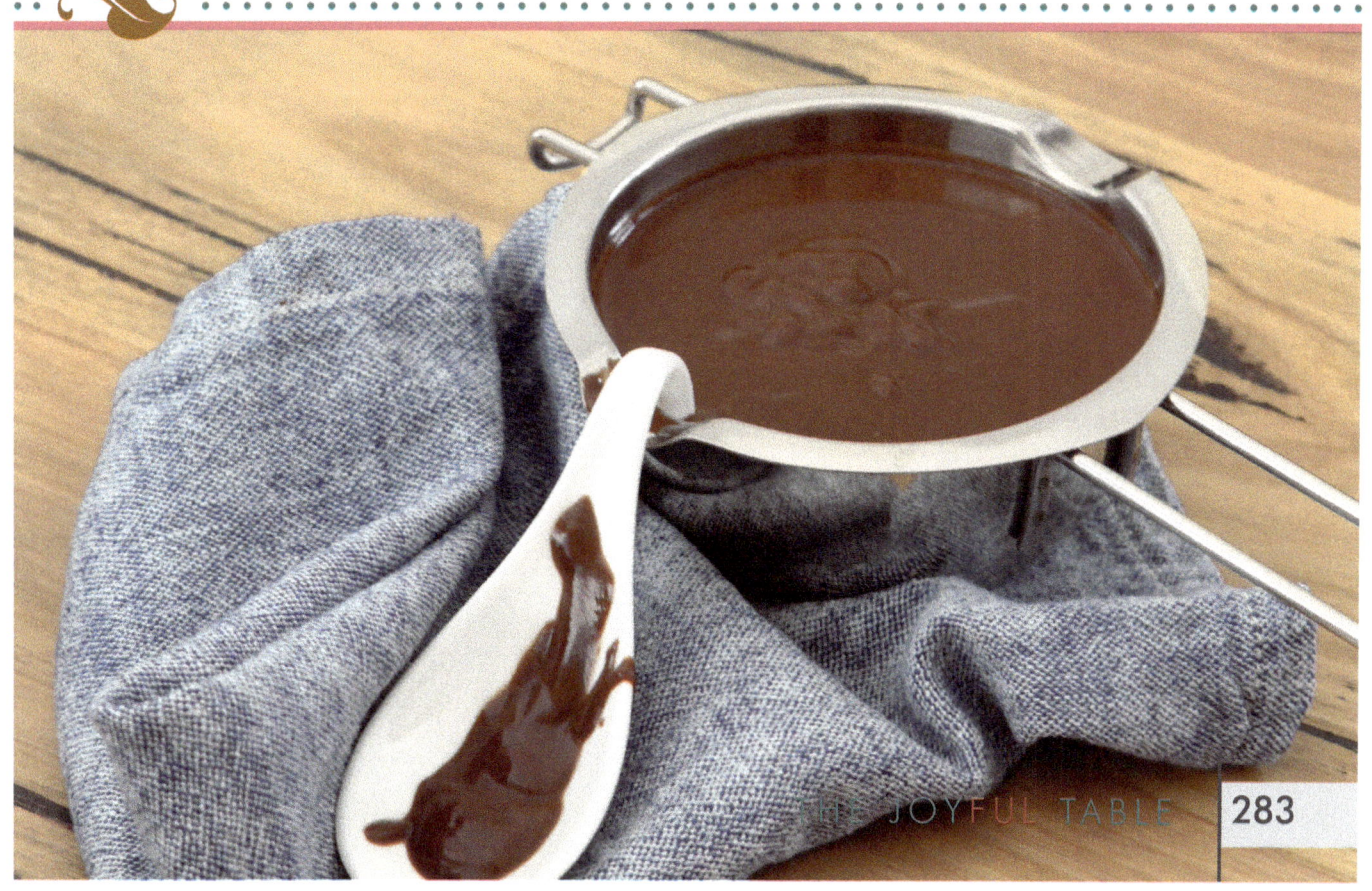

Cookie and Cake Glazes

Healthy icings for your paleo cookies, biscuits, cupcakes or buns. They are light in texture and can be poured over warm or allowed to cool and spread with a knife.

Prep time: 5 minutes Cooking time: 5 minutes Makes: ½ cup

Ingredients:

VANILLA GLAZE
- ¼ cup coconut milk or cashew milk
- ¼ cup coconut oil
- 1 tsp arrowroot flour
- 2 tsp honey
- 1 tsp vanilla extract

LEMON GLAZE
- ¼ cup coconut milk or cashew milk
- ¼ cup coconut oil
- 1 tsp arrowroot flour
- 1 Tbsp honey
- 1 tsp lemon juice, adjust to taste
- 1 tsp lemon zest

CINNAMON GLAZE
- ¼ cup coconut milk or cashew milk
- ¼ cup coconut oil
- 1 tsp arrowroot flour
- 2 tsp honey
- ¼ tsp ground cinnamon, adjust to taste

Method:

To a small saucepan add all the ingredients for your choice of glaze. Whisk continually, while heating over low heat until milk and oil have emulsified and slightly thickened. Do not allow too boil.

Once the mixture is all melted and combined, cool slightly then pour or spread.

If you would like it thicker, whisk in a little extra arrowroot flour.

Makes approximately ½ cup, if you are icing a large cake double your recipe.

TOPPINGS & SPREADS | 285

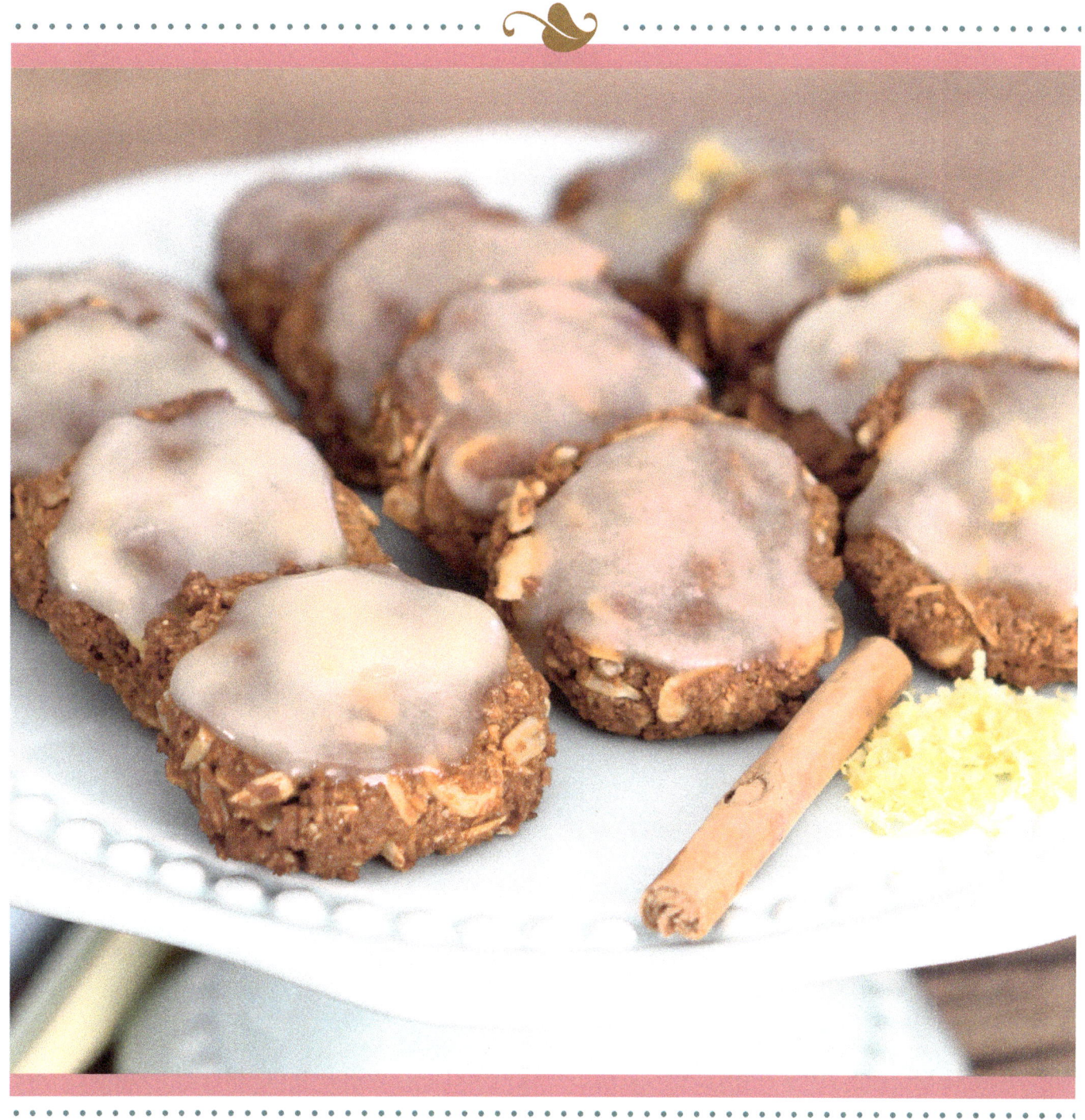

Marshmallow Frosting

A light and fluffy frosting that looks impressive on a chocolate cake. If you are decorating your cake with strawberries or fruit, you will need to place them before the marshmallow sets.

Prep time: 8 minutes   Cooking time: none   Makes: 3 cups

Ingredients:

- 2 tsp unflavoured gelatin, for setting
- 2 Tbsp filtered water
- ¼ cup 100% maple syrup, heated
- 2 egg whites, room temperature
- Pinch fine sea salt
- ½ tsp vanilla extract

Method:

Heat maple syrup in a saucepan, set aside. Add water to a small jug or cup and sprinkle over gelatin. Leave to soften. Set aside.

Add egg whites and salt to a medium stainless steal or glass bowl. Use an electric beater to whip egg whites. Beat until you have firm peaks.

Pour hot maple syrup into the gelatin mixture and stir quickly to dissolve the softened gelatin.

Slowly drizzle maple syrup/gelatin mixture into egg whites, while you continue to beat on high (the hot syrup will cook the eggs for you). Stop and add vanilla. Continue beating for a further 2 minutes to produce a lovely shiny frosting.

Once you have finished beating you will need to frost your cake within 5-10 minutes, as the mixture will set. Best to serve frosted cakes on the day. If you are decorating, place your extra toppings in place before marshmallow firms up.

TOPPINGS & SPREADS

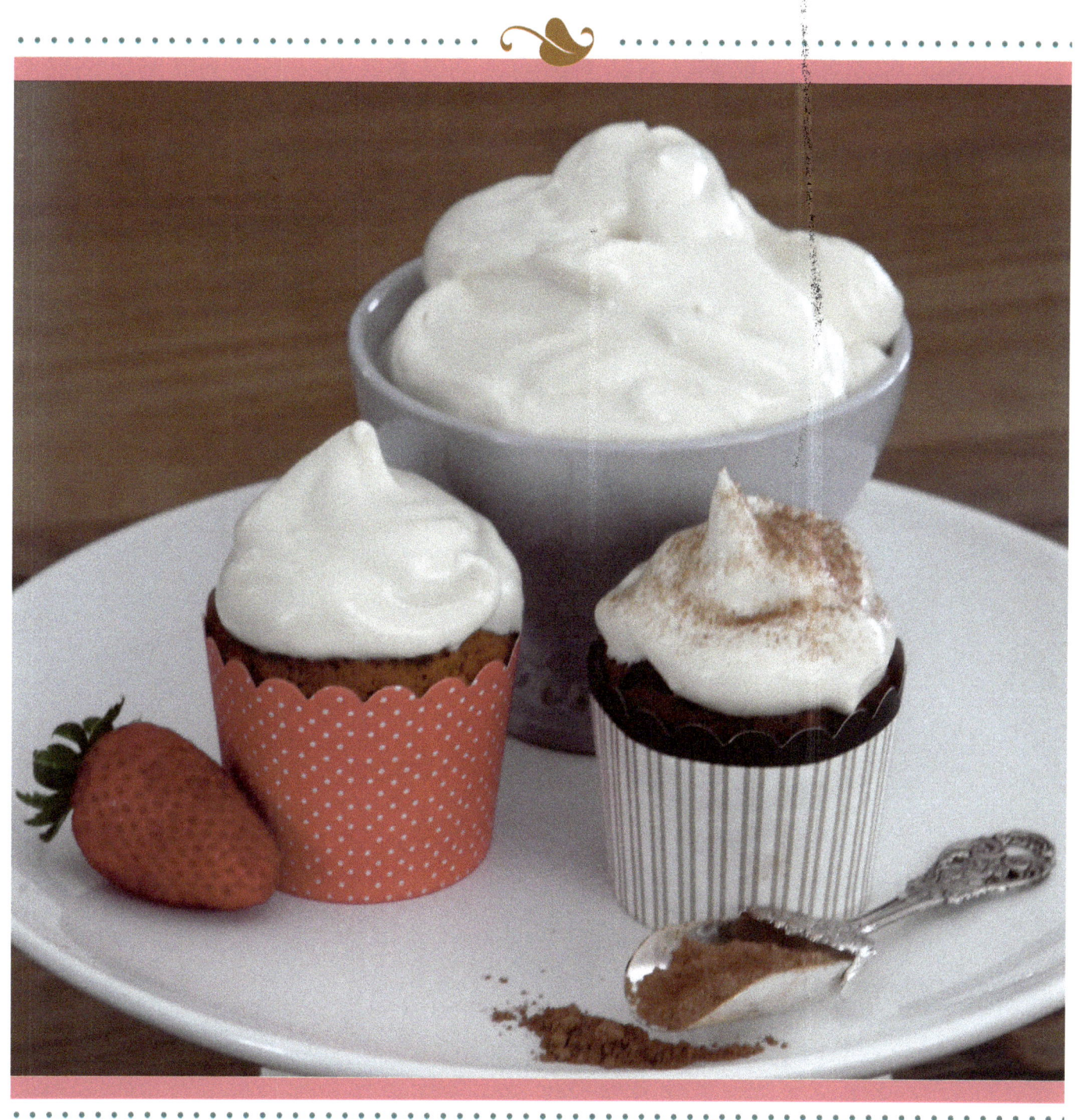

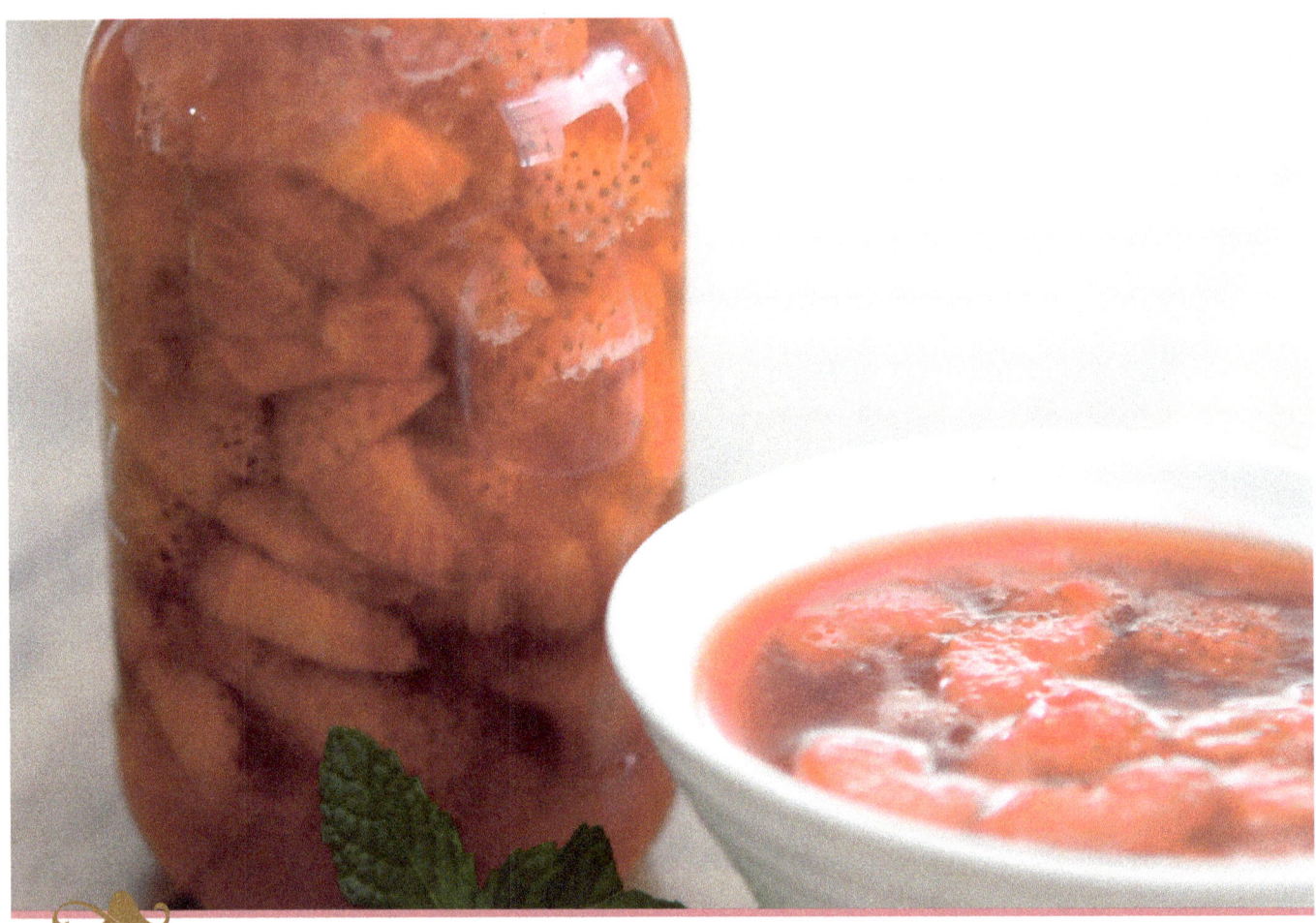

Strawberry Preserve

A preserve has lumps of fruit in it, not smooth like a jam or jelly. Delicious spread on grain free bread. It can be used in a flan or pie. This is a great way to get good gut healing gelatin into your diet too.

Prep time: 10 minutes Cooking time: 10 minutes Makes: 2 cups

Ingredients:

- 500g/1.1lb strawberries
- 1 Tbsp vinegar, to wash strawberries
- Juice of 1 small lemon
- 3 Tbsp 100% maple syrup
- 2 tsp unflavoured gelatin, for setting
- 2 Tbsp filtered water

Method:

Wash strawberries in a bowl of water with vinegar. (The vinegar will keep the strawberries fresh longer). Pat dry and chop strawberries.

To a medium saucepan add, strawberries, lemon juice and maple syrup. Bring to a gentle boil and simmer for 1 minute. Remove from heat.

Add water to a small bowl and sprinkle over gelatin. Let sit to soften a minute. Add 2 tablespoons of hot strawberry liquid from saucepan to the gelatin bowl. Mix to dissolve gelatin then pour into the saucepan, whisk through quickly for 30 seconds.

Pour into a sterilized glass jar with a sealed lid. Store in the fridge.

Toppings & Spreads

Fruity Chia Jam

The chia seeds create a lovely jelly texture. You can use fresh or frozen berries for this recipe.

Prep time: 5 minutes Cooking time: none Makes: 1 cup

Ingredients:

- 1½ cups of berries of choice (I normally use strawberries and blueberries together)
- 1 Tbsp honey
- 1 tsp vanilla extract
- 1½ Tbsp chia seeds

Method:

Place all ingredients into a blender and blend until combined. If you like pieces of fruit in your jam, keep aside a few berries and add at the end and just give a quick blend to break them up a little.

Pour into a glass jar or container and store sealed in the fridge. Jam will thicken from the chia seeds.

Keeps for 10 days in the fridge. (If using fresh berries, wash in water and vinegar, this will keep the fruit in the jam fresher for longer.)

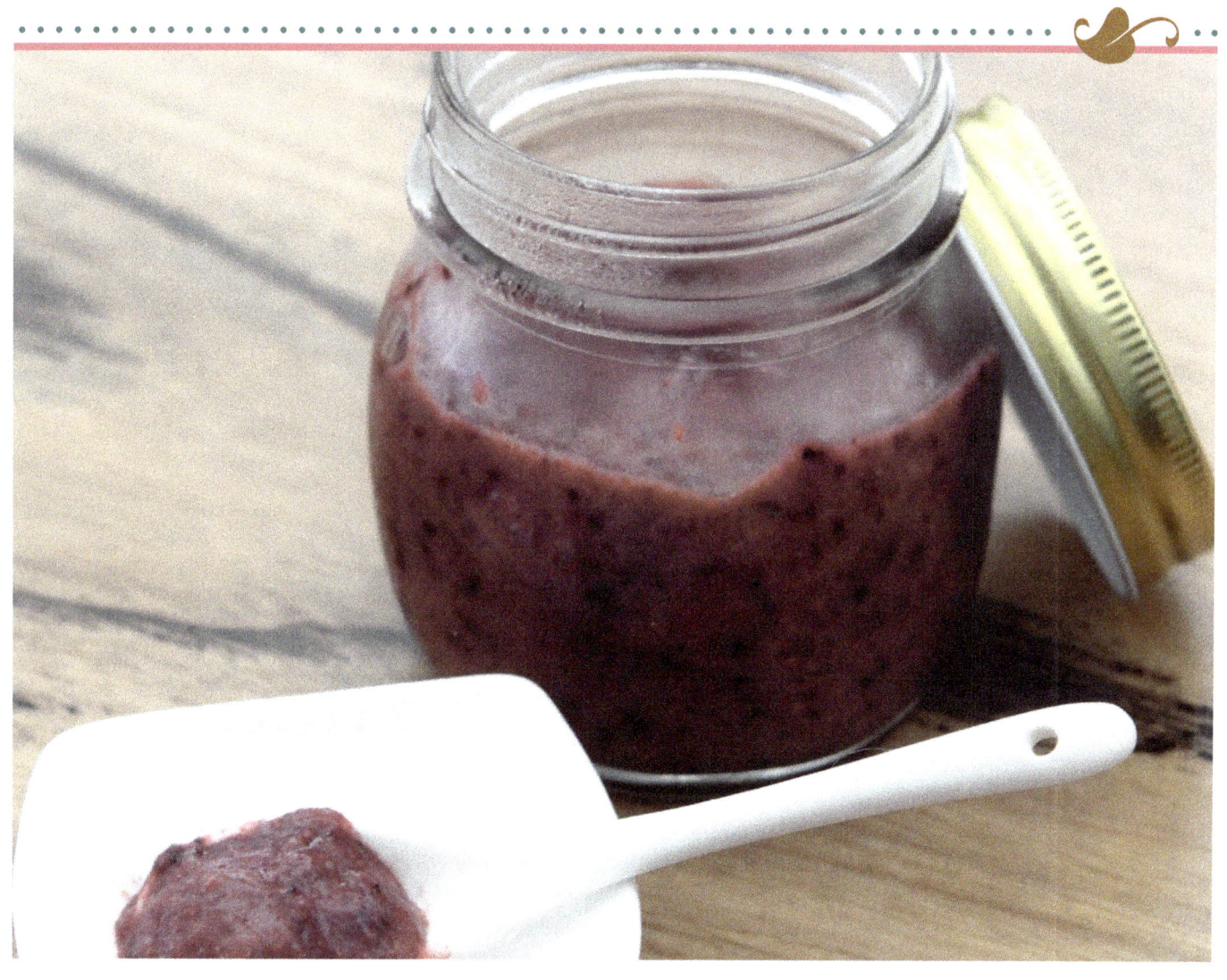

Blueberry Spread

I initially made this spread to pour over a cake but I have found endless uses for it. I used it in my thumbprint biscuits on page 231. My grandson has also found a way to eat it; straight from the jar! Pour over homemade ice cream or pancakes. It's best to use frozen blueberries, as they have a much stronger flavour and colour than fresh.

Prep time: 10 minutes Cooking time: 15 minutes Makes: 1 cup

Ingredients:

- 2 cups frozen blueberries
- Juice of ½ lemon
- 1½ Tbsp 100% maple syrup
- 2 tsp arrowroot flour
- 1-2 Tbsp filtered water to make arrowroot slurry

Method:

Add to a small saucepan, frozen blueberries, lemon juice and maple syrup. While heating, use the back of a spoon to smash the blueberries. You can leave it partly lumpy or smooth depending on your preference or use.

Mix arrowroot flour with a little water to make a smooth paste/slurry. Once the mixture starts to get hot, stir in the slurry. Stir until you have a gently simmer, continue stirring while simmering and thickening, approximately 3-4 minutes. Be careful not to over boil as arrowroot reverses its thickening properties when boiled for too long.

Remove from heat and let cool. Pour into a sterilized glass jar or container with a sealed lid. Store in the fridge.

TOPPINGS & SPREADS | 291

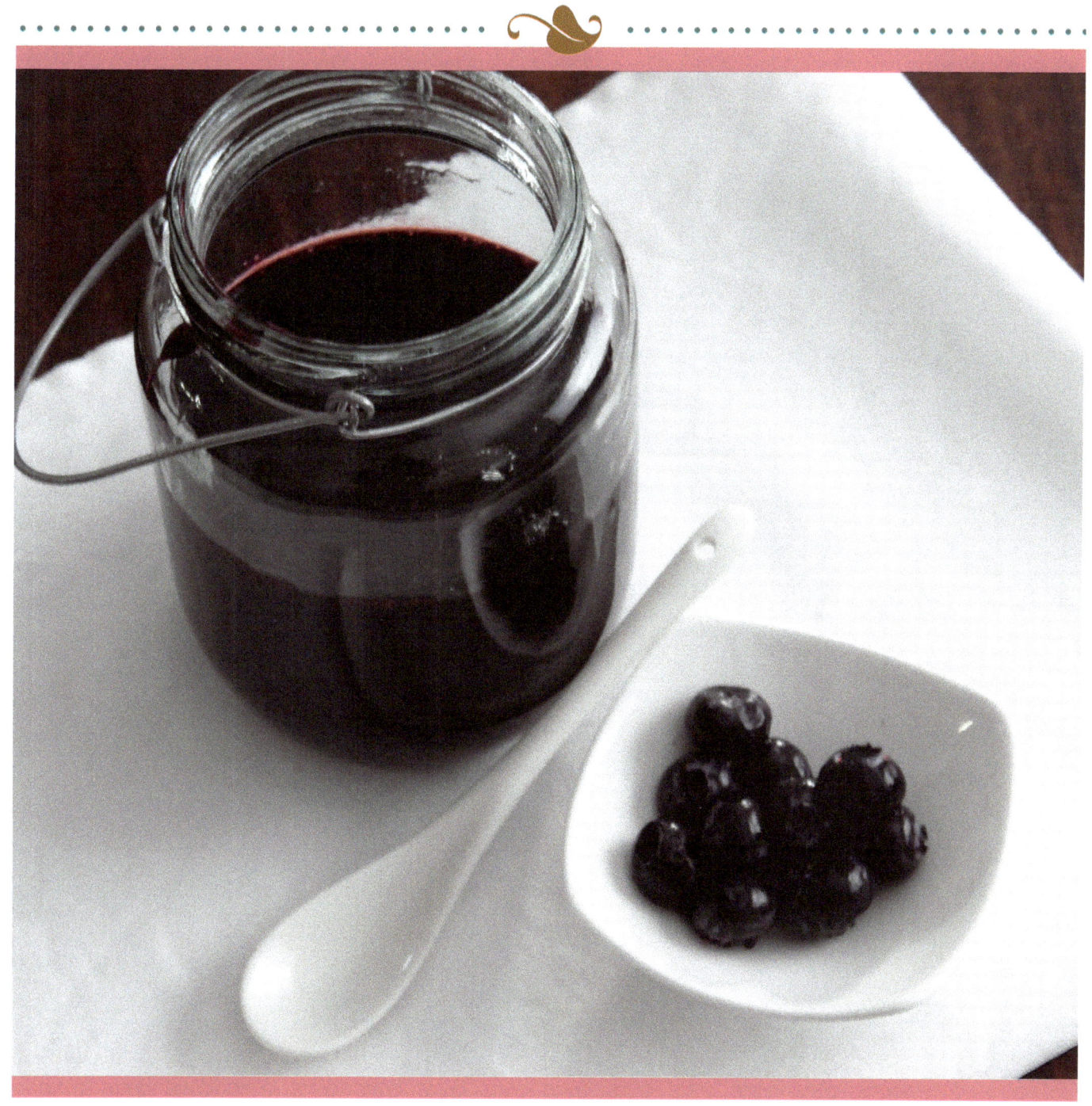

BASICS

Chicken Broth/Stock 295

Dairy Free Milks 297

Cashew Probiotic Cheeze 301

Cashew Sour Cream 302

Roasted Almond Butter 303

Sunflower Butter 304

Coconut Butter 304

Cashew Butter 306

Chocolate Cashew Butter 306

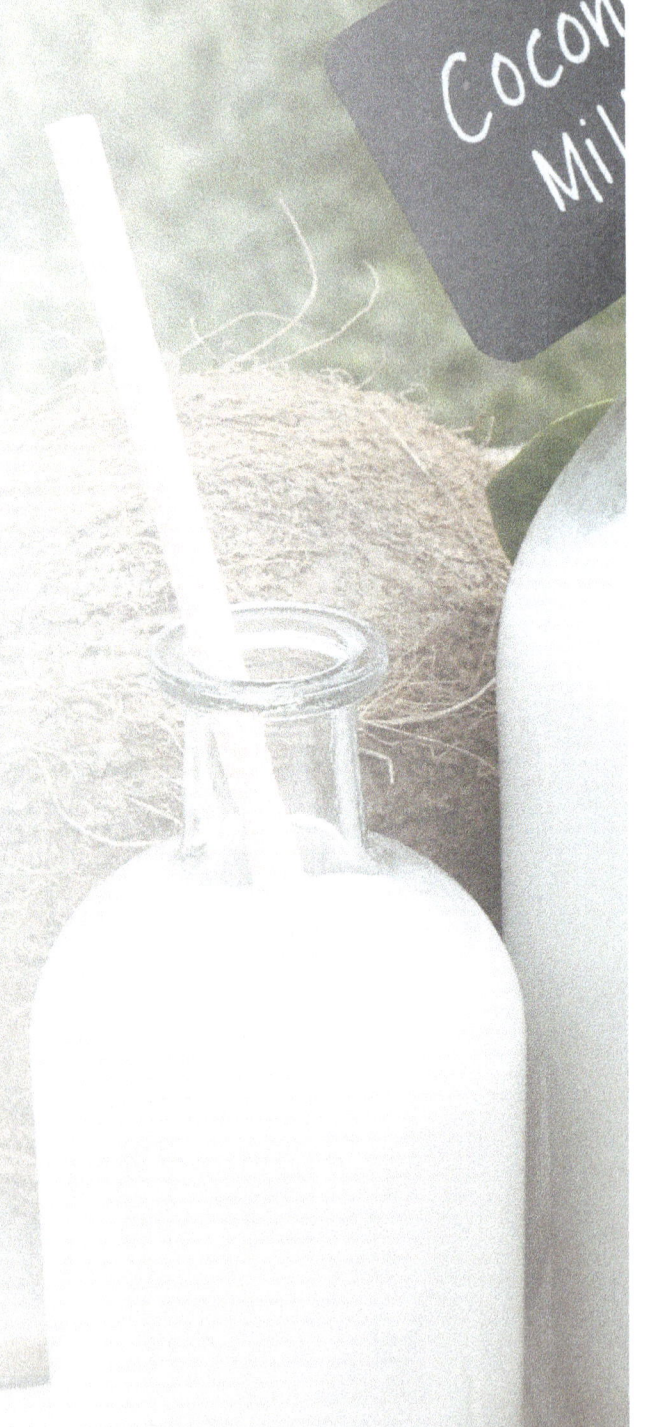

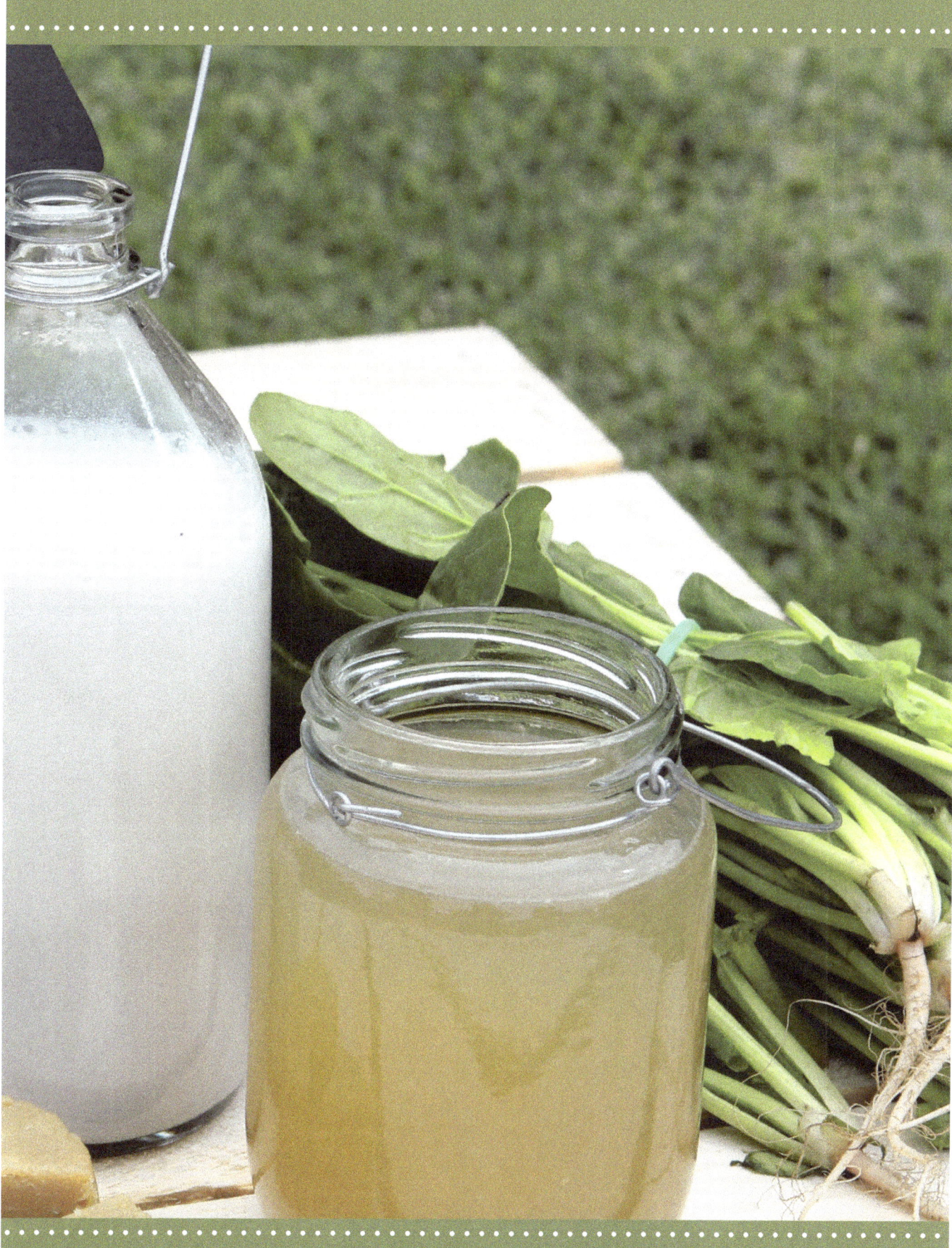

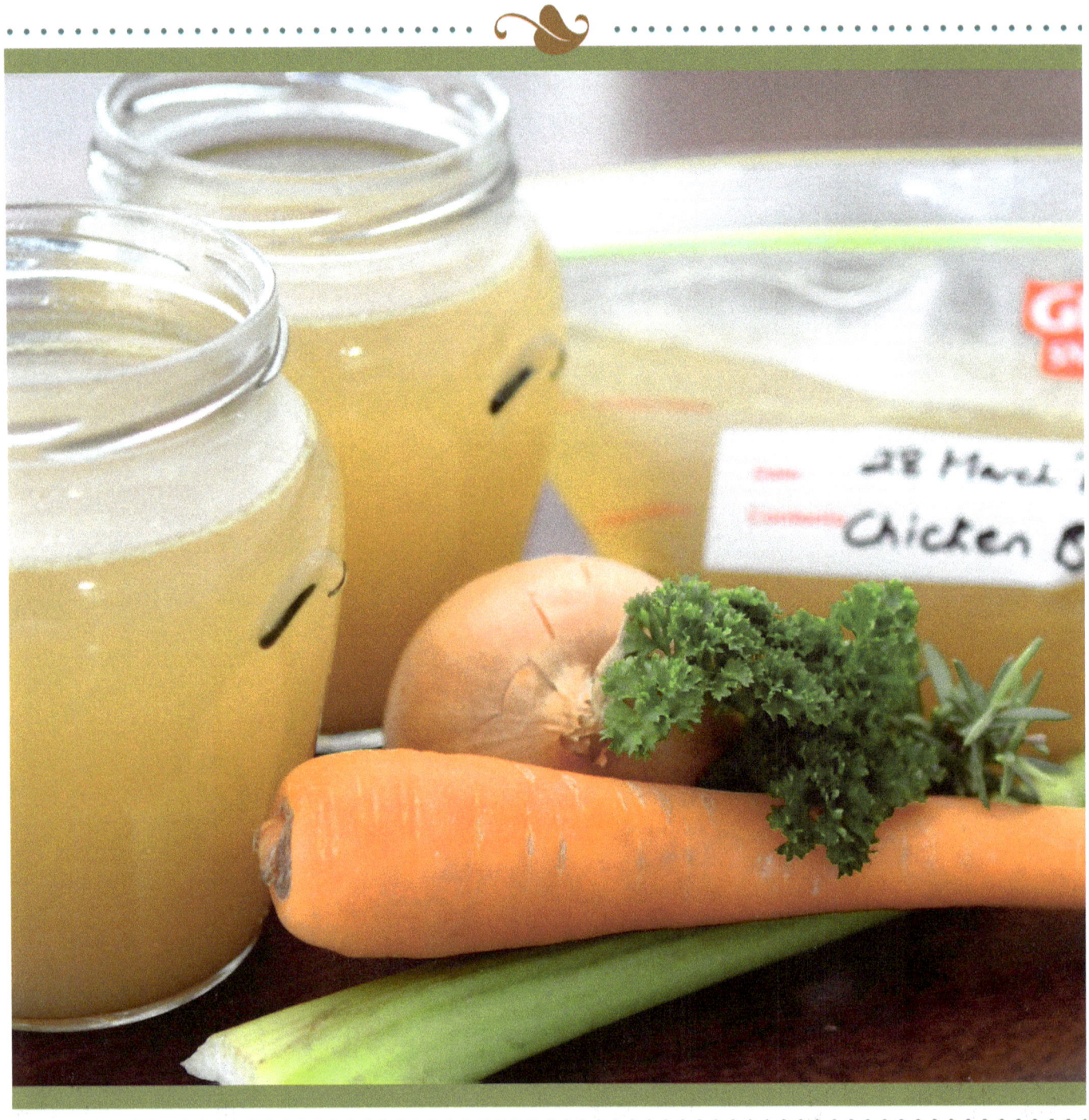

Chicken Broth/Stock

This delicious homemade chicken broth is excellent to drink when feeling unwell. Traditionally broth was made just from meat bones and simmered for hours to remove the gelatin, marrow and goodness from them. These days vegetables are also added to give extra flavour. By using a slow cooker, making your own broth/stock is so easy.

Prep time: 10 minutes Cooking time: 12 hours Make: 2 litres/8 cups

Ingredients:

- 2 free range chicken carcass, drumsticks etc. (with a little meat left on for flavour)
- 1 carrot, in chunks
- 1 onion, in chunks
- 1 celery stick, in chunks
- 2 cloves garlic, chopped
- 3 slices of lemon
- Handful of parsley
- Sprig of rosemary
- 1 Tbsp Apple Cider vinegar
- 1 Tbsp coconut aminos
- ½ tsp sea salt
- ¼ tsp ground pepper
- 2L/8 cups filtered water, plus extra

Method:

To a slow cooker or large soup pot add, chicken bones including any meat left on them. (The meat will add extra flavour but not necessary). Add remaining ingredients and water.

Cook covered on low for 12-14 hours. During cooking there may be some evaporation, top up broth with extra filtered water towards the end of cooking time.

Allow to cool down. Remove larger vegetables and bones with a slotted spoon, then strain broth through a fine metal sieve or muslin cloth.

Store broth in glass jars in the fridge for up to 4 days. If freezing store in glass jars or snap lock bags, leave a space at the top for expansion. Can be kept frozen for up to 3 months.

For Beef Broth/Stock:
Purchase soup bones or use meaty bones left from a roast and the above ingredients. Skim off scum from top if using raw bones. Once chilled scoop off any solidified fat.

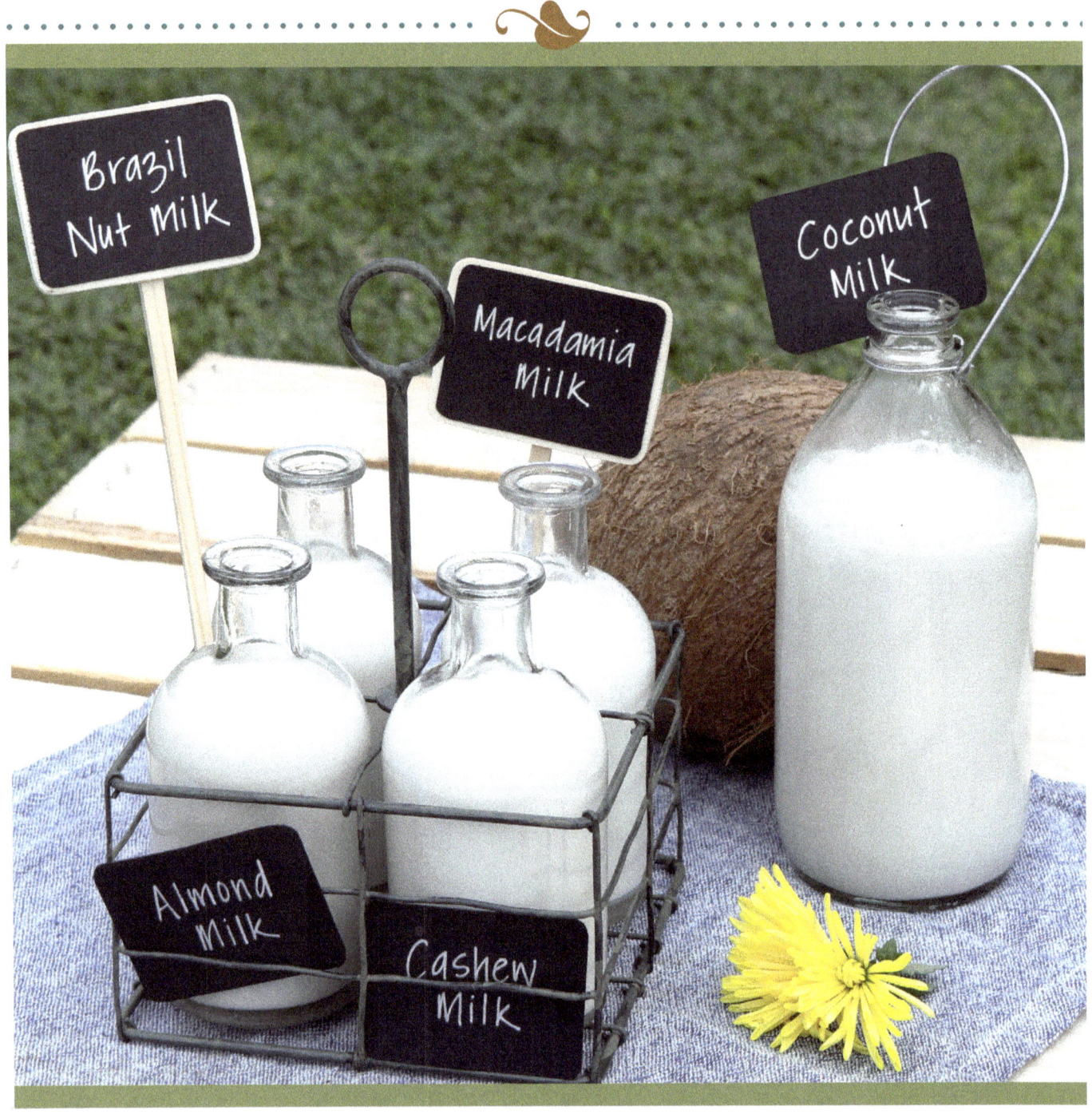

Dairy Free Milks

Nut and coconut milk are excellent alternatives to animal milk. Use them in smoothies, pour over grain free cereals and in your baking. Making your own milk means you don't get the sugars, gums, thickeners and preservative that many commercial nut milks contain. It is also cheaper and tastes better. These recipes all make 3-4 cups of milk. Depending on what I am using the milk for it can be stretched to be more economical. For drinking I like it creamier and use 1 cup of nuts to 3 cups of water and add a date or a little honey. For baking I use 1 cup of nuts to 4 cups of water and don't sweeten. You taste test and see what you prefer.

Prep time: 5 minutes plus soaking time
Cooking time: none Makes: 750ml-1 litre/3-4 cups

ALMOND MILK

Ingredients:

- 1 cup almonds
- 3-4 cups filtered water, plus soaking water
- Optional: 1-2 pitted Medjool dates or 1-2 tsp honey
- Pinch of sea salt

Method:

Soak almonds in water for at least 8 hours, drain and rinse well. Add to a blender with 1 cup of filtered water and date or honey if using. Blend for 30 seconds. Add remaining 2 or 3 cups of water and salt. Blend until mixed.

Strain milk using a nut milk bag (or muslin cloth) draped over a bowl, pour milk through the bag, making sure bag is secured. For large quantities divide and strain half at a time. Squeeze bag from the top down, wring all the liquid out leaving the pulp clumped together in the bag.

Transfer to a sealed glass bottle or jar (kept only for milk). Store in the fridge for 3-4 days, shake before each use.

Almond milk is alkalising to the body and packed with a huge amount of nutrition, including calcium.

CASHEW MILK

Ingredients:

- 1 cup cashews
- 3-4 cups filtered water, plus soaking water
- Optional: 1-2 pitted Medjool dates or 1-2 tsp honey
- Pinch of sea salt

Method:

Soak cashews in water for 1-2 hours, drain and rinse well. Add to a blender with 1 cup of filtered water and date or honey if using. Blend for 30 seconds. Add remaining 2 or 3 cups of water and salt. Blend until mixed. If you are using in baking there is no need to strain, that's why this is my preferred milk when cooking.

Strain milk using a nut milk bag draped over a bowl, pour milk through the bag, making sure bag is secured. For large quantities divide and strain half at a time. Squeeze bag from the top down, wring all the liquid out leaving the pulp clumped together in the bag.

Transfer to a sealed glass bottle or jar (kept only for milk). Store in the fridge for 5-6 days, shake before each use.

Bonus, cashew milk lasts longer than other nut milks and full of magnesium for strong bones.

....

MACADAMIA MILK

Ingredients:

- 1 cup macadamia nuts
- 3-4 cups filtered water
- Optional: 1-2 pitted Medjool dates or 1-2 tsp honey
- Pinch of sea salt

Method:

There is no need to soak macadamia nuts. Add to a blender with 1 cup of filtered water and date or honey if using. Blend for 30 seconds. Add remaining 2 or 3 cups of water and salt. Blend until mixed. If you are using in baking there is no need to strain. This is my preferred drinking milk. For drinking strain milk using a nut milk bag draped over a bowl, pour milk through the bag, making sure bag is secured. For large quantities divide and strain half at a time.

Squeeze bag from the top down, wring all the liquid out leaving the pulp clumped together in the bag.

Transfer to a sealed glass bottle or jar (kept only for milk). Store in the fridge for 3-4 days, shake before each use.

Full of heart healthy fats.

BRAZIL NUT MILK

Ingredients:

1 cup brazil nuts
3-4 cups filtered water, plus soaking water
Optional: 1-2 pitted Medjool dates or 1-2 tsp honey
Pinch of sea salt

Method:

Soak brazil nuts in water for 1 hour, drain and rinse well. Add to a blender with 1 cup of filtered water and date or honey if using. Blend for 30 seconds. Add remaining 2 or 3 cups of water and salt. Blend until mixed.

Strain milk using a nut milk bag draped over a bowl and pour milk through the bag, making sure bag is secured. For large quantities divide and strain half at a time.

Squeeze bag from the top down, wring all the liquid out leaving the pulp clumped together in the bag.

Transfer to a sealed glass bottle or jar (kept only for milk). Store in the fridge for 3-4 days, shake before each use.

This is a very creamy milk and a great support for thyroid function.

....

COCONUT MILK

Ingredients:

1 cup organic desiccated or shredded coconut, avoid coconut with preservatives
3-4 cups filtered water (1 cup to be boiling)
Pinch of sea salt

Method:

Add coconut to a blender with 1 cup of boiling water, let sit for 30 seconds to soften, then blend for 30-40 seconds. Add remaining 2 or 3 cups of water and salt. Blend until mixed.

Strain milk using a nut milk bag draped over a bowl and pour milk through the bag, making sure bag is secured. For large quantities divide and strain half at a time.

Squeeze bag from the top down, wring all the liquid out leaving the pulp clumped together in the bag.

Transfer to a sealed glass bottle or jar (kept only for milk). Store in the fridge for 3-4 days, shake before each use.

Full of vitamins and minerals, great for your heart, skin and immune and digestive systems, plus it's cheap to make and so creamy.

300 | BASICS

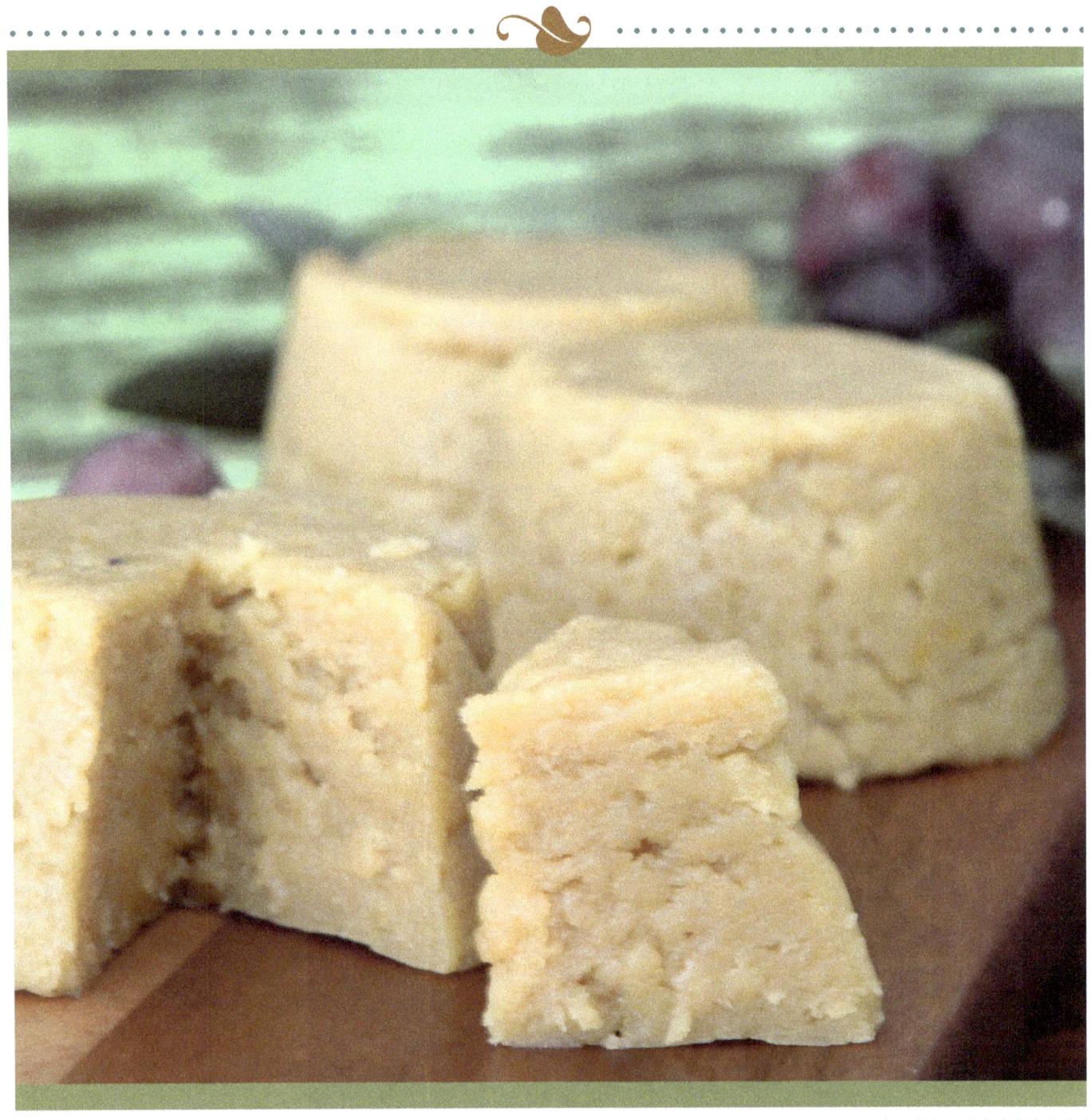

Cashew Probiotic Cheeze

I use a six-hole silicon muffin mold to shape the cheezes to look like small Brie or Camembert cheeses. Fermenting gives a slight sour taste which helps to counteract the sweetness of the nuts, plus you get the bonus of probiotics for good gut health.

Prep time: 10 minutes plus soaking & fermentation time
Cooking time: 1.5 hours Makes: 6

Ingredients:

- 4 cups raw cashew or macadamia nuts
- Filtered water and ½ tsp sea salt for soaking
- 2 good quality probiotic capsule (Acidophilus, non dairy brand)
- ¼ cup Nutritional Yeast Flakes
- 2 tsp fine sea salt

Method:

To a large bowl add, nuts, ½ teaspoon of sea salt and hot water. Let soak for 1 hour. Use a metal sieve to drain and rinse well.

Add half the nuts to a high-speed blender. Use tamper stick to help push nuts onto the blade until you have a smooth texture. Split in half the probiotic capsules, add powder to blender. Add second half of nuts. Blend nuts until smooth and silky.

Place nut mixture into a mason jar or glass bowl with space for the mixture to rise. Cover with a tea towel and place somewhere dark or in a cupboard to ferment for 20-24 hours. In hot weather the time can be reduced.

Cheeze will be ready when it has risen and become light and airy. The longer you ferment the sourer the cheeze (I like mine mild, 20 hours). Experiment with times and see what flavour you prefer.

When fermenting has finished, add Nutritional Yeast Flakes and sea salt, stir well to combine.

Use a silicone muffin pan and fill 6 muffin holes with cashew cheeze. Press cheeze mixture firmly into holes, making sure it is well compacted.

Place in a very cool oven at 50c/100f for 45 minutes to dehydrate. Remove from oven and carefully pop cheezes out. Place upside down on a lined baking tray. Return back to the oven and continue drying the cheezes out for a further 45 minutes. (If you have soaked your nuts longer there will be more moisture in them, so you will need to adjust the drying time.)

Remove and allow to cool to room temperature. Wrap each cheeze and place in the fridge. Once chilled you can slice and serve on grain free crackers or bread. The longer the cheeze is stored in the fridge the firmer it becomes and easier to slice. They will keep wrapped in the fridge for up to a month.

Cashew Sour Cream

Use Cashew Sour Cream in place of regular sour cream. Use for dips, serve a big dollop on top of grain free nachos or any recipe that calls for sour cream.

Prep time: 8 minutes plus soaking time Cooking time: none Makes: 1 cup

Ingredients:

- 1 cup raw cashews, soaked in filtered water and a pinch of sea salt for 30-60 minutes
- 2 Tbsp lemon juice
- 2 tsp Apple Cider vinegar
- ½ tsp fine sea salt
- ¼ cup filtered water

Method:

Drain and rinse soaked cashews well. Add to a high-speed blender, along with the remaining ingredients. Blend on high until smooth and creamy, with no grainy bits. Scrape down sides and blend again until your cream is smooth like the dairy version. Chill before serving.

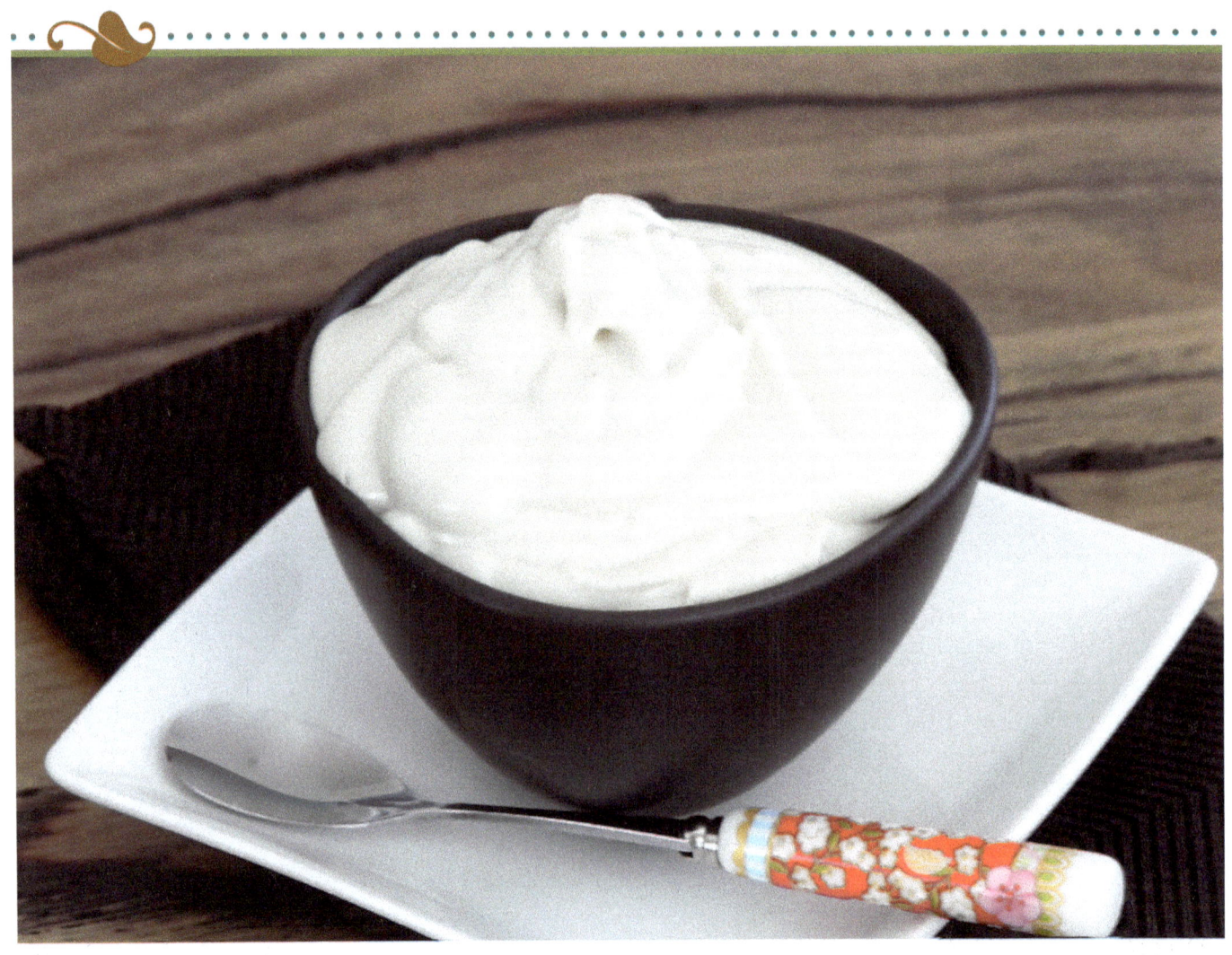

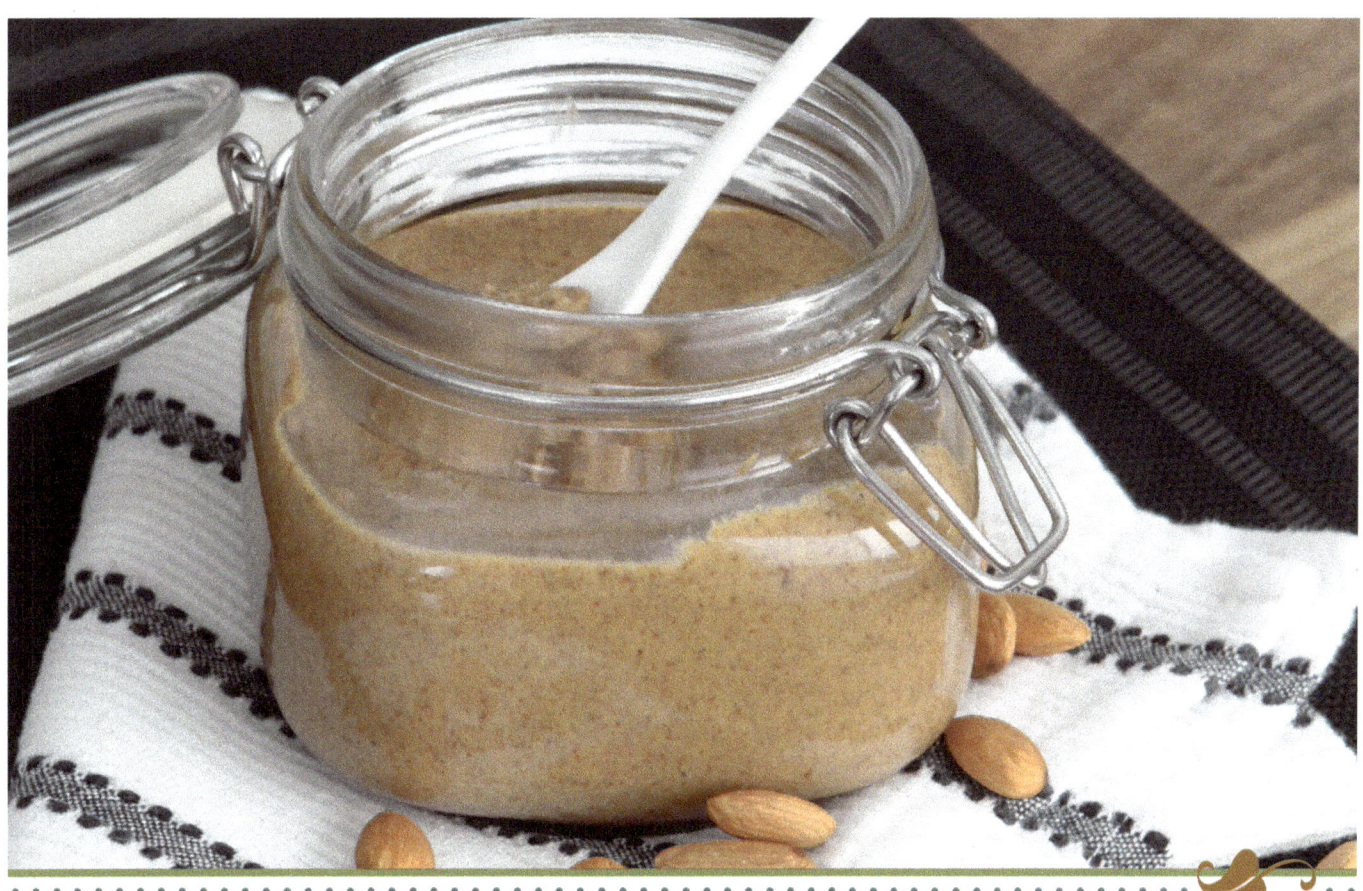

Roasted Almond Butter

Roasting the almonds gives a richer flavour. Add Almond Butter to recipes to help achieve a creamier and fudge like texture. Use it to fill your celery sticks for a healthy snack.

Prep time: 6 minutes Cooking time: 15 minutes Makes: 1¾ cup

Ingredients:

- 3 cups almonds
- ½ tsp fine sea salt, or to taste
- 1 Tbsp macadamia oil

Method:

Preheat oven to 160c/320f. Line a large baking tray with baking paper and spread nuts out evenly in a single layer. Roast until just changing colour, don't over roast, oil needs to remain in the nuts. Let cool.

Add the almonds to a food processor, blend until they become a fine meal.

Add salt and continue to process for a further 2 minutes. Consistency should be like a thick paste. Stop from time to time to scrap down sides and bottom of bowl.

Add oil, gradually through the chute of the processor lid while the processor is running. Process until you reach a smooth spreadable consistency. You can adjust processing time to reach your own personal preferred texture.

Store in a sealed glass jar in the fridge.

Sunflower Butter

Store bought Sunflower Butter is quite bland. The step of roasting the sunflower seeds gives an amazing flavour. Do not over roast or they will dry out. Oil needs to be left in the seeds to make a nice consistency. A great peanut butter substitute.

Prep time: 12 minutes Cooking time: 10 minutes Makes: 1 cup

Ingredients:

- 2 cups sunflower seeds
- 2 Tbsp macadamia nut oil
- ⅓ tsp fine sea salt

Method:

Preheat oven to 160c/320f. Line 2 large baking trays with baking paper and spread out one cup sunflower seeds per tray. Roast until just changing colour, this adds so much flavour, but don't over dry them. Let cool.

Add the seeds to a food processor, and blend until they become a fine meal.

Add oil gradually through the chute of the processor lid. Proccess until it comes together and looks like peanut butter. Stop often to scrape down sides and give the motor a rest.

Add the salt and blend for a further few minutes. It is ready when the blade looks like it's spinning around by itself and the butter is now creamy and collecting around the sides of bowl, it will be quite warm. If too dry, add extra oil.

Store in a sealed glass jar in the fridge.

Coconut Butter

Organic Coconut Butter is expensive, you can make it with a fraction of the cost. It adds creaminess to smoothies, gives flavour and texture to sweet baking.

Prep time: 12 minutes Cooking time: none Makes: 1¾ cups

Ingredients:

- 5 cups organic desiccated coconut
- 2 tsp vanilla extract
- ½ tsp fine sea salt

Method:

Add coconut to a food processor, process for 2–3 minutes, stop and scrape down sides of bowl.

Add vanilla and salt. Continue to process. Every couple of minutes stop to give the motor a rest and scrape down sides and bottom of bowl. It will take you a total of 9–10 minutes, depending on the size of your food processor to complete.

The Coconut Butter will be ready when you have a soft texture with liquid rising to the top.

Store in a sealed glass jar at room temperature.

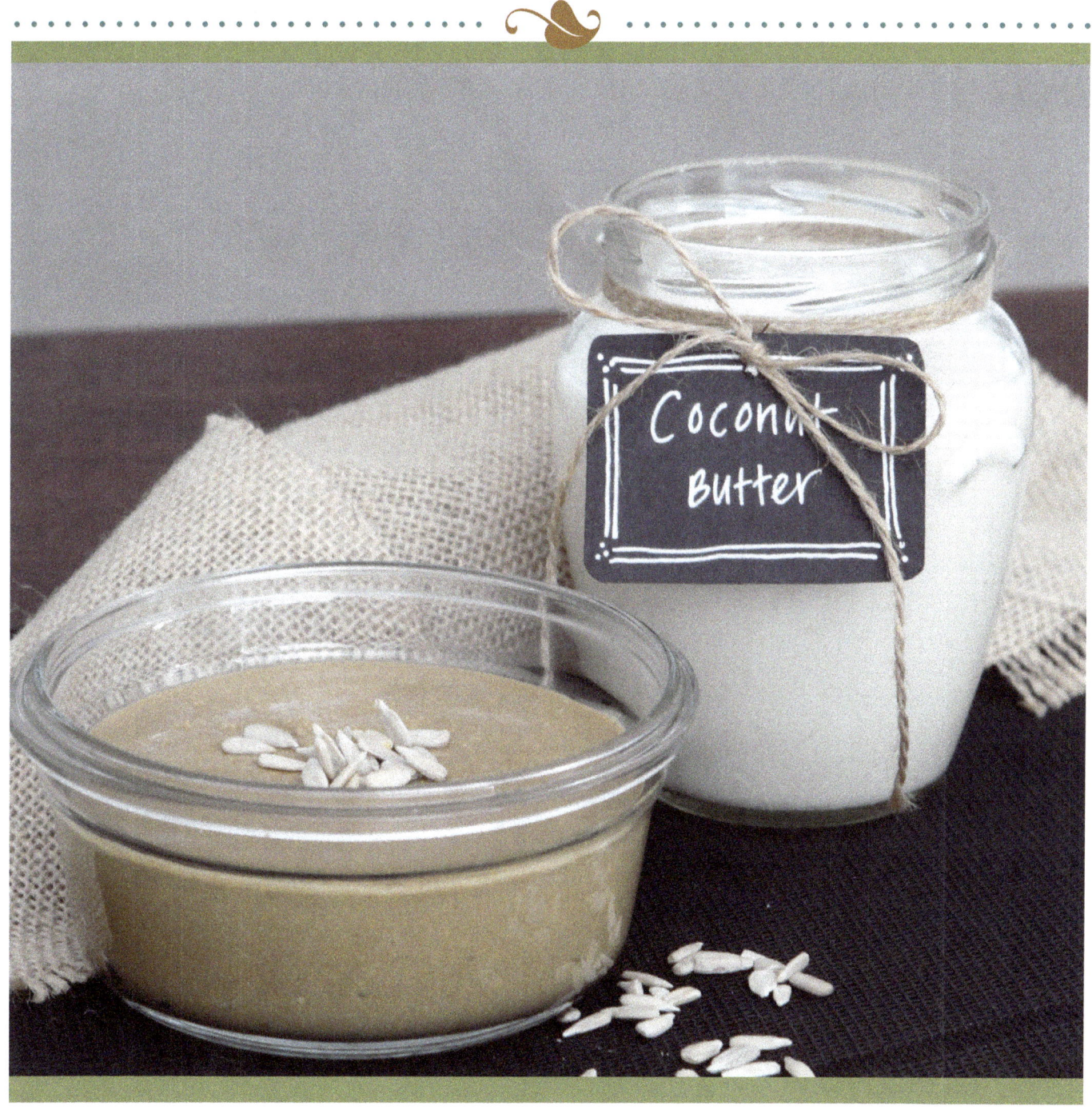

Cashew Butter

I have added Cashew Butter to a few recipes in my book, sometimes it is just convenient to purchase a jar, but if you are doing a lot of baking it's wiser to make your own. I prefer the taste and texture of my homemade Cashew Butter. There is something else you can make with it too, "Chocolate Cashew Butter". So delicious!! When I have reached my desired consistency, I remove half the Cashew Butter into a sealed jar and leave the other half in the food processor. I then go ahead and make my version of Cashew Nutella.

Prep time: 12 minutes
Cooking time: none   Makes: 2½ cups

Ingredients:

- 4 cups cashews
- ¼ tsp sea salt
- 1 Tbsp macadamia oil

Method:

To a food processor add the cashews and process until you have a nut meal consistency. Scrape down sides of bowl. Continue processing for a further 2 minutes. Add salt and continue to blend, stopping often to rest the motor and scrape down bowl. When the cashew butter consistency changes to a paste, pour the macadamia oil through the chute while the processor is running.

The Cashew Butter will be ready when you have a soft creamy consistency, it will be warm from the friction of the blade. Takes approximately 8-10 minutes, depending on the size of your food processor to complete.

Transfer to a sealed jar and store in the fridge.

Chocolate Cashew Butter

To the remaining half of Cashew Butter left in the processor bowl, add the following ingredients to enjoy a very yummy chocolate butter. Use it to spread on apple pieces or grain free bread but best of all eat with a spoon straight from the jar.

Prep time: 3 minutes
Cooking time: none   Makes: 1¼ cups

Ingredients:

- 1 cup cashew butter or 2 cups cashews made into butter
- 2 Tbsp coconut oil
- 2 Tbsp honey
- 2 Tbsp cacao powder
- 1 tsp vanilla extract
- ½ tsp sea salt

Method:

To the one cup of cashew butter in your food processor add, coconut oil, honey, cacao, vanilla and salt. Process for 1 minute to combined all ingredients well into a very smooth soft butter. If you would prefer it softer, just add a little extra coconut oil.

Transfer to a sealed jar, store in fridge. If Chocolate Butter becomes too firm, warm before spreading.

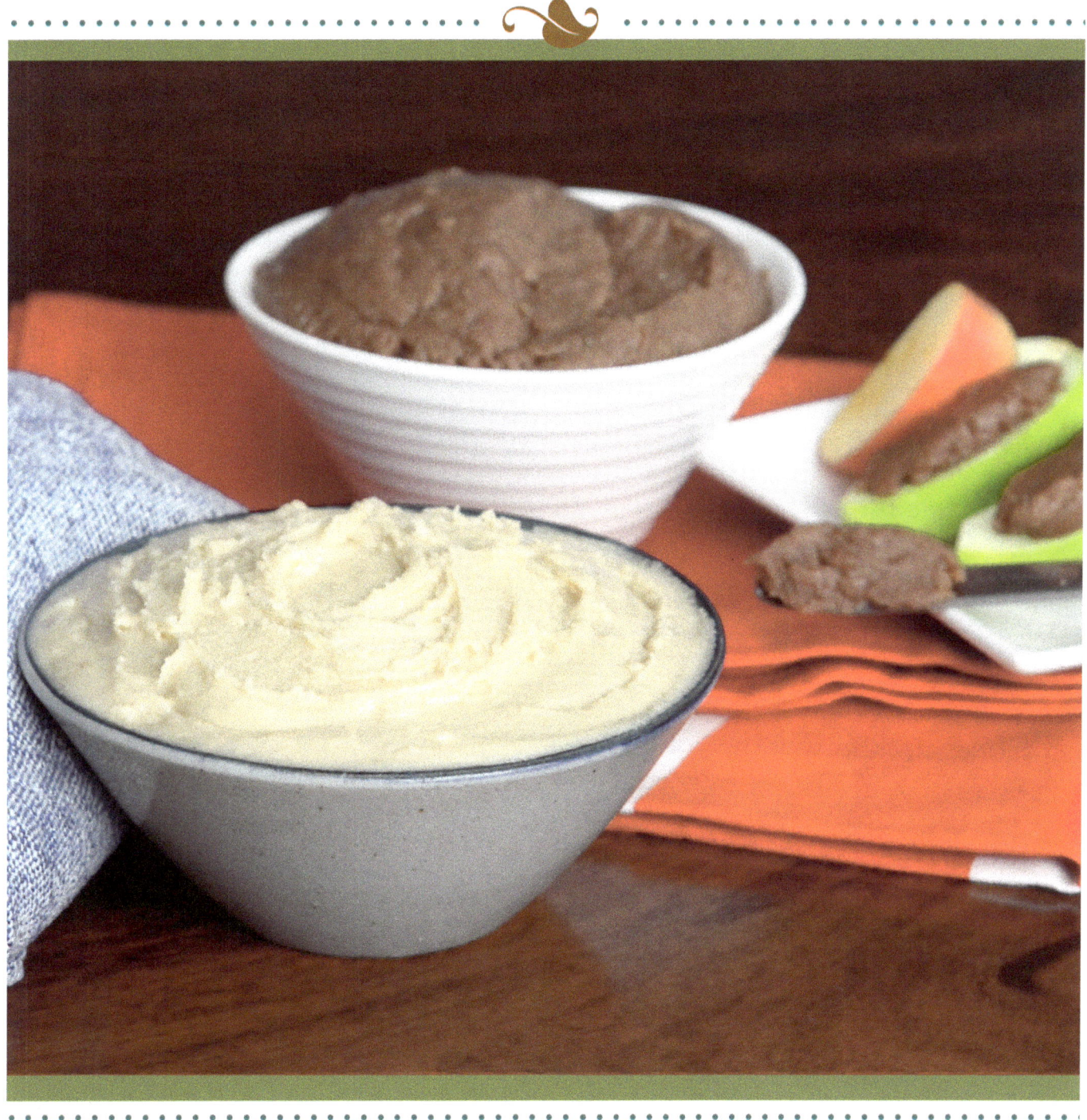

ACKNOWLEDGEMENTS

This book would not have been possible without the patience, support and love of my wonderful husband. You are a rare treasure, my love.

To my amazing sons and daughters in law. From taste testing to proof reading and listening to my constant chatter about my recipes, thank you with more love than you can imagine. Mark, thank you for trusting me with your fancy camera, knowing full well your mother had no idea what she was doing.

To my precious mother in law, you accepted your meals each day in wonder of what on earth I could be feeding you. I never tired of hearing you say, "I have no idea what you fed me but it was delicious." It always thrilled my heart. You played such a big part in the taste testing. You have gone to be with the Lord now, I just wish you could have seen the finished project.

To my gorgeous mother Dorothy. You have been so patient while I completed my book. Thank you for understanding and I can't wait to catch up on all our missed shopping days. I love you very much and I know if dad was still here, he would have been proud of my achievement.

To Pete and Elizabeth Taylor, for planting the seed back in 2012 and continuing to encourage me to publish my recipes.

To my lovely friends who accepted samples of my cooking and gave me their feedback.

Thank you…

INDEX

A

"anzac" biscuits   214, 225

aioli dipping mayo   118, 122

almond   12-14, 29, 34, 51, 66, 69, 73-74, 77-78, 80, 82, 86, 125, 148, 150, 172, 174, 182, 186, 192, 196, 198, 200, 212, 214, 217, 219, 221, 223, 225, 227, 229, 231, 233, 235, 237, 239, 241, 243, 245, 247, 249, 251, 253, 262, 273, 292, 297, 303

apple   8, 13, 19-20, 24, 85, 180, 184, 192, 202, 213, 256, 258, 269, 306

apple and mango chutney   202, 213

apple and pear crumble   256, 269

apple pie   85, 256, 258

asparagus   44, 47, 136, 138, 168

avocado   8, 16, 34, 56, 74, 93, 101, 118, 133, 136, 142, 144, 146, 150, 162

avocado dip   118, 133

B

banana   16, 24, 214, 217, 233, 270

banana and blueberry muffins   214

banana bread   214, 233

battered fish and seasoned fries   166, 198

beef   12, 56, 94, 136, 142, 148, 153-154, 158, 166, 168, 170, 172, 174, 178, 180, 202, 204, 225

beef stroganoff   166, 168

bircher style muesli   16

biscuits   214, 225, 231, 284, 290

bites   118, 126, 129, 131, 214, 255

blueberries   217, 239, 270, 290

blueberry chocolate chia puddings   256, 270

blueberry smoothie   16, 25

blueberry spread   231, 278, 290

blueberry thumbprint biscuits   214

bolognese with sweet potato pasta   166, 170

brazil nut   265, 299

bread   7, 55, 59, 62, 64, 66, 69-70, 73-74, 78, 133, 142, 184, 188, 214, 225, 233, 235, 288, 301, 306

breakfast sausages   16

broccoli   44, 48, 88, 97, 111, 114, 136, 140, 182, 190

broccoli salad   88, 97

brownies   214, 221, 280

buns   62, 70, 284

burgers   136, 160

butter   8, 11, 64, 66, 73-74, 118, 125, 128, 166, 188, 221, 237, 239, 251, 255, 292, 303-304, 306

butter balls   118, 128

THE JOYFUL TABLE | 309

C

cacao powder   10, 255, 265, 270, 273, 306

caesar dressing   202, 208

carrot   56, 91, 93, 98, 144, 164, 170, 178, 182, 190, 214, 243

carrot cake with lemon cream icing   214

cashew   12, 47, 64, 160, 221, 269, 278, 282, 292, 298, 301-302, 306

cashew butter   64, 221, 292, 306

cashew probiotic cheeze   292, 301

cashew sour cream   292, 302

cauliflower   44, 51-52, 60, 88, 111, 114, 116-117, 136, 162, 164, 168, 176, 178, 180, 182, 190, 202, 212

cauliflower and broccoli bake   88

cauliflower mash   88, 116, 176, 182

cauliflower rice   88, 117, 164, 190

chia   10, 24, 64, 125, 243, 256, 270, 278, 289

chicken   10, 52, 74, 114, 136, 140, 144, 146, 150, 154, 166, 186, 188, 190, 192, 202, 204, 210, 213, 292, 295

chicken and avocado caesar salad   136

chicken and broccoli frittata   136

chicken and leek pie   166, 186

chicken broth   52, 150, 292, 295

chinese cauliflower fried rice   136

chocolate   11, 16, 26, 126, 131, 214, 221, 223, 227, 229, 245, 249, 251, 256, 265, 270, 273, 278, 280-281, 283, 286, 292, 306

chocolate cashew butter   292, 306

chocolate chip cookies   214

chocolate coconut smoothie   16

chocolate dessert cake   256, 273

chocolate frosting   245, 249, 278, 280

chocolate ganache   221, 273, 278, 283

chocolate mousse cake with strawberry sauce   265

cinnamon   11, 19-20, 29, 38, 52, 55, 170, 214, 241, 247

cinnamon pecan rolls   214, 241

coconut   8, 10-11, 13-14, 16, 19-20, 24, 26, 29, 31, 37, 41, 47-48, 51-52, 55, 59-60, 62, 64, 69, 74, 77, 82, 85-86, 107, 118, 121, 125, 130, 138, 140, 144, 148, 150, 153-154, 156, 158, 160, 162, 164, 168, 170, 178, 182, 186, 188, 190, 192, 196, 198, 200, 204, 214, 217, 219, 221, 223, 225, 227, 231, 233, 235, 237, 241, 243, 245, 247, 249, 251, 253, 255, 258, 262, 265, 270, 273, 276, 282, 292, 297, 299, 304, 306

coconut butter   11, 292, 304

coconut rough bites   214, 255

coleslaw   88, 93

cookies   13, 214, 223, 227, 229, 284

cookie and cake glazes   278

corned silverside (beef)   166, 180

cranberry   166, 174

cranberry meatballs   166, 174

cream   3, 10-11, 20, 29, 44, 47-48, 51, 55-56, 60, 73, 77, 107, 114, 140, 149, 168, 190, 214, 221, 235, 237, 243, 247, 258, 261-262, 269, 278, 282, 290, 292, 302 cream of asparagus soup   44

cream of broccoli soup   44

cream of cauliflower soup   44

creamy zucchini noodles   136

crumbed chicken   166, 192, 213

crunchy nut fish   166, 196

cucumber   24, 88, 93, 98, 101-102, 188

cucumber and tomato salad   88

curried nut burgers   136, 160

curry   136, 148, 158, 160, 166, 190

curry pasties   136, 148

D

dairy free milks   292

damper   59, 62, 66

dates   13, 19, 125-126, 221, 227, 233, 239, 255, 266, 273, 276, 297-299

dip   66, 118, 133-134, 154, 184, 188, 198, 210, 229

dressing   8, 88, 91, 93, 97-98, 101-102, 111, 146, 192, 202, 208-209

E

egg   10, 12, 16, 29, 33-34, 69, 77, 80, 85-86, 98, 107, 136, 140, 149-150, 158, 160, 164, 172, 182, 186, 192, 198, 200, 202, 207, 229, 239, 241, 253, 261, 265, 286

egg and bacon toasts   136

egg burrito with leftovers   16

egg mayonnaise   150, 202, 207

english muffins with egg and avocado   16

F

fish   8, 12, 60, 108, 134, 144, 154, 164, 166, 196, 198, 200, 208, 210, 213

flaxseed meal   12

focaccia style bread   62, 69

frosting   245, 249, 273, 278, 280-281, 286

fruit   7-8, 10, 14, 19, 29, 77, 86, 118, 125, 219, 237, 245, 269-270, 274, 286, 288

fruit and nut fingers   118

fruity chia jam   278, 289

fruity nut scones   214, 239

G

"granola cereal" grain free   16

gingerbread cookies   214, 227

goji berry energy bites   118

grain free sandwich bread   55, 62

granola   16, 20

grated beetroot salad   88

gravy   66, 116, 172, 182, 184, 202, 204, 206

gravy (beef and chicken)   202

green banana smoothie   16

green beans and water chestnuts   88

green eggs and ham muffins   16

green thai curry chicken   166

H

ham and asparagus quiche   136

hamburger   62, 70, 94, 136, 158

hamburger buns   62

hamburger patties   94, 136, 158

hash browns   16, 38, 41

hazelnut sticky date pudding with caramel sauce   266

I

indian butter chicken   74, 166, 188

individual strawberry cheesecakes   256, 274

J

jaffa bites   118, 131

L

lamb   94, 154, 166, 182, 184

lamb and rosemary pies   166, 182

lamington cake   214, 249

layered salad   88, 98

leek   44, 52, 59, 166, 186

lemon   19, 88, 93, 102, 111, 113, 144, 164, 192, 196, 198, 214, 219, 243, 253, 256, 261, 290

lemon meringue pies   256, 261

lemon poppy seed muffins   214

loaf   62, 64, 66, 73, 166, 172, 194, 233, 235

M

macadamia   8, 23, 73, 82, 126, 186, 196, 198, 212, 217, 223, 245, 273, 278, 281, 298, 304, 306

macaroon and chocolate slice   214, 251

mango   8, 24, 136, 144, 192, 202, 213

mango and avocado salad   136

marshmallow frosting   273, 278, 286

marzipan cookies   214, 229

mayonnaise   93, 98, 150, 202, 207

meat   8, 11, 13-14, 24, 56, 74, 102, 108, 116, 136, 142, 144, 148-149, 156, 166, 168, 172, 178, 180, 182, 184, 204, 210, 295

mexican beef toasts   136

mexican shepherd's pie   166, 178

mini meat loaves   136, 156

mexican   133, 136, 153, 166, 178

muesli   16, 19, 23

muesli breakfast slice   16

muffins   10, 16, 34, 37, 214, 217, 219

mushroom gravy   202, 206

N

naan bread   62, 74, 188

nachos   78, 136, 142, 302

nut and seed mix   118

nut bars   118, 122

nutritional yeast flakes   12, 37, 138, 142, 153, 162, 192, 211, 301

nuts   9, 12, 19, 23, 47, 82, 97, 114, 121, 125-126, 154, 160, 196, 198, 211, 221, 223, 233, 235, 239, 243, 245, 247, 253, 270, 276, 281, 297-299, 301

O

orange and almond cake   214, 247

P

pancakes   16, 29, 136, 150, 290, 311

paleo satay chicken   136, 154

pear   256, 269

pie   12, 20, 62, 85-86, 138, 140, 166, 178, 182, 186, 256, 258, 261-262, 288

pie crust   62, 86, 138, 261

pistachio macaroons   214, 253

pizza base   62, 80

protein balls in coconut   118, 130

pumpkin   19, 23, 44, 55, 59, 70, 73, 82, 91, 118, 126, 133, 136, 153, 156, 188, 204

pumpkin "hummus"   118, 133

pumpkin soup   44, 55, 59, 73

pumpkin, spinach and feta toasts   136

R

rainbow salad   88, 91, 209

raspberry   256, 276

raw raspberry cheesecake   256, 276

roasted almond butter   292, 303

S

salad   8-9, 13, 74, 88, 91, 93-94, 97-98, 101-102, 136, 144, 146, 156, 158, 160, 186, 192, 194, 198, 200, 209

sandwich   55, 62, 64, 273

sauerkraut   88, 104

sauce   11-13, 60, 80, 114, 134, 142, 154, 156, 162, 164, 168, 170, 172, 174, 176, 178, 180, 182, 184, 188, 190, 194, 196, 200, 202, 204, 208, 211-212, 256, 265-266, 283

sausage   31

savoury pancakes   136, 150

scones   184, 214, 237, 239, 311, 313

seafood chowder   44, 60

seasoned fries   118, 122, 166, 198, 312

seed crackers   62, 82, 133

seeds   9-10, 12-13, 19, 23-24, 64, 66, 78, 82, 91, 101, 121, 125-126, 129, 153, 174, 196, 198, 219, 225, 239, 243, 270, 289, 304

sesame   13, 64, 66, 78, 82, 118, 126, 129, 153, 196, 198, 239

sesame snaps   118, 129

slice   16, 23, 42, 64, 69, 73, 107, 125-126, 140, 168, 180, 194, 214, 221, 233, 251, 269, 301

soup   44, 47-48, 51-52, 55-56, 59-60, 66, 73, 114, 168, 184, 190

spicy guacamole salsa   202, 210

spinach   37, 47, 62, 73, 78, 88, 91, 101, 133, 136, 142, 153, 192

spinach & feta loaf   62, 73

spinach flat bread   62, 78, 133, 142

strawberry   256, 262, 265, 274, 278, 288

strawberry crumble   256, 262

strawberry preserve   278, 288

sue's irish stew   166, 184

sunflower butter   292, 304

sunflower   9, 19, 23, 34, 82, 101, 172, 225, 239, 292, 304

swede   42, 48, 52, 55, 88, 107-108, 184

sweet potato   16, 38, 41, 44, 59-60, 88, 101, 107, 122,

134, 140, 148, 154, 156, 166, 170, 178, 192

sweet and sour meatballs   166, 176

sweet coconut piecrust   62, 258

sweet potato and spinach salad   88

sweet potato and vegetable soup   44

sweet potato hash browns   16, 41

sweet potato & onion hash browns   16

sweet swede   88, 108

T

taco   44, 56, 74

taco soup   44, 56

tahini dressing   91

tasty toasts   136, 152-153

thai fish cakes   166, 200

tomato   13, 31, 80, 88, 98, 102, 140, 153, 156, 170, 172, 178, 180, 182, 194, 196

tortillas   62, 77

traditional english meat loaf   166

turkey meatloaf   166, 194

V

vanilla cupcakes   214, 245

vanilla macadamia frosting   273, 278, 281

vegetable   7-9, 16, 42, 44, 59, 88, 107, 113, 133, 140, 156, 160, 178, 182, 207

vegetable and bacon slice   16

W

whipped cashew cream   269, 278, 282

white (cauliflower) sauce   202, 212

white (nut) sauce   202, 211

winter vegetable bake   88

wraps   62, 77

wraps, tortillas or crepes   62

Z

zucchini   111, 136, 160, 162, 168, 214, 235

zucchini bread   214, 235

www.ingramcontent.com/pod-product-compliance
Lightning Source LLC
Chambersburg PA
CBHW061810290426
44110CB00026B/2840